100 Cases for
MEDICAL DATA
INTERPRETATION

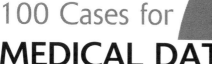

100 Cases for
MEDICAL DATA
INTERPRETATION

Editors:
Dr David C Howlett FRCP FRCR
Consultant Radiologist, Eastbourne District General Hospital and Honorary
Clinical Reader in Imaging and Electronic Learning at Brighton and Sussex
Medical School

Dr Nicola Gainsborough FRCP
Consultant Physician, Brighton and Sussex University Hospitals NHS Trust and
Honorary Senior Clinical Lecturer, Brighton and Sussex Medical School, UK

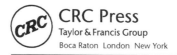

CRC Press
Taylor & Francis Group
Boca Raton London New York

CRC Press is an imprint of the
Taylor & Francis Group, an **informa** business

CRC Press
Taylor & Francis Group
6000 Broken Sound Parkway NW, Suite 300
Boca Raton, FL 33487-2742

© 2013 by Taylor & Francis Group, LLC
CRC Press is an imprint of Taylor & Francis Group, an Informa business

No claim to original U.S. Government works

Printed and bound by CPI Group (UK) Ltd, Croydon, CR0 4YY
Version Date: 20121211

International Standard Book Number: 978-1-4441-4904-3 (Paperback)

Visit the Taylor & Francis Web site at
http://www.taylorandfrancis.com

and the CRC Press Web site at
http://www.crcpress.com

Dedications

To Joanna and the children Tom, Ella, Robert, Miles and Christopher and also to Lara.

DCH

To David (DMW), with all my love and without whom this would not have been possible.

NG

Contributors

Clinical Chemistry: Dr Gifford Batstone, consultant Clinical Chemistry, Dr Gary Weaving, PhD, clinical biochemist, Royal Sussex County Hospital, Brighton.

Radiology: Dr Mo Faris, consultant radiologist Eastbourne District General Hospital, Dr Celine Inglis, core trainee Eastbourne District General Hospital, Dr Rasha Ameen, core trainee Eastbourne District General Hospital, Dr Jo Wade, core trainee Eastbourne District General Hospital

Haematology: Dr Joel Newman, specialty registrar haematology Eastbourne District General Hospital

Cardiology: Dr Steve Podd, research registrar cardiology – Eastbourne District General Hospital

Miscellaneous: Dr Fergus Chedgy, specialty trainee medicine Eastbourne District General Hospital

Contents

Foreword   *x*
Foreword   *xi*
Acknowledgements   *xii*
Abbreviations   *xiii*

SECTION 1: CLINICAL CHEMISTRY

Case 1:   Elderly woman with history of vomiting   3
Case 2:   Elderly man with shortness of breath   8
Case 3:   Woman with headache   13
Case 4:   Elderly man with a cough   20
Case 5:   Woman with abdominal pain   24
Case 6:   Depressed elderly man   28
Case 7:   Teenager with headache and vomiting   34
Case 8:   Man with severe vomiting   38
Case 9:   Man found semi-conscious   44
Case 10:   Young woman with aspirin overdose   48
Case 11:   Asthmatic male with cough   52
Case 12:   Man with renal failure   56
Case 13:   Teenager with colicky pain   61
Case 14:   Man with diabetes mellitus   66
Case 15:   Elderly man with dysuria   70
Case 16:   Middle-aged woman with tiredness   74
Case 17:   Middle-aged man with shortness of breath   78
Case 18:   Elderly woman admitted following a fall   82
Case 19:   Elderly man with nocturia   86
Case 20:   Man with severe headaches   90
Case 21:   Elderly confused woman   94
Case 22:   Middle-aged woman feeling tired   100
Case 23:   Woman with irregular periods   104
Case 24:   Man with painful knees   108

SECTION 2: RADIOLOGY

Case 25:   Woman with abdominal pain   115
Case 26:   Woman with cough and weight loss   122
Case 27:   Middle-aged woman with difficulty in swallowing 127
Case 28:   Young man with chest pain   132
Case 29:   Young woman with loss of vision   136
Case 30:   Middle-aged man with shortness of breath   141
Case 31:   Elderly woman with weight loss   146
Case 32:   Elderly woman with shortness of breath   151
Case 33:   Elderly woman with diabetes   156
Case 34:   Middle-aged woman with a cough   161
Case 35:   Man with a bloody cough   167
Case 36:   Middle-aged man with a cough   173
Case 37:   Elderly man with headache   179
Case 38:   Elderly man with pain in the hip   185
Case 39:   Woman with headache and vomiting   191
Case 40:   Elderly woman with epigastric pain   195
Case 41:   Elderly man with shortness of breath   200

Case 42: Woman with abdominal pain 204
Case 43: Middle-aged woman with swelling in hands and feet 210
Case 44: Middle-aged man with confusion 215
Case 45: Elderly woman with upper limb weakness 219
Case 46: Nasogastric feeding on the stroke unit 223

SECTION 3: HAEMATOLOGY

Case 47: Elderly woman with constipation 229
Case 48: Young woman with profound fatigue 234
Case 49: Middle-aged man with lethargy 237
Case 50: Teenager with chest pain 241
Case 51: Elderly woman with light-headedness 247
Case 52: Elderly woman with anaemia 252
Case 53: Middle-aged woman with anaemia 256
Case 54: Confused elderly woman 260
Case 55: Elderly woman with bruising 265
Case 56: Elderly man with hip pain 270
Case 57: Teenager with unexplained bruises 274
Case 58: Teenager with panic attacks 278
Case 59: Elderly man with nose bleeds 282
Case 60: Teenager with a swollen knee 286
Case 61: Woman with a heavy period 290
Case 62: Young woman with leg pain and swelling 294
Case 63: Elderly woman with fever and lethargy 298
Case 64: Woman with emergency hip repair 302
Case 65: Middle-aged woman with right-sided weakness 306
Case 66: Middle-aged man with increasing tiredness 310
Case 67: Elderly man with abnormal blood test results 314
Case 68: Middle-aged man with cellulitis 318

SECTION 4: CARDIOLOGY

Case 69: Elderly man with palpitations 325
Case 70: Elderly man with chest pain 331
Case 71: Middle-aged man with syncope 336
Case 72: Middle-aged woman with chest pain 339
Case 73: Middle-aged man with light headedness 341
Case 74: Young woman with palpitations 343
Case 75: Elderly woman with chest pain 348
Case 76: Elderly man with syncope 351
Case 77: Middle-aged woman with chest pain 353
Case 78: Young woman with syncope 358
Case 79: Middle-aged man with abdominal pain 361
Case 80: Elderly man with palpitations 365
Case 81: Elderly woman with fever and weight loss 367
Case 82: Young man with shortness of breath 372
Case 83: Young man undergoing army medical 376
Case 84: Woman with increasing shortness of breath 379
Case 85: Elderly man with atrial fibrillation 384
Case 86: Elderly man with kidney disease 388
Case 87: Young man with central chest pain 391
Case 88: Young man with palpitations 393

SECTION 5: MISCELLANEOUS

Case 89:   Elderly woman with COPD   398
Case 90:   Elderly man with increasing confusion   403
Case 91:   Elderly man with respiratory distress   409
Case 92:   Young woman with cough   414
Case 93:   Elderly man with progressive leg swelling   419
Case 94:   Woman suspected of attempted suicide   424
Case 95:   Man with chest pain and weight loss   429
Case 96:   Young woman with pain in her legs and back   432
Case 97:   Middle-aged man with severe headache   436
Case 98:   Middle-aged man with epigastric pain   440
Case 99:   Elderly woman with fever and mild confusion   444
Case 100: Elderly woman admitted following a fall   448

Bibliography   *452*
Index   *453*

Foreword

Part of the enduring fascination of medicine is the mental agility needed in clinical problem solving. It is a truism—but worth repeating—that no two patients are identical. But, it is equally true that there are patterns which are sufficiently consistent to enable us to make a diagnosis and start treatment. This book is about learning to recognise those patterns. Nicki Gainsborough and David Howlett are two of the most inspirational clinical teachers I have had the privilege to work with, and in this book they have put together a compendium of common and important clinical syndromes to help students recognise problems and what to do about them. One of the things that I particularly like is that the text goes beyond simply giving the *right* diagnosis and explains the underlying physiology and pathology behind each case. I am sure that this is critical: most students say that trying to simply memorise huge numbers of facts is a lost cause; understanding *why* a patient presents in a particular way is not only why medicine is so interesting but also helps to cement the information in one's memory. Oscar Wilde wrote that "Experience is the name everyone gives to their mistakes". This book will not substitute for experience but it will reduce the number of mistakes that are made as you accumulate your personal experience.

Professor Jon Cohen
Dean, Brighton and Sussex Medical School

Foreword

Case histories always interest and inform clinicians. They are almost like mini-detective stories. In my experience a surprising number suddenly appear relevant to one's recent past and future clinical experience. I congratulate the authors, both fellows of the Royal College of Physicians, on compiling these hundred cases ranging widely across the specialties, but concentrating on data from supporting departments.

They make compulsive reading, and the answers are comprehensive, backed up by expert contributions from radiology, cardiology, haematology and clinical chemistry. I really recommend medical students, trainees and consultants with an interest in acute and general medicine to read this book – they will find much to learn or jog their memories, and not just on the first, but on subsequent readings too. It could be a very useful form of CPD.

Sir Richard Thompson
President of the Royal College of Physicians, London

Acknowledgements

The editors would like to acknowledge Gifford Batstone and Gary Weaving of Royal Sussex County Hospital, Brighton, for their assistance in supplying normal reference ranges for use in the cases, and also Celine Inglis and Jo Wade for compiling the bibliography of recommended further reading. The editors would also like to thank Nicholas Taylor, medical illustrator at Eastbourne District General Hospital, for his invaluable help with creating the images within this book (see below for more information on Nick).

David C Howlett
Nicola Gainsborough

Nick Taylor

Nick brings over 30 years' experience as a medical photographer to the preparation of the images for this book. Employed since 1980 in various hospitals across the south east, including Guy's, Royal Sussex County, Brighton and, currently, Eastbourne District General, he has been involved in the publication of numerous images for articles, journals and textbooks.

A member for many years of the Institute of Medical Illustrators and registered medical illustration practitioner, he has recently been awarded honorary membership of the Royal College of Radiologists through his expertise and involvement in providing the images for the College Fellowship anatomy examination.

Collaboration with Brighton and Sussex Medical School enabled Nick to be involved in compiling the images for many hundreds of on-line e-learning cases. Auditing of student access and use of the facility have been presented at national and international conferences.

Running a one-man department at Eastbourne District General Hospital, Nick aids the research across the Trust in providing the whole clinical and educational illustration service used by the clinicians – this has resulted in many conference prize-winning posters and videos produced from the department.

In addition to the medical publications, Nick has received acknowledgment in illustrating many Eastbourne local history books, as well as being co-author in a couple.

Abbreviations

ACTH	adrenocorticotropic hormone
ALP	alkaline phosphatase
ALT	alanine aminotransferase
APTT	activated partial thromboplastin time
AST	aspartate transaminase
BNP	brain natriuretic peptide
CT	computed tomography
DEXA	dual energy x-ray absorptiometry
ESR	erythrocyte sedimentation rate
FLAIR	fluid-attenuated inversion recovery
GGT	gamma-glutamyltransferase, gamma-GT
HDL	high-density lipoprotein
LDH	lactate dehydrogenase
LDL	low-density lipoprotein
MCH	mean corpuscular haemoglobin
MCHC	mean corpuscular hemoglobin concentration
MCV	mean corpuscular volume
MIBI	methyl-isobutyl-isonitrile
MRI	magnetic resonance imaging
MSU	midstream specimen of urine
PTH	parathyroid hormone
PSA	prostate-specific antigen
STEMI	segment elevation myocardial infarction
TSH	thyroid-stimulating hormone
VLDL	very-low-density lipoprotein
WCC	white cell count

SECTION 1: CLINICAL CHEMISTRY

Case 1: Elderly woman with history of vomiting

Case 2: Elderly man with shortness of breath

Case 3: Woman with headache

Case 4: Elderly man with a cough

Case 5: Woman with abdominal pain

Case 6: Depressed elderly man

Case 7: Teenager with headache and vomiting

Case 8: Man with severe vomiting

Case 9: Man found semi-conscious

Case 10: Young woman with aspirin overdose

Case 11: Asthmatic male with cough

Case 12: Man with renal failure

Case 13: Teenager with colicky pain

Case 14: Man with diabetes mellitus

Case 15: Elderly man with dysuria

Case 16: Middle-aged woman with tiredness

Case 17: Middle-aged man with shortness of breath

Case 18: Elderly woman admitted following a fall

Case 19: Elderly man with nocturia

Case 20: Man with severe headaches

Case 21: Elderly confused woman

Case 22: Middle-aged woman feeling tired

Case 23: Woman with polycystic ovary syndrome

Case 24: Man with painful knees

CASE 1: ELDERLY WOMAN WITH HISTORY OF VOMITING

History

A 63-year-old retired woman presented to A&E with a 3-week history of nausea and vomiting which had become worse in the past 3 days such that she could no longer 'keep anything down'. She also complained of feeling 'close to collapsing'. She was a smoker of 20 cigarettes per day for 40 years and consumes 5 units alcohol/week. She had no history of recent weight loss and was on no medication.

Examination

Pulse 85 beats per minute, blood pressure (BP) 140/70 mmHg, no postural drop, heart sounds normal. No abdominal localizing signs. Nothing else found on examination.

Investigations

		Reference range
Sodium	118 mmol/L	135–145 mmol/L
Potassium	4.1 mmol/L	3.2–5.1 mmol/L
Urea	2.4 mmol/L	1.7–8.2 mmol/L
Creatinine	52 µmol/L	44–80 µmol/L
Bicarbonate	20 mmol/L	22–29 mmol/L
Chloride	90 mmol/L	96–108 mmol/L
Cortisol	237 nmol/L	171–536 nmol/L (9 a.m.)
Osmolality	245 mmol/kg	275–295 mmol/kg
Urine		
Osmolality	564 mmol/kg	400–1400 mmol/kg
Sodium	136 mmol/L	No reference range

Liver function tests (LFT), clotting and bone profile were normal. Chest radiograph reported as normal.

In view of her biochemistry consistent with syndrome of inappropriate antidiuretic hormone (SIADH) production, her history of vomiting and normal chest x-ray findings, a magnetic resonance image (MRI) of her head was undertaken (Figure 1.1). This showed a large pituitary-based mass with suprasellar extension (see arrow, coronal T1-weighted post-contrast image) and chiasmal displacement.

Formal visual field testing was also undertaken (Figure 1.2).

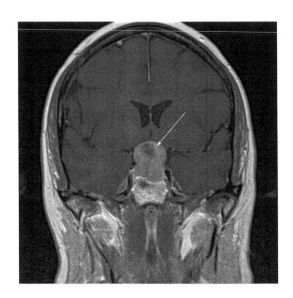

Figure 1.1

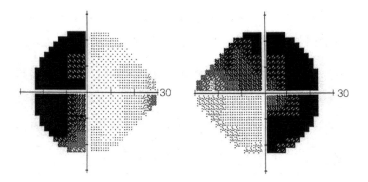

Figure 1.2

Further investigation findings

		Reference range
Cortisol	509 nmol/L	171–536 nmol/L (9 a.m)
Thyroid-stimulating hormone (TSH)	3.91 mU/L	0.3–4.2 mU/L
Free thyroxine (fT4)	7.4 pmol/L	12–22 pmol/L
Free tri-iodothyronine (fT3)	2.8 pmol/L	3.1–6.8 pmol/L
Luteinizing hormone (LH)	1.0 IU/L	7.7–59 IU/L (menopausal)
Follicle-stimulating hormone (FSH)	1.9 IU/L	26–135 IU/L (menopausal)
Prolactin	15 262 mL U/L	102–496 mL U/L

QUESTIONS

1. Which conditions may cause this degree of hyponatraemia?
2. What is the most likely cause of the hyponatraemia based on laboratory and clinical information?
3. What medical conditions may be associated with SIADH?
4. What visual field deficit is seen on the above visual field test?
5. Which of the endocrine test results are abnormal in this woman?
6. What medical conditions and drug therapy may be associated with an elevated prolactin?
7. What drugs are suitable for treatment of microadenomas causing hyperprolactinaemia?

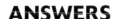

ANSWERS

1. The following conditions may commonly cause this degree of hyponatraemia: acute renal failure, adrenal insufficiency (Addison's disease), cirrhosis with ascites, use of thiazide diuretics, severe vomiting and the syndrome of inappropriate ADH secretion (SIADH). Causes of profound hyponatraemia are best categorized by the overall clinical fluid status of the patient:

    - Hypovolaemic (decreased extracellular volume)
      - Renal losses (diuretics, salt-losing nephropathy)
      - Non-renal losses (vomiting, diarrhoea)
      - Adrenal insufficiency (Addison's disease)
    - Euvolaemic
      - Excess fluid replacement (5 per cent dextrose for example)
      - Syndrome of inappropriate ADH secretion
      - Hypothyroidism
      - Psychogenic polydipsia (excess water consumption)
    - Hypervolaemic (increased extracellular volume)
      - Congestive cardiac failure
      - Nephrotic syndrome
      - Cirrhosis with ascites

2. The most likely cause of the hyponatraemia in this patient based on laboratory and clinical information is the syndrome of inappropriate antidiuretic hormone secretion (SIADH). Hyponatraemia with a low plasma osmolality and inappropriately high urine osmolality and urine sodium levels is typical of SIADH. The normal physiological response to a low sodium would be to retain sodium avidly (urine sodium <10 mmol/L) and excrete a dilute urine (urine osmolality <50 mmol/kg). Addison's disease is probably excluded by the normal cortisol, even though this is not as high as might be expected in the presence of her current illness. Additionally, hyperkalaemia would be expected in Addison's disease. Severe vomiting sufficient to cause hyponatraemia would usually be associated with a metabolic alkalosis and probably hypokalaemia. Acute renal failure is excluded by her normal creatinine and urea. Cirrhosis is excluded by normal examination, international normalized ratio (INR) and LFT.

3. SIADH may be associated with many neurological conditions (such as meningitis, encephalitis, head trauma, intracerebral haemorrhage, primary or secondary cerebral tumour), pneumonia, tumours such as small cell lung cancer, and the possibility of acute intermittent porphyria should be considered in appropriate clinical circumstances. In acute cardiac failure, the secretion of ADH is an appropriate physiological response to a diminished circulating volume.

4. The visual field deficit shown is a bitemporal hemianopia, caused by a pituitary lesion at the optic chiasm pressing upwards on the optic nerve fibres from the nasal halves of the retina which cross at the optic chiasm. The visual pathways are shown in Figure 1.3.

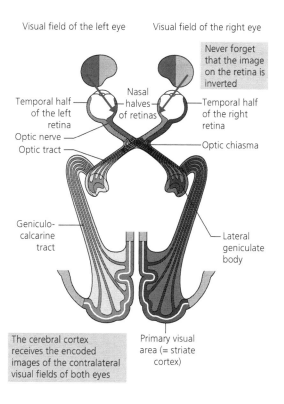

Visual field of the left eye   Visual field of the right eye

Never forget that the image on the retina is inverted

Nasal halves of retinas

Temporal half of the left retina

Temporal half of the right retina

Optic nerve
Optic tract

Optic chiasma

Geniculo-calcarine tract

Lateral geniculate body

The cerebral cortex receives the encoded images of the contralateral visual fields of both eyes

Primary visual area (= striate cortex)

Figure 1.3

5. In this particular woman, the TSH is inappropriate for her low fT4 and fT3. An exceedingly high TSH would be anticipated for these fT4 and fT3 concentrations. She is hypothyroid due to a lack of TSH stimulating the release of thyroid hormones. Her LH and FSH are very low for a post-menopausal woman. Post-menopause, as there is very little oestrogen production by the ovaries and therefore no suppression of gonadotrophin secretion, values of LH and FSH are typically >50 IU/L. Hence, these values are inappropriately low. Compression of the pituitary tends to adversely affect trophic factors differentially. Thus, TSH and gonadotrophin secretion fall before adrenocorticotropic hormone (ACTH) and hence cortisol.

6. Elevated prolactin may be due to physiological factors, such as emotional stress, pregnancy and breast feeding; drugs especially dopaminergic antagonists such as chlorpromazine, risperidone, domperidone and metaclopramide; pituitary tumours; polycystic ovary syndrome; and severe thyroid failure. The higher the prolactin the greater the likelihood that a tumour is present: concentrations of more than 2000 mIU/L are suggestive of microadenoma whereas values >6000 mIU/L are more likely to indicate a macroadenoma.

7. Dopamine agonists, such as cabergoline or bromocriptine, are suitable for treatment of prolactin-secreting pituitary tumours and may act to shrink large tumours, avoiding the need for surgery.

CASE 2: ELDERLY MAN WITH SHORTNESS OF BREATH

History

A 78-year-old male presents to his GP with a 3-month history of increasing shortness of breath when walking and swelling of his ankles. On examination, his jugular venous pressure is raised 6 cm, there is ankle oedema and scattered crepitations at both bases. On the presumptive diagnosis of cardiac failure, his GP organizes blood tests including brain natriuretic peptide (BNP).

Investigations

		Reference range
Sodium	142 mmol/L	135–146 mmol/L
Potassium	4.3 mmol/L	3.2–5.1 mmol/L
Urea	10.8 mmol/L	1.7–8.3 mmol/L
Creatinine	110 µmol/L	62–106 µmol/L
Bilirubin	21 µmol/L	<21 µmol/L
Total protein	72 g/L	66–87 g/L
Albumin	41 g/L	34–48 g/L
Alanine aminotransferase (ALT)	62 U/L	<41 U/L
Alkaline phosphatase (ALP)	120 U/L	40–129 U/L
Haemoglobin (Hb)	15.6 g/dL	13.5–18.0 g/L
NT-proBNP	1965 ng/L	>400 ng/L (intervention level)

On the basis of the BNP result, the patient is referred for echocardiography which demonstrates a reduced ejection fraction, but no other abnormalities.

His GP commences treatment with ramipril and adds a loop diuretic to help control his ankle oedema. On follow up, the patient reports improved exercise tolerance, but complains that his ankle oedema has not improved. Repeat electrolytes are undertaken two months after starting treatment.

His GP decides to change his diuretic to spironolactone. At about the same time, the patient learns of the role of sodium in cardiac failure and decides to reduce his salt intake by using LoSalt in cooking.

	After two months on treatment	Follow-up tests	Reference range
Sodium	140 mmol/L	139 mmol/L	135–145 mmol/L
Potassium	4.1 mmol/L	7.3 mmol/L	3.2–5.1 mmol/L
Urea	11.3 mmol/L	11.8 mmol/L	1.7–8.3 mmol/L
Creatinine	114 µmol/L	120 µmol/L	62–106 µmol/L

QUESTIONS

1. Which conditions or treatments may be associated with a high NT-proBNP?
2. Which conditions or treatment might be the cause of his elevated ALT?
3. What laboratory tests would you consider in the initial investigation of a patient who exhibited a persistently increased isolated ALT of about 100 U/L over a three-month period?
4. Which medical conditions may be associated with elevations of serum potassium?
5. Which drugs may cause an elevated serum potassium?

ANSWERS

1. NT-proBNP levels may be raised with left ventricular hypertrophy, myocardial ischemia, tachycardia, right ventricular overload, hypoxaemia (including pulmonary embolism), renal dysfunction (glomerular filtration rate (e-GFR) <60 mL/min/1.73m^2), sepsis, chronic obstructive pulmonary disease (COPD), diabetes, age >70 years, cirrhosis of the liver, obesity. Treatment with diuretics, ACE (angiotension converting enzyme) inhibitors, beta-blockers, angiotensin II receptor antagonists (ARBs) and aldosterone antagonists can all reduce serum concentrations of natriuretic peptides.

2. ALT varies throughout the day, and is also higher in people of Hispanic or Black African origin. In addition, there is a relationship with body mass index (BMI), although this of course is also linked with non-alcoholic fatty liver disease risk (NAFLD). Liver enzymes may be elevated in cardiac failure due to increased pressure in the hepatic vein. However, this is normally associated with an increase in alkaline phosphatase and gamma-glutamyl transpeptidase (GGT). Isolated elevations of ALT may indicate chronic liver disease and persistent elevations over a 6-week period are an indication for further tests to exclude treatable causes of liver disease. The use of statins may cause a raised ALT and it is likely that this patient with heart failure will be taking a statin.

   ALT is a much more liver-specific enzyme than aspartate aminotransferase (AST) which is also prevalent in red cells, skeletal muscle, cardiac muscle and kidney, as well as liver.

   Marked increases in serum ALT (5–10× upper limit of reference range) are usually associated with:

   - circulatory failure (shock) and hypoxia
   - acute viral or toxic hepatitis

   More moderate increases (up to 5× upper limit of reference range) may be found in:

   - chronic viral infections
   - cirrhosis
   - cytomegalovirus (CMV) infection
   - liver congestion secondary to cardiac failure
   - cholestatic jaundice
   - alcoholic liver disease
   - non-alcoholic fatty liver disease (NAFLD)
   - inherited causes of liver disease (haemochomatosis, Wilson's disease, alpha-1 antitrypsin deficiency
   - coeliac disease

   In addition a wide range of drugs may cause an elevation of ALT including analgesics (especially when taken in excess), cholesterol-lowering drugs (e.g. statins), some antibiotics (e.g. sulphonamides), anti-tuberculosis drugs (e.g. isoniazid), anti-fungal drugs (e.g. fluconazole), anti-epileptics (e.g. phenytoin), anti-depressants (e.g. tri-cyclis).

3. The investigation of a persistently elevated ALT level is important as early intervention allows treatments which will prevent progression to cirrhosis. The two major routes are viral infections (more frequent in those who have lived in areas where these virus diseases are endemic) and inherited metabolic conditions. If gamma-GT is not included within LFT, this should be requested together with full blood count (FBC) and fasting glucose concentration.

   a. Viral infections: hepatitis A, B, C and CMV (Cytomegalovirus)
   b. Inherited/metabolic: alpha-1 anti-trypsin; iron, transferrin and ferritin (haemachromatosis); copper and caeruloplasmin (Wilson's disease)

4. Acute renal failure, Addison's disease, metabolic acidosis of any aetiology, tumour lysis syndrome may all be associated with hyperkalaemia.

5. ACE inhibitors, angiotensin receptor blockers and digoxin may cause an elevated potassium.

   In this case, the hyperkalaemia was probably due to two factors: first, the switch to spironolactone and second, the patient increasing his potassium intake through use of LoSalt, in which sodium salts are largely replaced by potassium salts.

   The causes of hyperkalaemia may be divided into those associated with (1) renal and (2) non-renal causes:

- Renal causes:
  - Insufficient sodium exchange
    - o Glomerular dysfunction – acute and chronic renal failure
    - o Sodium depletion
  - Decreased sodium/potassium exchange
    - o Mineralocorticoid deficiency – Addison's disease, congenital adrenal hyperplasia, renal tubular acidosis type IV
  - Drugs
    - o Angiotensin-converting enzyme inhibitors
    - o Spironolactone
    - o Potassium-sparing diuretics
    - o Angiotensin receptor blockers
- Non-renal causes:
  - *In vitro* effects
    - o Haemolysis
    - o Leukocytosis or thrombocytosis
    - o Delayed sample separation
  - Increased input
    - o Dietary – natural or supplements
    - o Intravenous

- – Redistribution
  - o Acidosis
  - o Hypoxia
  - o Severe tissue damage, including tumour lysis syndrome
  - o *In vivo* haemolysis
  - o Drugs, e.g. digoxin
  - o Familial hyperkalaemic periodic paralysis

CASE 3: WOMAN WITH HEADACHE

History

A 35-year-old female presented to her GP with headache. He found nothing significant apart from a history of recurrent urinary tract infections and an elevated blood pressure (BP) of 185/99 mmHg. Her body mass index (BMI) was 25. He arranged for further measurements of BP, a mid-stream urine (MSU) sample for urinary infection and blood for electrolytes in view of possible renal failure.

Laboratory results

MSU, negative
Full blood count, normal

Investigations

		Reference range
Sodium	144 mmol/L	135–146 mmol/L
Potassium	3.0 mmol/L	3.2–5.1 mmol/L
Urea	3.5 mmol/L	1.7–8.3 mmol/L
Creatinine	75 μmol/L	44–80 μmol/L

Repeat BP measurements confirmed her hypertension and in view of her hypokalaemia she was referred for further investigation. She commenced ramipril 10 mg od.

The hospital physician confirmed hypertension and arranged for repeat electrolytes, random urine potassium and resting and ambulant renin and angiotensin levels. He also enquired whether there was a family history of hypertension. Ramipril was stopped for three days prior to the tests and it was checked that she was not taking oral contraception.

Results

		Reference range
Sodium	143 mmol/L	135–146 mmol/L
Potassium	2.9 mmol/L	3.2–5.1 mmol/L
Urea	3.7 mmol/L	1.7–8.3 mmol/L
Creatinine	72 μmol/L	44–80 μmol/L
Chloride	94 mmol/L	96–108 mmol/L
Bicarbonate	40 mmol/L	22–29 mmol/L
Calcium (adjusted)	2.35 mmol/L	2.15–2.55 mmol/L
Magnesium (adjusted)	0.94 mmol/L	0.65–1.05 mmol/L
Urine potassium	64 mmol/L	

	Resting	Reference range	Ambulant	Reference range
Plasma renin activity (PRA)	0.35 nmol/h/L	0.5–2.2 nmol/h/L	0.68 nmol/h/L	1.2–4.4 nmol/h/L
Aldosterone	672 pmol/L	100–500 pmol/L	1450 pmol/L	600–1200 pmol/L
Aldosterone/ PRA ratio	1920		2100	

Aldosterone/renin ratio	
<80	Conn's unlikely
80–200	Conn's not excluded
>200	Conn's likely

A magnetic resonance image (MRI) of her adrenal glands was undertaken and showed a probable adenoma of the left adrenal gland.

Venous blood catheter studies were undertaken which revealed a three-fold difference in aldosterone levels between the left and right adrenals. On the basis of this, she was referred for surgery.

QUESTIONS

1. What is the mechanism of her hypokalaemia?
2. What conditions and drug therapies are associated with hypokalaemia?
3. What is her anion gap and does this explain her high bicarbonate level?
4. What is the significance of the urine potassium level?
5. Which drugs affect plasma renin and aldosterone measurements?
6. Why did the physician enquire about a family history of hypertension?
7. Describe the clinical use of renin and aldosterone measurements?

ANSWERS

1. Aldosterone acts on the cells of the distal renal tubule and promotes the exchange of sodium for either potassium or hydrogen ions. Potassium is almost totally reabsorbed from the glomerular filtrate in the proximal tubule and therefore aldosterone provides the major route for adjusting potassium excretion. Aldosterone secretion is increased by hyperkalaemia, thus providing a regulatory route. It is also the end of the renin–angiotensin cascade and provides a route for sodium (and water) reabsorption. The excessive secretion of aldosterone in Conn's syndrome leads to an enhanced exchange process with the sodium reabsorption promoting hypertension and the potassium exchange leading to hypokalaemia. In addition, as there is a competition between potassium and hydrogen ions in the process, there is an increased exchange of sodium with hydrogen ions. The hydrogen ion is generated by a process that also generates bicarbonate. The bicarbonate follows the sodium into the plasma with the net effect of elevating the serum bicarbonate concentration. Hence, the hypokalaemia is accompanied by a metabolic alkalosis (see Figure 3.1).

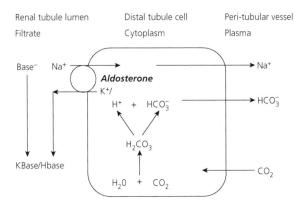

Figure 3.1

2. The causes of hypokalaemia may be divided into those of direct renal origin and those which are non-renal. Renal causes of hypokalaemia may be divided into:

   a. Increased sodium/potassium exchange, for example,
      i.   Conn's syndrome
      ii. Secondary hyperaldosteronism
      iii. Ectopic adrenocorticotropic hormone (ACTH) production
      iv. Carbenoxolone therapy
      v.   Excessive liquorice consumption
      vi. Inherited conditions, e.g. Bartter's, Liddle's and Gitelman's syndromes
   b. Excess sodium available for exchange, for example,
      i.   Excessive saline infusion
      ii. Loop diuretics

  c. Decreased sodium/hydrogen ion exchanged, for example,
    i.   Carbonic anhydrase inhibitors
    ii. Renal tubular acidosis (types I and II)
  d. Impaired proximal renal tubular reabsorption
    i.   Fanconi syndrome
    ii. Hypomagnesaemia

Non-renal causes may be divided into:

  a. Redistribution, for example,
    i.   Glucose and insulin
    ii.   Catecholamines
    iii. Familial hypokalaemic periodic paralysis
  b. Intestinal loss, for example,
    i.   Prolonged vomiting
    ii.   Diarrhoea/small bowel fistula loss
    iii. Purgative abuse

In alkalosis and pyloric stenosis, both renal and non-renal factors are involved in hypokalaemia.

3. Her anion gap is normal at 12 mmol/L and therefore her high bicarbonate is likely to be due to a secondary rather than a primary phenomenon. The mechanism is that once the potassium has been significantly reduced by aldosterone, a sodium/hydrogen pump in the nephron becomes more active leading to increased excretion of hydrogen ions. The hydrogen ions that are exchanged for sodium are generated by carbonic anhydrase in the renal tubule epithelium causing increased production of bicarbonate. The increased bicarbonate and the excreted hydrogen combine to generate a metabolic alkalosis.

4. The finding that the urine potassium is greater than 20 mmol/L in the presence of significant hypokalaemia indicates that the potassium loss is of renal origin.

5. The following drugs influence measurements of renin (PRA) and aldosterone and must be stopped before sampling if the results are to be interpretable.

Drug	Effect on PRA and aldosterone	Duration
Spironolactone	Increase PRA	Stop for 6 weeks before testing
Oestrogens	Increase PRA	Stop for 6 weeks before testing
Angiotensin-converting enzyme (ACE) inhibitors	Increase PRA, decrease aldosterone	Stop for 2 weeks before testing
Other diuretics	Increase PRA	
Beta-blockers	Decrease PRA	
Calcium-channel blockers	Decrease aldosterone	

6. In this context, it was the possibility of familial hypertension, such as the glucocorticoid suppressible hyperaldosteronism, that prompted the question. This presents in young adults with hypertension, hypokalaemia and suppressed plasma renin activity (features caused by the excess activity of aldosterone secretion), and is distinguished from other forms of primary hyperaldosteronism by its autosomal dominant mode of inheritance and the reversal of all its clinical and biochemical abnormalities by the administration of small doses of the synthetic glucocorticoid dexamethasone. It is also characterized by abnormally elevated levels of 18-hydroxycortisol and 18-oxocortisol, the excretion of which also falls to normal following dexamethasone administration.

7. The interpretation of renin and aldosterone results must be undertaken with regard to the clinical features:

Diagnosis	Features	Aldosterone/ PRA	Effect of upright posture	
			PRA	Aldosterone
Normal		Aldosterone/ PRA <500–800	Increase	Increase
Primary hyperaldosteronism. Prevalence: 0.5–2% in general, but 5-12% in hypertension centres. (a) Unilateral adenoma, (b) bilateral nodular hyperplasia	Hypertension and sustained hypokalaemia; kaliuria and metabolic alkalosis	Low PRA which is suppressed by markedly increased aldosterone; aldosterone/ PRA >2000	No change	Decrease
Glucocorticoid suppressible hyperaldosteronism	Suppression of aldosterone after dexamethasone for 48 h		No change	Decrease
Bartter's/Gitelman's syndrome; autosomal recessive resistance of the vasculature to the pressor action of angiotensin II	Secondary hyperaldosteronism. This resistance is associated with an increase in PRA with juxtaglomerular apparatus (JGA) hyperplasia. There is reduced K^+ without hypertension	Increased PRA, increased aldosterone		

Diagnosis	Features	Aldosterone/ PRA	Effect of upright posture	
			PRA	Aldosterone
Renal artery stenosis (RAS)	Measurement of PRA in renal vein from both kidneys can assist in the diagnosis of renal artery stenosis as asymmetrical measurement indicates unilateral correctable stenosis. Peripheral measurement is of no value since levels may be normal or raised			
Renin secreting tumour	Hypertensive patients with ↑↑↑ PRA and in whom chronic renal failure and RAS have been excluded			

CASE 4: ELDERLY MAN WITH A COUGH

History

A 67-year-old male former coal miner has a long history of early morning productive cough. He presented to his GP feeling generally unwell complaining of lower back pain. He was taking thiazide diuretics to control mild hypertension. His appetite was poor due to dyspepsia, but with no apparent weight loss, and he controlled his dyspepsia with milk and over-the-counter antacids. On direct questioning, he admitted to taking 20 units of alcohol per week and had recently stopped smoking. He had smoked 20 cigarettes per day for 50 years.

Examination

He was apyrexial with a blood pressure of 135/80 mmHg and regular pulse at 75 beats per minute. His chest was clear. The mobility of his back was limited by pain and there was discomfort on palpation of his lower lumbar spine.

Investigations

		Reference range
Sodium	138 mmol/L	135–145 mmol/L
Potassium	3.4 mmol/L	3.2–5.1 mmol/L
Urea	8.2 mmol/L	1.7–8.3 mmol/L
Creatinine	107 µmol/L	62–106 µmol/L
Bilirubin	23 µmol/L	Up to 21 µmol/L
Total protein	72 g/L	66–87 g/L
Albumin	32 g/L	34–48 g/L
Globulin	40 g/L	18–36 g/L
Alanine transaminase (ALT)	58 U/L	<41 U/L
Alkaline phosphatase (ALP)	176 U/L	40–129 U/L
Calcium	2.94 mmol/L	2.15–2.55 mmol/L
Adjusted calcium	3.11 mmol/L	2.15–2.55 mmol/L

He was referred to medical outpatients, and plain film radiology of his lumbar spine, together with a chest x-ray, were organized. Further investigations revealed:

		Reference range
IgG	16.2 g/L	6–16 g/L
IgM	1.5 g/L	0.5–2.0 g/L
IgA	3.4 g/L	0.8–4.0 g/L

		Reference range
Serum protein electrophoresis	Monoclonal band detected at 3.8 g/L	
Immunofixation	IgG/lambda band	
Free lambda light chain	66 mg/L	6–26 mg/L
Free kappa light chain	11 mg/L	3–20 mg/L
Kappa:lambda ratio	0.17	0.26–1.65
Parathyroid hormone (PTH)	3.2 ng/L	15–65 ng/L
Vitamin D	45 nmol/L	50–120 nmol/L
Prostate-specific antigen (PSA)	4.8 µg/L	<4.0 µg/L
Free T4	16.3 pmol/L	12–22 pmol/L
Thyroid-stimulating hormone (TSH)	4.7 mU/L	0.3–4.2 mU/L
GGT	75 U/L	10–71 U/L
Cortisol (time not stated)	578 nmol/L	171–536 nmol/L (9 a.m.)
PTH-related peptide (PTHrP)	9.3 pmol/L	<2 pmol/L

The chest film confirmed a mass in his right lung and lumbar spine x-ray showed a destructive lesion in his L4 vertebral body.

Cells obtained at bronchoscopy were typical of small cell carcinoma.

QUESTIONS

1. What might be causing his hypokalaemia?
2. What might be causing his raised alkaline phosphatase?
3. What is the significance of the monoclonal band and related findings?
4. What additional investigations may be undertaken concerning myeloma?
5. What is the most likely cause of his hypercalcaemia?
6. What medical conditions are associated with hypercalcaemia and through what mechanism?
7. What is the role of PTHrP in generating his hypercalcaemia?

ANSWERS

1. Hypercalcaemia is associated with a mild metabolic alkalosis and hence a tendency to hypokalaemia. However, in this case, the possibility of cortisol excess associated with ectopic adrenocorticotropic hormone (ACTH) production may need to be considered. The cortisol measurement had no time associated with the request and, if it were a midnight sample, might be considered elevated.

2. Although bone metastases, as demonstrated on x-ray, is the most likely cause, he does show a rather high ALT and gamma-glutamyl transpeptidase (gammaGT) indicating the possibility of mild obstruction of his biliary tree possibly due to hepatic metastases. In addition, the generation of a placental-like alkaline phosphatase has been associated with tumours, especially lung cancer.

3. The elevated IgG and the presence of a band on electrophoresis indicates the high probability of the presence of a monoclonal protein. This is confirmed by immunofixation as the band consists of only one type of heavy chain (G in this case) and one type of light chain (lambda in this case). The presence of a band does not necessarily indicate the patient has myeloma. Bands of this nature from patients with no significant changes in the bone marrow are termed MGUS (monoclonal gammopathy of unknown significance). Patients with these types of monoclonal bands are monitored on a regular basis as about 1 per cent per annum will transform to become myeloma.

4. The additional investigations will include a urine sample for Bence Jones protein and bone marrow examination for plasma cell changes. Bence Jones protein is detected by electrophoresis and immunofixation to determine if the light chain is kappa or lambda. The importance is that there is a risk of renal dysfunction associated with the presence of excess free light chains in the urine. The suppression of the immunoglobulins not associated with the monoclonal band is also an indication that the band is due to myeloma.

5. The most likely cause of his hypercalcaemia is bony metastases, although the humoral effects of PTHrP (see below) and myeloma need to be considered.

6. The possible causes of hypercalcaemia in this patient are myeloma, milk-alkali syndrome and thiazide diuretics, as well as carcinoma of the lung.

   Myeloma is associated with hypercalcaemia and, although this is often associated with bony lesions, it is primarily due to increased osteoclastic bone resorption caused by potent cytokines expressed or secreted locally by the myeloma cells, such as the receptor activator of nuclear factor-κB ligand (RANKL).

   Thiazide diuretics reduce urinary calcium excretion. Although the main action of thiazides is to block the sodium/chloride co-transporter, the effect on intracellular sodium appears to stimulate sodium/calcium exchange. Thiazides are likely to exacerbate hypercalcaemia due to other causes.

Hypercalcaemia may be caused by excessive intake of milk and alkaline antacids – milk/alkali syndrome. The increase in serum bicarbonate influences the handling of calcium by the kidney at a number of points leading to increased calcium reabsorption.

7. PTHrP has a number of autocrine and paracrine functions, including chondrocyte function and mammary gland differentiation. However, in the context of tumour hypercalcaemia, the circulating concentrations are much higher than normal and its main effect is its ability to bind to PTH receptors, mimicking the normal effects of PTH.

CASE 5: WOMAN WITH ABDOMINAL PAIN

History

A 33-year-old female complained to her GP of bouts of abdominal discomfort and lethargy. On direct questioning, she admitted to rather loose stools at times and slight weight loss. On examination, nothing abnormal was discovered apart from pallor. Her body mass index (BMI) was calculated as 18 (ideal range, 18.9–25).

Investigations

		Reference range
Sodium	138 mmol/L	135–146 mmol/L
Potassium	2.9 mmol/L	3.2–5.1 mmol/L
Urea	1.6 mmol/L	1.7–8.3 mmol/L
Creatinine	46 µmol/L	44–80 U/L
Calcium (adjusted)	2.12 mmol/L	2.15–2.55 mmol/L
Phosphate	0.85 mmol/L	0.87–1.45 mmol/L
Alkaline phosphatase (ALP)	108 U/L	35–104 U/L
Haemoglobin (Hb)	11.8 g/dL	13.5–18 g/dL
Mean corpuscular volume (MCV)	78 fL	76–100 fL
Mean corpuscular haemoglobin (MCH)	27 pg	27–32 pg
Mean corpuscular haemoglobin concentration (MCHC)	31 g/L	31–36 g/L
Ferritin	10 µg/L	13–150 µg/L
C-reactive protein (CRP)	<5 mg/L	<5 mg/L
Faecal calprotectin	40 µg/g	<50 µg/g

The chemical pathologist signing out results phoned the GP and suggested the possibility of malabsorption as the cause of the biochemical findings. The GP recalled the patient and discovered that the patient's brother was taking a gluten-free diet and that the patient herself tended to avoid wheat products.

Additional tests were organized yielding the following:

		Reference range
IgA	2.5 g/L	0.8–2.8 g/L
IgA TTG	9	Negative <4
		Borderline 4–10
		Positive >10

		Reference range
IgA endomyseal Ab	Positive	
25 OH Vitamin D	35 nmol/L	50–120 nmol/L
Parathyroid hormone (PTH)	75 ng/L	15–65 ng/L
Iron	4.5 µmol/L	5.4–28.6 µmol/L
Transferrin	3.8 g/L	2.0–3.6 g/L
Transferrin saturation	2%	5–50%
Vitamin B12	320 ng/L	197–866 ng/L
Folate	4.8 µg/L	4.6–18.7 µg/L

QUESTIONS

1. Why is her serum potassium slightly low?
2. Explain the findings related to calcium metabolism.
3. What conditions are associated with hypocalcaemia?
4. Why was the faecal calprotectin measured? What are the causes of an elevated concentration?
5. Why did the laboratory measure CRP when a ferritin was requested?
6. Why do you think the IgA tissue transglutaminase test was only borderline high?
7. Taking the clinical sensitivity and specificity of IgA tissue transglutaminase antibody testing in adults as 93 and 96 per cent, respectively, calculate the likelihood ratios of a positive test and a negative test.
8. What method can be used to calculate the post-test probability of coeliac disease based on a clinical supposition of a 50 per cent pre-test probability as in this case?

ANSWERS

1. The most likely explanation is chronic diarrhoea, although in malabsorption syndromes hypomagnesaemia may be a contributing factor (see Case 3).

2. The patient has a borderline low calcium with slightly high alkaline phosphatase and rather high parathormone. These three may be associated with either a high phosphate level, as in chronic renal failure, or a low phosphate as in this patient with malabsorption syndrome. In addition, her vitamin D level is also rather low thus exacerbating her hypocalcaemia and the parathormone and alkaline phosphatase responses. The primary cause of her hypocalcaemia is failure to absorb calcium from the gut.

3. Causes of hypocalcaemia (adjusted calcium is that which allows for changes in calcium due to high or low albumin levels):
   a. Drug induced
      i. Enzyme-inducing agents, e.g. phenytoin
   b. Hypocalcaemia, usually with hypophosphataemia
      i. Vitamin D deficiency – rickets and osteomalacia
      ii. Malabsorption states
   c. Hypocalcaemia, usually with hyperphosphataemia
      i. Chronic renal failure
      ii. Hypoparathyroidism – idiopathic, autoimmune, surgical removal, congenital
      iii. Pseudohypoparathyroidism (rare)
      iv. Parathormone resistance (rare)
   d. Other causes
      i. Acute pancreatitis
      ii. Severe hypomagnesaemia
      iii. Rapid cell breakdown – tumour lysis syndrome, rhabdomyolysis
      iv. Hypercalciuric hypocalcaemia – autosomal dominant condition (rare)
      v. High calcitonin levels (rare)

4. Calprotectin is produced by neutrophils and elevated concentrations in faeces are associated with inflammation in the intestine. Faecal calprotectin is used as a marker for inflammatory bowel disease. In this patient, it was assessed to determine the possibility of inflammatory bowel disease and to differentiate this from the possibility of irritable bowel syndrome. The negative predictive value of this test for the exclusion of inflammatory bowel disease is about 90 per cent. Conditions which cause an elevated faecal calprotectin are Crohn's disease, ulcerative colitis and bowel cancer. It is normal in coeliac disease.

5. Ferritin is one of the acute-phase reactant proteins as is CRP. Therefore, if the CRP is raised, it can be anticipated that the ferritin level will be higher than when the CRP is normal. Hence, in inflammatory conditions leading to an elevated CRP, iron deficiency cannot be excluded even if the ferritin level is up to 100 µg/L.

6. The clinical and biochemical information points to a diagnosis of coeliac disease. However, the antibody levels will only be positive if the patient is taking gluten as a regular part of their diet. This lady was taking very little gluten at the time of the test and the results were therefore those of a coeliac patient taking a gluten-free diet. Indeed, measurements may be used to assess compliance with the gluten-free diet.

7. Taking the sensitivity and specificity of IgA tissue transglutaminase antibody testing in adults as 93 and 96 per cent, respectively, the likelihood ratios of a positive test and a negative test for coeliac disease are as follows:

    a. LR+ = sensitivity/(1–specificity): LR+ = 23.25
    b. LR– = (1–sensitivity)/specificity: LR– = 0.073

    Likelihood ratios for a positive test of 10 or more and for a negative test of 0.1 or less are regarded as clinically useful. A likelihood ratio of 1.0 is equivalent to a 50:50 option – thus, no predictive value.

8. Fagan's nomogram is used and links the pre-test probability of a condition with the probability when a specific test has been undertaken. It emphasizes the need for a pre-test probability if a test result is to be interpreted effectively – even if this is simply a population-based probability. The post-test probability in this patient was about 97 per cent. On the basis of this, the patient declined an intestinal biopsy and took a strict gluten-free diet.

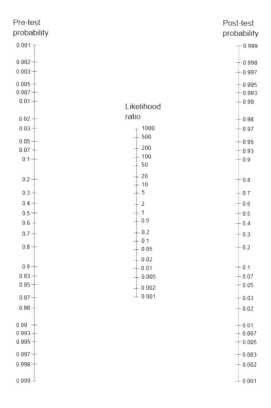

CASE 6: DEPRESSED ELDERLY MAN

History

A 65-year-old man with a history of psychotic depression who has been treated with lithium, olanzapine, diazepam, amlodipine for hypertension and simvastatin for hypercholesterolaemia was found to have abnormal thyroid function tests on routine monitoring. His lithium concentrations were in the therapeutic range. Thyroid function tests returned to normal on thyroxine replacement at a dose of 100 µg/day. He was admitted having become increasingly erratic in his behaviour and unsteady on walking. He was confused and unable to give a history.

Examination

He was dehydrated, pyrexial 38.3°C, blood pressure (BP) 152/88 mmHg, pulse 80 beats per minute regular, respiratory rate 21 per minute, oxygen saturation 90 per cent on air and evidence of right basal pneumonia. He commenced treatment with augmentin and clarithromycin, in addition to intravenous fluids. As a result of his initial blood tests, a fluid balance chart was started. This indicated that he was producing urine at a rate of 240 mL/h. Serum and urine osmolality were requested and on the basis of the results lithium treatment was stopped. As a result, his serum sodium slowly returned to normal. He received a course of electroconvulsive therapy (ECT) for his depression. During the admission, a bone profile was undertaken which showed hypercalcaemia and a raised parathormone (PTH) concentration.

Investigations

	Admission results	On stopping lithium	Reference range
Free thyroxine fT4	18.9 pmol/L		12–22 pmol/L
Thyroid-stimulating hormone (TSH)	4.2 mIU/L		0.3–4.2 mIU/L
Lithium	0.7 mmol/L	<0.1 mmol/L	0.4–1.0 mmol/L (therapeutic range)
Prolactin	654 mIU/L		86–324 mIU/L
Sodium	168 mmol/L	136 mmol/L	135–146 mmol/L
Potassium	3.6 mmol/L	4.2 mmol/L	3.2–5.1 mmol/L
Urea	9.8 mmol/L	8.7 mmol/L	1.7–8.3 mmol/L
Creatinine	129 µmol/L	134 µmol/L	62–106 µmol/L
e-GFR	52 mL/min/1.73m^2	49 mL/min/1.73m^2	>60 mL/min/1.73m^2
Total protein	67 g/L		66–87 g/L
Albumin	36 g/L		34–48 g/L
Haemoglobin (Hb)	14.7 g/dL		13.5–18.0 g/dL

	Admission results	On stopping lithium	Reference range
White blood count (WBC)	$14.0 \times 10^9/L$		$4.0–11.0 \times 10^9/L$
C-reactive protein	98 mg/L		<5 mg/L
Serum osmolality	341 mmol/kg		275–295 mmol/kg
Urine osmolality	363 mmol/kg		
Urine sodium on saline infusion	117 mmol/L		
Calcium (adjusted)	2.56 mmol/L	2.68 mmol/L	2.15–2.55 mmol/L
Phosphate	0.63 mmol/L	0.56 mmol/L	0.87–1.45 mmol/L
Alkaline phosphatase (ALP)	88 U/L	98 U/L	40–129 U/L
Magnesium (adjusted)	0.78 mmol/L	0.82 mmol/L	0.65–1.05 mmol/L
25OH Vitamin D		14 nmol/L	50–120 nmol/L
PTH	166 ng/L	183 ng/L	15–65 ng/L

A parathyroid radioisotope MIBI (methoxy-isobutyl isonitrile) scan was arranged which demonstrated uptake within a solitary right-sided parathyroid adenoma (Figure 6.1). In view of his clinical state, it was agreed to monitor his serum calcium and parathormone.

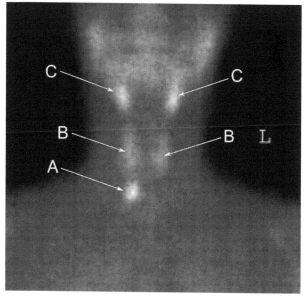

Figure 6.1 Frontal image from the MIBI scan. Note focus of pathological uptake in the right-sided adenoma (A) and (C) submandibular glands, (B) Normal uptake in right and left thyroid lobes. Courtesy of Dr David Sallomi.

QUESTIONS

1. What is the link between lithium therapy and hypothyroidism?
2. What other drugs may interfere with thyroid function tests?
3. What is the probable cause of his elevated prolactin?
4. What are the possible explanations of his serum sodium concentration and high urine outputs?
5. What are the causes of diabetes insipidus?
6. What is the potential link between his therapy and hypercalcaemia?
7. What are the potential causes of his hypercalcaemia?

ANSWERS

1. Lithium increases intrathyroidal iodine content and inhibits the coupling of iodo-tyrosine molecules to form T4 and T3. It also inhibits the release of T4 and T3. The hypothyroidism may be associated with goitre and is more common in iodine deficiency areas. Overall, the incidence is up to 30 per cent of patients treated with lithium, with women being affected more often than men.

2. A number of drugs have effects on thyroid function, but not all of them are clinically significant. Increased thyroxine disposal is associated with anti-epileptics (phenytoin, carbamazepine) and selective serotonin reuptake inhibitors (SSRI) (sertraline), although these are rarely significant if using fT4 and fT3 assays. Interference with thyroxine metabolism is seen during treatment with amiodarone (interferes with T4 to T3 conversion and interference with TSH synthesis), lithium (interferes with T4 synthesis and release), β-blockers (T4 to T3 conversion, but little clinical effect). Interferon-related thyroid disease includes destructive thyroiditis, Grave's thyrotoxicosis and hypothyroidism – the prevalence is variable at 1–35 per cent, with an average about 15 per cent and females affected more than males.

   In addition, there are a number of drugs which inhibit the absorption of thyroxine: antacids, proton pump inhibitors, bile acid sequestrants and phosphate-binding agents used in chronic renal failure.

3. Antipsychotic drugs, such as olanzapine, are the most likely cause of an elevated prolactin other than pituitary adenomas. The major routes for drug-induced hyper-prolactinaemia are: dopamine receptor antagonists (e.g. phenothiazines, risperi-done), dopamine depletion (e.g. methyl dopa, reserpine), hormones (e.g. oestrogens, anti-androgens), other drugs including tricyclic antidepressants, opiates and cime-tidine. Dopamine is the major route for inhibition of prolactin secretion and hence the mechanism of action of some of these drugs.

4. The most likely causes of hypernatraemia associated with a high urine output are an osmotic diuresis, or impairment of antidiuretic hormone (ADH) function. The most frequent cause of this pattern due to osmotic effects is, of course, diabetes mellitus, but other osmotic factors such as mannitol infusions are capable of caus-ing similar effects. The impairment of ADH function is termed diabetes insipidus.

5. Diabetes insipidus (DI) may be divided into those cases which are caused by pitui-tary problems (cranial DI) and those associated with failure of the target for ADH and hence termed nephrogenic DI. The differential diagnoses for DI are psychogenic polydipsia, diuretic abuse and, in this case, the possibility of a very high rate of intravenous therapy.

   The causes of cranial DI include cerebral trauma, infection and infiltrative condi-tions, especially cerebral tumours. Nephrogenic DI may be due to chronic renal fail-ure, interstitial nephritis, hypercalcaemia, hypokalaemia and drugs, such as lithium and demeclocycline.

The definitive test to differentiate between DI and psychogenic polydipsia is the water deprivation test. If at the end of the test there is no evidence of normal ADH activity, as judged by a urine osmolality that does not reach 650 mmol/kg, then DDAVP (a synthetic ADH) is given. If in response to DDAVP, the urine osmolality rises to >650 mmol/kg, then this indicates a cranial cause for DI, but if the urine osmolality remains below 300 mmol/kg, then nephrogenic causes need to be considered.

Condition	Urine osmolality following water deprivation	Urine osmolality following water deprivation and DDAVP
Normal	>650 mmol/kg	N/A
Cranial DI	<300 mmol/kg	>650 mmol/kg
Nephrogenic DI	<300 mmol/kg	<300 mmol/kg

Figures provide typical results.

In this case, the response to stopping lithium therapy indicated the cause as lithium-induced diabetes insipidus, albeit exacerbated by his gastrointestinal condition and hypercalcaemia.

6. The potential causes of his hypercalcaemia may also have been a response to lithium, but as the hypercalcaemia persisted following lithium cessation, this together with the elevated PTH and positive MIBI scan indicate hyperparathyroidism. An elevated PTH is an appropriate response to hypocalcaemia but is inappropriate in hypercalcaemia when it should be suppressed – this indicates PTH as the primary cause of hypercalcaemia.

7. There is a wide range of causes of hypercalcaemia: malignancy (bony metastases, solid tumour humoral effects, myeloma), hyperparathyroidism (primary, tertiary and lithium induced), elevated bone turnover (thyrotoxicosis, immobilization with Paget's disease), elevated vitamin D (vitamin D toxicity, granulomatous conditions, such as sarcoid), drugs (thiazides), milk-alkali syndrome, familial hypocalciuric hypercalcaemia, other endocrine conditions (acromegaly, Addison's disease) and rare conditions, e.g. berylliosis.

CASE 7: TEENAGER WITH HEADACHE AND VOMITING

History

A 17-year-old female, a known insulin-dependent diabetic for nine years, presented in A&E with a headache and vomiting. She had been on antibiotics for the past few days for an 'ear infection'. There was no evidence of neck stiffness, but tenderness behind her right ear.

Investigations

		Reference range
Sodium	138 mmol/L	135–146 mmol/L
Potassium	4.0 mmol/L	3.2–5.1 mmol/L
Urea	6.0 mmol/L	1.7–8.3 mmol/L
Creatinine	97 µmol/L	44–80 µmol/L
Bicarbonate	11.6 mmol/L	22–29 mmol/L
Chloride	100 mmol/L	96–108 mmol/L
Glucose	27.1 mmol/L	3.2–6.0 mmol/L (fasting)
Osmolality	331 mmol/kg	275–295 mmol/kg
Total protein	89 g/L	66–87 g/L
Albumin	49 g/L	34–48 g/L
Alkaline phosphatase (ALP)	303 U/L	35–104 U/L
GGT	44 U/L	6–42 U/L
pH	7.32	7.35–7.42
$PaCO_2$	3.12 kPa	4.5–6.1 kPa
PaO_2	13.96 kPa	12–15 kPa
Base excess	−12.9 mmol/L	±2 mmol/L
Oxygen saturation	95.4%	

The patient received the following fluid replacement:

Normal saline	1 L stat
Normal saline	1 L over 1 hour
Normal saline + 20 mmol K	1 L over 2 hours
Normal saline	1 L over 4 hours
Plus insulin 10 units i.v. over 2 hours	

QUESTIONS

1. What clinical symptoms and signs would you expect with this presentation and why?
2. What is the anion gap in this patient and what is the significance of a high value?
3. What are the main causes of a high anion gap?
4. Comment on the fluid replacement schedule prescribed.
5. What are the possible causes of her vomiting and headache?
6. What explanation can you provide for the alkaline phosphatase?

ANSWERS

1. The patient may complain of drowsiness, fever, sweating, headache, ear ache, nausea, vomiting and thirst. Her pulse would be rapid due to infection, vomiting and diabetic ketoacidosis (DKA). Her blood pressure (BP) may well be low due to her dehydration, vomiting, poor oral intake and possible underlying sepsis. Dehydration is likely to be present and is due to her osmotic diuresis secondary to her hyperglycaemia. Her hyperventilation is a response to her metabolic acidosis to reduce her PCO_2 and hence the balance between PCO_2 and HCO_3, see below She is likely to smell ketotic due to high levels of acetoacetate. Please note that in alcoholic ketosis, there is no ketotic smell as the ketones present are nearly all as 3OH-butyrate. Even in DKA, there is more 3OH-butyrate than acetoacetate and hence this is a better measure of ketosis. Pyrexia may be associated with DKA, but in this case it is likely related to acute infection which precipitated her DKA. The same applies to her leukocytosis.

2. Anion gap:

    Normal: $[Na + K] - [Cl + HCO_3] = 19$
    This case: $[138 + 4] - [100 + 12] = 30$

    The anion gap is the balance between the major cations and anions. The difference is explained by the presence of ions such as sulphate, phosphate and charged proteins, such as albumin. A high anion gap indicates the presence of anions not normally present in significant quantities.

3. Causes of a high anion gap (mnemonic 'Dr Maples')
    D, DKA
    R, renal failure
    M, methanol
    A, alcoholic ketosis
    P, paracetamol poisoning
    L, lactic acidosis
    E, ethylene glycol
    S, salicylate poisoning

A rational approach to abnormal acid/base presentations is to take each element in order (mnemonic ARMAC):
    A – Acidosis or alkalosis – look at pH/hydrogen ion concentration
    R – Respiratory – look at $PaCO_2$
    M – Metabolic – look at bicarbonate
    A – calculate the Anion gap
    C – assess Compensatory processes

The findings in metabolic acidosis is a primary reduction in bicarbonate followed by hyperventilation reducing the $PaCO_2$ and restoring the balance of bicarbonate to CO_2:

  40 nmol/L = 180.1 × (5.3 kPa/24 mmol/L)

  40 nmol/L = 180 × 0.22

  [H+] = 180.1 × (respiration/metabolism)

- Acute metabolic acidosis

  60 nmol/L = 180.1 × (5.3 kPa/16 mmol/L) [5.3/16 = 0.33]

- Compensated metabolic acidosis

  40 nmol/L = 180.1 × (3.5 kPa/16 mmol/L) [3.5/16 = 0.22]

4. Using saline, rather than Hartman's, as the initial fluid replacement is reasonable in view of the history of vomiting. The potassium replacement is inadequate in view of her initial potassium level which is lower than anticipated in DKA – probably associated with her vomiting. Treatment with insulin will cause potassium to enter cells and without adequate replacement hypokalaemia will occur. Remember that serum potassium decreases by 0.3 mmol/L for each 100 mmol loss of total body potassium (loss of total body potassium may be via gastrointestinal secretion or renal loss). A patient with hypokalaemia will usually require 80 mmol/day of potassium replacement to restore the serum potassium to normal. In this case, as insulin causes potassium to enter cells, a larger amount may be required.

5. It is important to check for any history of head injury and to check for neck stiffness, photophobia, petechial, purpuric skin rash as an indication of meningitis. In this case, it is probably due to her ear infection. Computed tomography confirmed evidence of right-sided mastoiditis with no bone destruction and this was treated with intravenous antibiotics. Intracerebral abscess as a complication of middle ear infection may also be associated with decreased cognitive function, headache and drowsiness without necessarily being associated with focal neurological signs.

6. The most likely cause for the raised alkaline phosphatase is that she is still growing and this is reflected in her alkaline phosphatase which is of bone orgin. A hepatic cause is unlikely as her gamma-glutamyl transpeptidase (gammaGT) is normal. One other possibility in a young woman complaining of vomiting is placental alkaline phosphatase in pregnancy (check pregnancy test).

CASE 8: MAN WITH SEVERE VOMITING

History and examination

A 30-year-old man arrived in A&E with a 1-week history of severe vomiting. He had been taking antacids for dyspepsia for some time, but this week the antacids did not seem to be working. He had been unable to 'keep even fluids down' and was feeling rather faint and unwell. On examination, he showed epigastric discomfort, his pulse was 100 beats per minute and blood pressure (BP) 110/65 mmHg, and he was afebrile.

Investigations

		Reference range
Sodium	146 mmol/L	135–146 mmol/L
Potassium	2.7 mmol/L	3.2–5.1 mmol/L
Chloride	83 mmol/L	96–108 mmol/L
Bicarbonate	41 mmol/L	22–29 mmol/L
Urea	28.2 mmol/L	1.7–8.3 mmol/L
Creatinine	132 µmol/L	62–106 µmol/L
Hydrogen ion	31 nmol/L	35–45 nmol/L
PaO_2	15.1 kPa	12–15 kPa
$PaCO_2$	7.2 kPa	4.5–6.1 kPa
Total protein	89 g/L	66–87 g/L
Albumin	50 g/L	34–48 g/L
Haematocrit (Hct)	0.497 L/L	0.35–0.47 L/L
Serum osmolality	330 mmol/kg	275–295 mmol/kg
Urine osmolality	660 mmol/kg	
Urine sodium	11 mmol/L	

QUESTIONS

1. What observations may be of value in determining the degree of salt and water lost by this patient?
2. What was the most likely tonicity of his fluid loss – this may be hypertonic (higher electrolyte concentration than plasma), isotonic (same electrolyte concentration as plasma) or hypotonic (lower electrolyte concentration than plasma)?
3. What is the electrolyte content of the fluid the patient is losing through vomiting?
4. Which laboratory findings indicate the extent of his fluid loss and the nature of that loss?

5. Is there evidence here that the patient is about to develop acute tubular necrosis of the kidneys – acute renal failure?
6. What pattern of acid/base disturbance is demonstrated in his results?
7. Why is the potassium level low? What factors contribute to the hypokalaemia?
8. What fluids would you use to restore the patient's extracellular fluid volume? How much potassium would you give i.v. in the first 24 hours?
9. How would you assess that an appropriate fluid replacement was being delivered?

ANSWERS

1. In addition to pulse and blood pressure postural drop, loss of skin elasticity, increased respiratory rate, thirst, low urine volume and high urine concentration are useful markers of excessive fluid loss, especially isotonic fluid loss.

2. Upper gastrointestinal fluid loss is isotonic. Isotonic fluid loss causes symptoms of shock at lower volumes of loss than water. A comparison of fluid loss and symptoms is given below:

   a. 2 litres isotonic rapid loss – shock
   b. 2 litres isotonic slow loss – mild dehydration
   c. 4 litres isotonic slow loss – severe dehydration
   d. 6 litres isotonic slow loss – shock
   e. 0.5 litre water loss – thirst
   f. 2 litres water loss – mild dehydration
   g. 10+ litres water loss – severe dehydration

   The reason for this is the size of fluid compartment from which the fluid is being taken. Figure 8.1 indicates the volumes of plasma, interstitial fluid and intracellular water. The combination of plasma and interstitial volumes gives the extracellular fluid volume and the intracellular and extracellular, the total body water volume. These figures are for a young 70-kg person.

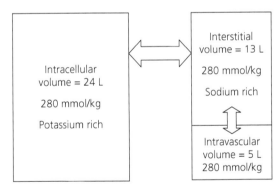

Figure 8.1

Isotonic fluid loss is taken just from the 18 litres of extracellular fluid (namely, interstitial and intravascular spaces), whereas water loss is taken from the 42 litres of total body water. Hence the symptoms of shock are present only following a much greater fluid loss if this is hypotonic.

A rapid pulse, low BP, a BP postural drop and a raised respiratory rate will occur more quickly with a loss of isotonic fluids than hypotonic fluid. Loss of skin elasticity indicates that the interstitial space has been affected by the fluid loss. A low urine volume and a high urine concentration together with thirst may be seen with all fluid loss; however thirst is noted more with hypotonic fluid loss.

3. The electrolyte content of his fluid loss through vomiting is shown in comparison with other gastrointestinal losses in the table below.

Intestinal secretion	Sodium (mmol/L)	Potassium (mmol/L)	Chloride (mmol/L)	Bicarbonate (mmol/L)
Gastric	20–60	14	140	0–15
Biliary	145	5	105	30
Pancreatic	125–138	8	56	85
Small bowel	140	5	125	30
Large bowel	60	15	40	–

In a young person, the gastric fluid will have a low sodium concentration and zero bicarbonate with the ionic difference being filled by hydrogen ions – about 105 mmol/L.

4. The extent of fluid loss may be assessed in previously fit people by the increase in haematocrit, total protein and albumin concentrations. However, where there is a background chronic disease, anaemia and hypoproteinaemia make interpretation more difficult. While it may indicate fluid depletion, an elevation in creatinine is also affected by pre-existing renal function. In dehydration, the urea tends to be raised more than creatinine.

5. Although both the urea and creatinine are raised, the plasma and urine osmolalities indicate the kidney tubules are capable of concentrating urine, and the low urine sodium shows that tubular reabsorption of sodium is effective. The risk of acute renal failure is high when:

a. Urine and plasma osmolalities are very similar values
b. Hyponatraemia with urine sodium >30 mmol/L, namely, inappropriate sodium loss
c. Percentage FENa >1 per cent in acute renal failure: (urine sodium/plasma sodium] × [plasma creatinine/urine creatinine] × 100% (FENa is the fractional excretion of sodium).

6. He shows a metabolic alkalosis with some respiratory compensation. This is the typical pattern seen with high loss of gastric fluid. The loss of hydrogen ions leaves an excess of bicarbonate in serum as normally this fluid would be reabsorbed and the effect on acid/base balance neutral. To compensate, there is a reduction in respiratory rate leading to retention of CO_2, although if there is pain and fear this is minimized by the hyperventilation associated with these factors.

7. There are a number of factors causing the hypokalaemia. Although gastric fluid contains 5–20 mmol/L of potassium, this is not the major reason for the hypokalaemia, although it does contribute. Poor kidney perfusion causes the release of renin, which then activates the angiotensin system and through this the secretion of aldosterone from the adrenal cortex. Aldosterone promotes the retention of sodium through the exchange of sodium for potassium or hydrogen ions (see Figure 8.2).

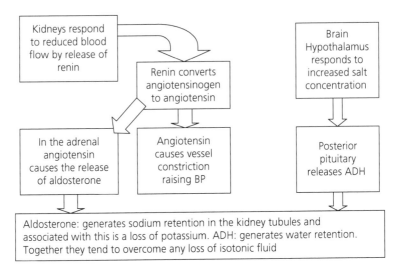

Figure 8.2

In this case, the ability to exchange sodium for hydrogen ions is limited by the relatively low hydrogen ion concentration. Furthermore, the exchange of sodium for hydrogen ions in the renal tubules generates bicarbonate, which is already in excess in plasma. Hence in this context, the exchange of sodium is mostly for potassium, thus generating the hypokalaemia.

Note: As the plasma potassium falls in the extracellular fluid, potassium leaves the intracellular space to compensate. For this reason, the amount of potassium lost to cause a fall in plasma potassium is considerable – usually a fall of plasma potassium by 0.3 mmol/L represents a loss of 100 mmol of potassium from the body. It is important to recognize this when replacing potassium intravenously.

8. Isotonic saline will be the major fluid infused in the first 24 hours. A 2:1 ratio of normal saline to 5% dextrose will probably be appropriate. Although Hartmann's solution is used extensively to cover loss from small bowel, the high chloride loss in this case requires the use of saline initially.

   The initial plasma potassium of 2.7 mmol/L indicates that the patient is at least 200 mmol deficient in potassium (100 mmol per 0.3 mmol/L fall in plasma potassium). This should not be replaced immediately as time must be given for equilibration between extracellular and intracellular spaces. However, more than 40 mmol will be required in the first 24 h and in a fit young person 100 mmol in 24 h is reasonable.

9. When pushing isotonic i.v. fluids into a patient with shock, it is important to monitor the physiological effects. These are pulse and BP – as an increase in BP will increase renal perfusion, there will be an increase in urine volume. So an increase in urine output is an indication of the adequacy of fluid replacement. Monitoring the jugular venous pressure (JVP) is important to ensure fluid replacement is not too vigorous and risking cardiac failure – especially important in the elderly.

However, it will be important to check the electrolyte levels but more to ensure that potassium replacement is appropriate. When the kidneys are better perfused, the plasma urea and creatinine will fall, but only when the urine volume has increased sufficiently to excrete the high level of urea in the total body water. Skin turgor will return to normal when the extracellular fluid volume is replete.

CASE 9: MAN FOUND SEMI-CONSCIOUS

History

The emergency service is called to a flat where a 25-year-old man is reported as being found semi-conscious. He is a diabetic wearing a warning bracelet. He has a history of poor control of his glycaemia and is well known to A&E.

On admission to the department, he has a Glasgow Coma Score (GCS) of 8, blood pressure 115/75 mmHg, pulse 95 per minute, respiratory rate 12 per minute. His chest was clear, his abdomen soft and there was no localizing neurology. As his blood glucose by stick reading was 17.1 mmol/L, an infusion of saline was commenced and sliding scale insulin regimen prepared.

Investigations

		Reference range
Sodium	143 mmol/L	135–146 mmol/L
Potassium	4.2 mmol/L	3.2–5.1 mmol/L
Urea	12.3 mmol/L	1.7–8.3 mmol/L
Creatinine	115 µmol/L	62–106 µmol/L
Bilirubin	28 µmol/L	<21 µmol/L
Albumin	40 g/L	34–48 g/L
Total protein	76 g/L	66–87 g/L
Alanine aminotransferase (ALT)	120 U/L	<41 U/L
Alkaline phosphatase (ALP)	135 U/L	40–129 U/L
Gamma-glutamyl transferase (gamma-GT)	85 U/L	10–71 U/L
pH	7.29	7.35–7.42
PaO$_2$ on 100% oxygen	47 kPa	
PaCO$_2$	7.10 kPa	4.5–6.1 kPa
Bicarbonate	25.1 mmol/L	22–29 mmol/L
Base excess	−2.3 mmol/L	−2/+1
Oxygen saturation	94%	
COHb (carboxyhaemoglobin)	5.5%	0–2%
Ethanol	1.3 g/L	(UK legal driving limit 0.8 g/L)
3OH (hydroxyl) butyrate	1.4 mmol/L	<0.6 mmol/L
Lactate	6.1 mmol/L	0.5–2.2 mmol/L

		Reference range
Opiate screen	Strong positive	
Salicylate	<5 mg/L	(0–20 mg/L negative)
Paracetamol	<5 mg/L	(>300 mg/L toxic, therapeutic range 10–20 mg/L at 2 hours post-dose)

QUESTIONS

1. Is the pattern of blood gases consistent with a diagnosis of diabetic ketoacidosis?
2. What findings support the diagnosis of diabetic ketoacidosis in this case?
3. Describe the pattern of blood gases in this patient?
4. What conditions may cause the pattern of liver function tests found in this patient?
5. What are the possible explanations of his COHb level?
6. What are the possible causes of his elevated lactate?

ANSWERS

1. No, the blood gas pattern does not support the diagnosis of diabetic ketoacidosis (DKA). In DKA, the bicarbonate would be low and the $PaCO_2$ reduced as part of the compensatory mechanism.

2. The GCS score is not typical of a patient with a blood glucose of 17.1 mmol/L. In DKA, the respiratory rate is elevated, whereas in this patient it is depressed. Both of these clinical factors indicate there is another critical problem. The elevated blood glucose and 3OH butyrate together with a raised urea lend some support to the diagnosis of DKA. Although the 3OH butyrate is above normal and indicates poor diabetic control, it is not at a concentration expected in DKA, however there is an alternative explanation for his raised 3OH butyrate. Excessive alcohol (ethanol) intake may cause an elevation of 3OH butyrate. The blood alcohol of 1.3 g/L in this patient may be compared with the legal limit for driving of 0.8 g/L. It seems likely that his peak alcohol was much higher. Blood alcohol concentrations of 2 g/L are associated with confusion, values of 3 g/L with stupor, 4 g/L with coma and 5 g/L may be fatal. In extreme cases, the accumulation of 3OH butyrate may lead to alcoholic ketosis. This potentially fatal condition may be missed as there may not be a ketotic odour and Ketostix test may be negative. (Ketostix measure acetoacetate not 3OH butyrate and it is the latter that is raised in alcoholic ketosis.) Alcoholic ketosis usually responds to an infusion of dextrose. An elevated urea is common in DKA secondary to the dehydration associated with glycosuria.

3. His pH shows he has an acidosis and the high $PaCO_2$ indicates this is respiratory in origin. In the presence of an elevated $PaCO_2$, there would normally be a compensatory increase in bicarbonate which is not found in this case. This is probably due to the metabolic effects of his diabetes, alcohol intake and use of opiates generating a production of metabolic acids (lactate and 3OH butyrate) which offset the anticipated compensatory rise in bicarbonate, hence the bicarbonate level is within normal limits as is the base excess.

4. The pattern of liver function tests (LFT) shows elements of both obstruction (elevated alkaline phosphatase (ALP) and gamma-glutamyl transferase (gamma-GT)) and cellular damage/destruction (elevated alanine aminotransferase (ALT) and aspartate transaminase (AST)). In acute viral hepatitis, the predominant feature would be the elevation of ALT indicating liver cell damage as being the major factor associated with mild hyperbilirubinaemia. In obstruction of the biliary duct, the predominant features would be an elevation of alkaline phosphatase and gamma-GT with a much lesser elevation of ALT. The blood ethanol in this case with the LFT pattern indicates the effects of long-term alcohol excess. The possibility of this being due to non-alcoholic fatty liver disease, which is associated with diabetes, needs consideration. However, the elevations of ALT and AST are higher than that found in simple non-alcoholic fatty liver disease, but may be found when this has progressed to fibrotic changes. Similarly, if DKA is associated with very elevated triglycerides then fatty liver may be present, however hyperbilirubinaemia would be unlikely.

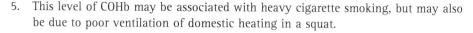

5. This level of COHb may be associated with heavy cigarette smoking, but may also be due to poor ventilation of domestic heating in a squat.

6. The elevation in lactate is due to poor oxygenation of tissues and is associated with the opiate-induced respiratory depression. Blood lactate is also elevated in paracetamol poisoning and if co-codamol has been taken, then both paracetamol concentration in the blood and a positive screening test for opiates will be present. Another possibility is the effect of carbon monoxide which is associated with lactic acidosis, as is diabetic ketosis. Lactic acidosis is a metabolic acidosis and is defined as a blood lactate concentration above 5 mmol/L, while values between the upper limit of normal and 5.0 mmol/L are termed lactic acidaemia. The causes of lactic acidosis may be divided into those associated with (1) hypoxic and (2) non-hypoxic causes.

    a. Hypoxic causes include ischemia, e.g. cardiac arrest; global hypoxia, e.g. carbon monoxide poisoning; respiratory failure, e.g. chronic obstructive pulmonary disease (COPD); and regional hypoperfusion, e.g. mesenteric ischemia.
    b. Non-hypoxic causes include delayed clearance, e.g. liver failure; pyruvate dehydrogenase dysfunction, e.g. sepsis and alcoholic and diabetic ketosis; uncoupled oxidative phosphorylation, e.g. salicylate, ethylene glycol and metformin; accelerated aerobic glycolysis, e.g. sepsis, seizures and high fructose loads.

    Treatment of lactic acidosis is primarily the removal of the underlying cause plus ensuring adequate oxygenation, and that perfusion is adequate.

CASE 10: YOUNG WOMAN WITH ASPIRIN OVERDOSE

History

Following a family row, a 21-year-old female is brought to A&E with a history that she had recently ingested 'at least 50' tablets believed to be enteric-coated 300-mg aspirins. She appears confused and complains of nausea, abdominal pain and tinnitus.

On suspicion of salicylate poisoning, blood gases are measured and blood samples sent to the laboratory.

Investigations

	Admission	8 hours later	Reference range
pH	7.55	7.28	7.35–7.42
PaCO$_2$	4.0 kPa	3.2 kPa	4.5–6.2 kPa
PaO$_2$	12.0 kPa	14.5 mmol/L	12.0–15.0 kPa
Sodium	140 mmol/L	142 mmol/L	135–146 mmol/L
Potassium	3.2 mmol/L	5.5 mmol/L	3.2–5.1 mmol/L
Urea	3.7 mmol/L	5.2 mmol/L	1.7–8.3 mmol/L
Creatinine	69 µmol/L	73 µmol/L	44–80 µmol/L
Chloride	100 mmol/L	102 mmol/L	96–108 mmol/L
Bicarbonate	20 mmol/L	17 mmol/L	22–29 mmol/L
Salicylate	310 mg/L		(0–20 mg/L negative, 20–200 mg/L therapeutic)
Paracetamol	<5 mg/L		(Therapeutic range 10–20 mg/L at 2 hours post-dose)
Glucose	8.8 mmol/L		
Lactate	2.2 mmol/L	6.8 mmol/L	0.5–2.2 mmol/L

Initial treatment was activated charcoal and in addition an intravenous 1 L of 5% dextrose infusion with 40 mmol potassium was commenced.

QUESTIONS

1. What pattern of disturbance is shown in the first set of blood gases?
2. Describe the reason(s) for your answer.
3. What change in serum calcium may be anticipated?
4. What clinical conditions are associated with a respiratory alkalosis?
5. Calculate the anion gap for the second set of laboratory tests and comment on the reasons for the change.

ANSWERS

1. The first set of blood gases shows predominantly a respiratory alkalosis as shown by the elevated pH with a low $PaCO_2$ and borderline low bicarbonate indicating a small degree of renal compensation.

2. Salicylate toxicity initially will create a pure respiratory alkalosis because of direct stimulatory effects on the respiratory centre of the cerebral medulla. This is characterized in the blood gases by a decrease in the partial pressure of dissolved CO_2 accompanied by an elevated pH and normal to slightly low concentration of serum bicarbonate. Compensatory mechanisms of renal bicarbonate retention do not respond sufficiently rapidly to move the pH towards normal.

3. The alkalosis may induce tetany due to a fall in ionized calcium, although total (adjusted) serum calcium may remain within normal limits. The mechanism is through increased binding of calcium to albumin when the pH is increased.
   Note also the increased blood glucose. Salicylate poisoning uncouples oxidative phosphorylation which can cause hypoglycaemia. However, increased glucose-6-phosphatase activity and hepatic glycogenolysis can also cause hyperglycaemia if large amounts of salicylate are ingested.

4. A respiratory alkalosis may be associated with a range of clinical conditions which may be grouped by causative mechanisms as shown below:

   - Hyperventilation, e.g. anxiety state
   - Exogenous agents increasing respiratory drive, e.g. salicylate, theophylline, catecholamines
   - Hypoxia in early pulmonary disease, e.g. asthma, pulmonary embolus
   - Increased cerebral respiratory drive, e.g. head injury, stroke, meningitis
   - Non-cerebral increase in respiratory drive, e.g. heat exposure, hepatic failure

5. The anion gap may be calculated as (sodium concentration + potassium concentration) – (chloride concentration + bicarbonate concentration). The reference range is 10–20 mmol/L. This difference is due to the presence of phosphate, sulphate and proteins, such as albumin. In the second set of results, the anion gap is $(142 + 5.5) - (102 + 17) = 27.5$ mmol/L. The high lactic acid is the major cause of this, although there is a small input from salicylate itself. The rise in lactate is due to the effect of salicylate in uncoupling mitochondrial function so that metabolism relies on the conversion of glucose to pyruvate and lactate. Hence, lactate levels rise in the serum and a respiratory alkalosis is overcome by a metabolic acidosis. This patient has moderately severe salicylate poisoning, levels >500 mg/L indicate severe poisoning and >700 mg/L may be lethal. She is exhibiting clinical features of salicylate poisoning (note tinnitus). In severe cases hypotension, pulmonary oedema, marked heart block and marked hyperthermia may occur.

Paracetamol levels must also be checked as this may also have been taken and salicylate levels may need to be repeated after 2 hours as salicylate absorption can continue during this time. Treatment depends on severity. More severe salicylate poisoning may require urine alkalinization with bicarbonate/potassium chloride and dialysis may be needed with very high salicylate levels.

CASE 11: ASTHMATIC MALE WITH COUGH

History

A male aged 58 years, weight 56 kg, body mass index (BMI) 22 (ideal range, 18.9–25), has had mild asthma for many years controlled by inhaled steroids and bronchodilators. Following an upper respiratory tract infection, he develops a cough with purulent sputum. His GP arranges his admission to hospital, largely because of his confused state.

Examination

He has widespread quiet wheeze and bilateral basal consolidation; temp 35.8°C; pulse 95 beats per minute; respiratory rate 27 per minute. He is increasingly confused and scores 6/10 on AMT (Abbreviated Mental Test score).

In A&E, samples were taken for routine tests and a dextrose infusion commenced prior to transfer to the medical assessment unit where blood tests were repeated 6 h later.

	In A&E	6 hours later	Reference range
Glucose		7.5 mmol/L	
Sodium	144 mmol/L	130 mmol/L	135–146 mmol/L
Potassium	4.5 mmol/L	5.2 mmol/L	3.2–5.1 mmol/L
Urea	4.8 mmol/L	10.8 mmol/L	1.7–8.3 mmol/L
Creatinine	71 μmol/L	105 μmol/L	62–106 μmol/L
Albumin	30 g/L	24 g/L	34–48 g/L
Total protein	69 g/L	62 g/L	66–87 g/L
Globulin	39 g/L	36 g/L	18–36 g/L
Haemoglobin	13.5 g/dL	12.8 g/dL	13.5–18.0 g/dL
White cell count	17.6×10^9/L	23.3×10^9/L	$4.0–11.0 \times 10^9$/L
IgG		17.8 g/L	6–16 g/L
IgA		1.5 g/L	0.8–4.0 g/L
IgM		2.1 g/L	0.5–2.0 g/L
C-reactive protein (CRP)		275 mg/L	<5 mg/L
Iron		4.5 μmol/L	8.1–28.6 μmol/L
Transferrin		1.7 g/L	2.0–3.6 g/L
Transferrin saturation		42%	5–50%
Ferritin		853 μg/L	30–400 μg/L
Ft4 (free throxine)		9.2 pmol/L	12–22 pmol/L
TSH (thyroid-stimulating hormone)		2.1 mIU/L	0.3–4.2 mIU/L

Liver function tests (LFT) were normal. He was commenced on intravenous antibiotics. Blood culture was undertaken. Blood gases revealed that he was acidotic and his lactate was 4.2 mmol/L.

QUESTIONS

1. What are clinical indications of sepsis?
2. What are laboratory indications of sepsis?
3. What is the significance of the change in the electrolyte pattern? Explain your conclusion.
4. Explain the findings related to iron metabolism.
5. Why is his blood glucose raised?
6. Explain the thyroid function tests.
7. What is the mechanism for the fall in serum albumin?
8. What is the significance of the increased serum lactate?

ANSWERS

1. The clinical indicators of sepsis include hyperthermia >38.3°C or hypothermia <36°C, tachycardia >90 beats per minute, tachypnoea >20 breaths per minute, and frequently an acutely altered mental state. The acute change in mental state was the trigger the GP saw that initiated the transfer to hospital, although the other clinical indicators are positive.

2. The laboratory indicators of sepsis are leukocytosis (white cell count >12 000 × 10⁹/L) or leukopenia (white cell count <4000 × 10⁹/L), hyperglycaemia (plasma glucose >6.7 mmol/L) and an elevated CRP (usually >150 mg/L).

3. The rise in creatinine is greater than 26 μmol/L indicating acute kidney injury even though the values remain within the reference intervals. By the criteria shown below he is at stage 1 of acute kidney injury.

Stage	Serum creatinine criteria	Urine output criteria
1	Increase >26 μmol/L within 48 hours or increase >1.5–1.9 × reference serum creatinine	<0.5 mL/kg/h for >6 consecutive hours
2	Increase >2.0–2.9 × reference serum creatinine	<0.5 mL/kg/h for >12 hours
3	Increase >3 × reference serum creatinine or increase >354 μmol/L or commenced on renal replacement therapy irrespective of stage	<0.3 mL/kg/h for >24 hours or anuria for 12 hours

The most common causes of acute kidney injury are (mnemonic P-STOP):

P, poor perfusion (check pulse, blood pressure, respiratory rate)
S, sepsis which leads to poor perfusion
T, toxins often drugs
O, obstruction – requires renal tract ultrasound
P, parenchymal renal disease

e-GFR is not of value in the diagnosis of acute kidney injury as the rate of change in creatinine may be rapid. e-GFR is designed to detect chronic renal disease.

4. The fall in transferrin and iron with low normal transferrin saturation but raised ferritin is typical of the response to sepsis. The rise in ferritin is part of the acute-phase response with increased production by the liver. The mechanism for the fall in iron levels is through the increased production of hepcidin by the liver. Hepcidin inhibits ferroportin on the basal side of enterocytes thus reducing iron absorption from the gut. Please note that reference ranges for iron are based on 9 a.m. samples. Serum iron changes through the day with a diurnal pattern similar to that of cortisol.

5. Hyperglycaemia is part of the metabolic response to injury. It occurs because of glucose mobilization via glycogenolysis and gluconeogenesis induced by high circulating levels of glucagon and catecholamines and the inhibition of insulin secretion (probably catecholamine mediated) in the early stages of the metabolic response to injury. At later stages in the metabolic response to injury, insulin

resistance dominates the metabolic response. Insulin resistance is the condition where insulin becomes relatively ineffective in the uptake of glucose by tissues. The cellular mechanism involves inappropriate phosphorylation of the insulin receptor substrate leading to reduction of the signalling process that increases the production of glucose receptors. This occurs when circulating and tissue fatty acid levels are elevated.

6. The pattern of low fT4 with no compensatory TSH response may lead to consideration of pituitary failure. However, this pattern is also part of the response to injury and sepsis. A serum cortisol estimation is useful in differentiating the two conditions. Cortisol secretion is increased in sepsis, whereas in pituitary failure it will be inappropriately normal or low.

7. The fall in serum albumin may be a dilutional effect due to intravenous fluid therapy, but the decrease in total protein concentration can be attributed to the fall in albumin alone. The major cause of hypoalbuminaemia in sepsis is an increase in the transcapillary escape rate (TCER). Normally there is a dynamic equilibrium between the TCER tending to transfer albumin into the interstitial space and the hydrostatic pressure (HP) generating a return to the circulation (see Figure 11.1). This equilibrium is disturbed in sepsis leading to a low serum albumin. Please note that even in healthy people more albumin is in the interstitial space than the intravascular space.

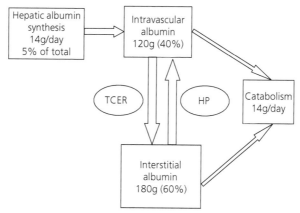

Figure 11.1

8. A lactate concentration of greater than 4 mmol/L due to sepsis is a serious prognostic indicator associated with increased mortality and morbidity. The probability of death within 3 days is five times greater when the lactate concentration is greater than 4.0 mmol/L compared with values between 2.5–3.9 mmol/L.

CASE 12: MAN WITH RENAL FAILURE

History

A 55-year-old male was diagnosed as having polycystic kidneys when about 30 years old. He moved his employment to another part of the country and did not make arrangements for follow up of his renal condition. He presented to his GP with general malaise and was found to have a blood pressure (BP) of 185/115 and also a positive urine stick test for albumin and blood.

Investigations

		Reference range
Haemoglobin (Hb)	10.8 g/dL	13.5–18.0 g/dL
White blood cells (WBC)	10.9 × 10⁹/L	4.0–11.0 × 10⁹/L
Mean corpuscular volume (MCV)	73 fL	76–100 fL
Mean corpuscular haemoglobin concentration (MCHC)	24 g/L	31–36 g/L
Iron	4.0 µmol/L	8.1–28.6 µmol/L
Transferrin	1.7 g/L	2.0–3.6 g/L
Transferrin saturation	4%	5–50%
Ferritin	35 µg/L	30–400 µg/L
C-reactive protein (CRP)	9.5 mg/L	<5 mg/L
Sodium	137 mmol/L	135–146 mmol/L
Potassium	6.3 mmol/L	3.2–5.1 mmol/L
Urea	21.7 mmol/L	1.7–8.3 mmol/L
Creatinine	352 µmol/L	62–106 µmol/L
e-GFR (glomerular filtration rate)	17 mL/min/1.73m²	>60 mL/min/1.73m²
Bicarbonate	13 mmol/L	22–29 mmol/L
Albumin	30 g/L	34–48 g/L
Calcium (adjusted)	1.79 mmol/L	2.15–2.55 mmol/L
Phosphate	2.63 mmol/L	0.87–1.45 mmol/L
Alkaline phosphatase (ALP)	175 U/L	40–129 U/L
PTH (parathormone)	235 ng/L	15–65 ng/L
Glucose (fasting)	6.3 mmol/L	3.2–6.0 mmol/L
Cholesterol	8.5 mmol/L	<5.0 mmol/L
High-density lipoprotein (HDL) cholesterol	0.9 mmol/L	>1.0 mmol/L

		Reference range
Low-density lipoprotein (LDL) cholesterol	6.0 mmol/L	<3.0 mmol/L
Triglyceride	3.2 mmol/L	0.8–1.7 mmol/L
Urine albumin:creatinine ratio	75 mg/mmol	<30 mg/mmol
Vitamin B12	250 ng/L	197–866 ng/L
Folate	6.2	4.6–18.7 µg/L

QUESTIONS

1. At which stage of renal failure do you consider him to be and which of the findings fit with that stage?
2. What type of anaemia does he have and what is the cause of his anaemia?
3. What acid-base disturbance do you suspect and why?
4. Explain the causes of his low calcium and high phosphate and PTH levels.
5. Explain the reason for his lipid abnormality.

ANSWERS

1. His e-GFR indicates he has stage 4/severe renal failure based on the criteria listed below:

Stage	Description	e-GFR
1	Normal	>90
2	Early renal insufficiency	60–89
3	Chronic renal failure	30–59
4	Severe renal failure	15–29
5	End-stage renal failure	<15

He demonstrates the following features of chronic kidney disease (CKD): high creatinine and urea, anaemia, hypocalcaemia, hyperphosphataemia, raised alkaline phosphatase, raised PTH and raised triglyceride.

Stage of CKD	Metabolic features
2	Elevated urea and creatinine with some increase in PTH
3	Calcium absorption decreased, lipoprotein lipase decreased, malnutrition, anaemia (erythropoietin decreased)
4	Elevated triglyceride, elevated phosphate, metabolic acidosis, hyperkalaemia
5	Marked elevation of urea and creatinine and more marked expression of other features

2. He shows the features of a microcytic hypochromic anaemia typical of iron deficiency. His transferrin is rather low due to loss through the glomerulus as part of his proteinuria. Anaemia may be due to lack of factors required for erythropoiesis (iron, B12 and folate), loss of red cells (bleeding and haemolysis) and failure of production.

In most cases of CKD, the major causes of anaemia are 'toxic' effects on the marrow and failure of production of erythropoietin. In most types of CKD, there is an inverse correlation between the haemoglobin level and the level of erythropoietin. Erythropoietin is normally produced by interstitial fibroblasts in the kidney in close association with peritubular capillary and tubular epithelial cells in response to oxygen deficiency.

It is currently recommended that the management of anaemia should be considered in patients with CKD when their haemoglobin level is less than or equal to 11 g/dL in adults.

Treatment with erythropoiesis-stimulating agents (ESA) should be offered to people with anaemia of CKD who are likely to benefit in terms of quality of life and physical function.

In people with anaemia of CKD, treatment should maintain stable Hb levels between 10.5 and 12.0 g/dL through adjusting treatment, typically when Hb rises above 12.0 or falls below 11.0 g/dl.

People receiving ESA maintenance therapy should be given iron supplements to keep their:

a. Serum ferritin levels between 200 and 500 µg/L in both
b. Haemodialysis and non-haemodialysis patients, **and** either
c. Transferrin saturation level above 20 per cent (unless ferritin is greater than 800 µg/L) **or**
d. Percentage hypochromic red cells (%HRC) less than 6 per cent (unless ferritin is greater than 800 µg/L).

In polycystic kidney disease, erythropoietin production is not depleted at the early stages of CKD because the cysts are associated with the cells which produce erythropoietin.

3. Based on the low bicarbonate and level of CKD, he has a chronic metabolic acidosis. The acidosis is due to the accumulation of organic acids together with anions, such as phosphate and sulphate. The elevated phosphate also supports the role of this anion in the acidosis.

4. Secondary hyperparathyroidism develops in chronic kidney disease because of the following factors:

a. Hyperphosphataemia
b. Hypocalcaemia
c. Decreased renal synthesis of 1,25-dihydroxycholecalciferol (1,25-dihydroxyvitamin D, or calcitriol)
d. Intrinsic alteration in the parathyroid gland, which gives rise to increased PTH secretion, as well as increased parathyroid growth
e. Skeletal resistance to PTH

Calcium and calcitriol are primary feedback inhibitors; hyperphosphataemia is a stimulus to PTH synthesis and secretion.

Phosphate retention begins in early chronic kidney disease; when the glomerular filtration rate (GFR) falls, less phosphate is filtered and excreted, but serum concentrations do not rise initially because of increased PTH secretion, which promotes renal phosphate excretion. Thus, there is a compensatory mechanism to keep the serum phosphate within reference limits. However, as the GFR falls further toward chronic kidney disease stages 4–5, hyperphosphataemia develops from the inability of the kidneys to excrete the patient's dietary intake of phosphate. At this stage, drugs to bind phosphate in the gut are useful.

Hyperphosphataemia suppresses the renal hydroxylation of inactive 25-hydroxyvitamin D to the active 1,25-hydroxyvitamin D (calcitriol), so serum calcitriol levels are low when the GFR is less than 30 mL/min. Increased phosphate concentration also effects PTH concentration by its direct effect on the parathyroid gland.

Hypocalcaemia develops primarily from decreased intestinal calcium absorption because of low plasma calcitriol levels. Low serum calcitriol levels, hypocalcaemia, and hyperphosphataemia have all been demonstrated to independently trigger PTH synthesis and secretion. In CKD, particularly in the more advanced stages, PTH secretion is linked to hyperplasia of the parathyroid glands. The persistently elevated PTH levels exacerbate hyperphosphataemia from bone resorption of phosphate. Hence, there may be multiple elements causing hyperphosphataemia.

5. The predominant mechanism responsible for increased concentration of triglyceride is delayed catabolism. The reduced catabolic rate is linked to two routes: first, to diminished lipoprotein lipase activity as a consequence of the downregulation of the enzyme gene; and second, the presence of lipase inhibitors such as apolipoprotein C-III which is found in increased amounts in triglyceride-rich lipoproteins in CKD.

It has also been suggested that secondary hyperparathyroidism is involved in the impaired catabolism of triglyceride-rich lipoproteins. Increased hepatic production of triglyceride-rich lipoproteins may also play a contributory role in the pathogenesis of dyslipidaemia in renal disease through the insulin resistance found in CKD promoting hepatic very-low-density lipoprotein (VLDL) production.

CASE 13: TEENAGER WITH COLICKY PAIN

History

A 16-year-old female presents with severe intermittent colicky pain over the previous 4 hours. The pain radiates from the left loin into her groin. There is no previous history of similar pain and she is otherwise healthy.

Examination

She is apyrexial, blood pressure (BP) 116/80 mm/Hg, pulse 80 beats per minute. No localizing abdominal tenderness was found on palpation. A urine dipstick test was positive for blood. Within a few hours, she passed a small stone which was sent to the laboratory for analysis.

Following the passage of the stone, she was allowed home and arrangements made for a follow-up appointment and further blood tests organized. Figure 13.1 is an axial unenhanced image from a computed tomography (CT) urogram through the kidneys – a large left-sided renal calculus is present (arrow).

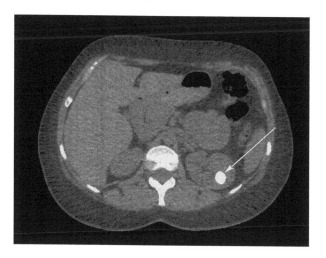

Figure 13.1

Investigations

	Initial findings	Follow-up findings	Reference range
Sodium	142 mmol/L	144 mmol/L	135–146 mmol/L
Potassium	2.8 mmol/L	2.6 mmol/L	3.2–5.1 mmol/L
Creatinine	65 µmol/L	67 µmol/L	44–80 µmol/L
Urea	3.7 mmol/L	3.9 mmol/L	1.7–8.3 mmol/L
C-reactive protein (CRP)	<5 mg/L		<5 mg/L

	Initial findings	Follow-up findings	Reference range
Chloride		112 mmol/L	96–108 mmol/L
Bicarbonate		17 mmol/L	22–29 mmol/L
Calcium (adjusted)		2.27 mmol/L	2.15–2.55 mmol/L
Albumin		40 g/L	34–48 g/L
Phosphate		1.05 mmol/L	0.85–1.45 mmol/L
Alkaline phosphatase		175 U/L	35–104 U/L

Liver function tests, full blood count normal white cell count normal – no leukocytosis.

When she was followed up in the Outpatient Department, the results of analysis of her renal stone were available – its composition was calcium phosphate.

QUESTIONS

1. What is the explanation of her alkaline phosphatase being above the reference limit?
2. In what sex and at what age are renal stones most common?
3. What chemical compositions of renal stones do you know and how frequently are they found in a general population?
4. What conditions do you associate with a calcium phosphate stone?
5. What does this electrolyte pattern suggest?
6. What is the reason for your answer?
7. How do you calculate the anion gap?
8. If you were suspicious that she had renal tubular acidosis, what next investigations would you undertake?
9. What confirmatory tests may be used?

ANSWERS

1. The reference range provided is for adults. In healthy adolescents, the alkaline phosphatase may be as high as 185 U/L due to bone growth – although in a female placental alkaline phosphatase should also be considered. If there was any concern that the alkaline phosphatase was of liver origin, a gamma-GT analysis is indicated.

2. Renal stones are more common in men and most stone formers have their first stone at between 30 and 40 years. However, because of the frequency of recurrent stone formation (50 per cent relapse in 5–10 years), the prevalence increases with age. So the possibility of either a metabolic cause or congenital malformation of the renal system should be considered when calculi are found in young people.

3. About 80 per cent of renal calculi contain calcium, 5–10 per cent contain uric acid, which indicates the relative rarity of other stone types. Some stones are mixtures of compounds such as calcium oxalate with calcium phosphate (35–40 per cent of stones) or uric acid with calcium oxalate (5 per cent).

Compound	Percentage of calculi
Calcium oxalate containing	40–60
Calcium phosphate containing	20–60
Uric acid	5–10
Magnesium ammonium phosphate	5–15
Cystine	1.0–2.5
Ammonium urate	0.5–1.0
Rare	
Silica, xanthine, dihydroxyadenine, indinivar, triamterene, homogentisic acid	<1

In a person of this age, renal stones of any type are unusual and an inherited cause, such as cystinuria and renal tubular acidosis, must be considered. Pure calcium phosphate calculi are relatively uncommon, especially at the age of this patient.

4. Calcium phosphate stones are associated with hyperparathyroidism and renal tubular acidosis.

5. The pattern of results suggests renal tubular acidosis (RTA).

6. The typical pattern for this condition is a low serum bicarbonate concentration with raised chloride and low potassium with a normal anion gap.

7. There are a number of methods, but $(Na + K) – (Cl + HCO_3)$ is probably the best. A normal anion gap is about 10–20 mmol/L. There is a balance between positively charged ions, such as sodium and potassium, and negatively charged ones, such as chloride and bicarbonate. Sodium and potassium provide 90 per cent of cations with calcium and magnesium providing the rest. Chloride and bicarbonate provide

80 per cent of anions with the other 20 per cent being from proteins, urate, phosphate, sulphate, lactate and other organic ions. It is these ions that are responsible for the anion gap. In this case, the anion gap is $(144 + 2.6) - (17 + 112) = 18$ mmol/L. This indicates that the acidosis is not due to any excess of metabolic anions and is therefore associated with the handling of bicarbonate in the kidney.

8. An early morning urine sample for pH is the next investigation. The urine pH varies between 4.8 and 7.5 through the day, being more alkaline after meals and acid following overnight fasting. The urine pH will be greater than 5.5 in type I (distal) RTA with hypokalaemia, but less than 5.5 in the rarer types II and IV RTA and in normal individuals.

9. An ammonium chloride load test or furosemide test may be used to help confirm the diagnosis and differentiate between the different types of renal tubular acidosis. Measurement of urinary citrate excretion may also be of value. These tests may also be used to help differentiate the different types of RTA as shown below:

	Classic distal RTA, type I	Proximal RTA, type II	Type IV RTA
Urine pH	>5.5	<5.5	<5.5
Urine anion gap	Positive	Negative	Positive
Fraction bicarbonate excretion	<5–10%	>15%	5–15%
Furosemide test	Abnormal	Normal	Normal
Urine citrate	Low	High	High
Urine calcium	Normal or high	Normal	Normal
Nephrolithiasis	Common	Rare	Rare
Metabolic bone disease	Rare	Common	Rare
Other tubular defects	Rare	Common	Rare
Plasma potassium	Normal or low	Normal or low	High

CASE 14: MAN WITH DIABETES MELLITUS

History

A 56-year-old male with type 2 diabetes mellitus presented with a 2–3-week history of lethargy and ankle oedema with watery diarrhoea for the previous ten days. In addition, he reported that his blood glucose had been about 22 mmol/L and that this had been associated with thirst and urinary frequency. There was no history of shortness of breath or chest pain. Current drug therapy was furosemide, metformin, rosiglitazone, atorvastatin and dihydrocodeine. He took no alcohol and had nearly 90 pack-years of cigarette smoking until stopping about two years previously.

Apyrexial, pulse 96 beats per minute regular, blood pressure (BP) 120/80 mmHg. His jugular venous pressure (JVP) was raised at +3 cm and there was bilateral pitting oedema of his legs (below knee). His chest was clear and a systolic murmur was noted. He showed no pigmentation, but appeared cyanosed.

Laboratory tests showed marked changes compared with those reported three months previously:

	Admission results	3 months pre-admission	Reference range
Sodium	145 mmol/L	143 mmol/L	135–146 mmol/L
Potassium	1.2 mmol/L	3.4 mmol/L	3.2–5.1 mmol/L
Bicarbonate	53.8 mmol/L	32.3 mmol/L	22–29 mmol/L
Chloride	81 mmol/L	99 mmol/L	96–108 mmol/L
Urea	13.3 mmol/L	9.1 mmol/L	1.7–8.3 mmol/L
Creatinine	106 µmol/L	94 µmol/L	62–106 µmol/L
Glucose (fasting)	11.3 mmol/L	8.2 mmol/L	<6.0 mmol/L
Troponin T	18.3 ng/L		<14 ng/L
Creatine phosphokinase (CPK)	175 U/L		30–170 U/L
pH	7.64		7.35–7.42
$PaCO_2$	6.39 kPa		4.5–6.1 kPa
PaO_2	8.97 kPa		12.0–15.0 kPa
Bilirubin	34 µmol/L		<21 µmol/L
Total protein	58 g/L		66–87 g/L
Albumin	32 g/L		34–48 g/L
Alanine aminotransferase (ALT)	55 U/L		<41 U/L
Alkaline phosphatase (ALP)	145 U/L		40–129 U/L

	Admission results	3 months pre-admission	Reference range
Gamma-glutamyl transferase (GGT)	120 U/L		10–71 U/L
Cortisol (random)	2750 nmol/L		171–536 nmol/L at 09.00 h

His electrocardiogram (ECG) showed mild ST depression.

Despite oral and intravenous potassium, his serum potassium remained about 2 mmol/L and glucose poorly controlled.

A 9 a.m. serum cortisol following dexamethasone 1 mg at midnight was 3320 nmol/L and following dexamethasone 2 mg each day for 2 days was 2970 nmol/L (expected response: cortisol <50 nmol/L). Adrenocorticotropic hormone (ACTH) level was later reported as 358 ng/L (reference range, <50 ng/L at 9 a.m.).

Cranial magnetic resonance imaging (MRI) indicated no abnormality of his pituitary fossa and was unremarkable. A chest radiograph on admission showed a right hilar mass and he proceeded to computed tomography (CT) of chest and abdomen which confirmed a 5-cm soft tissue lesion seen at the right hilum. Several nodular lesions were seen in both lungs. Below the diaphragm multiple hypodense, round lesions were present in a slightly enlarged liver (the largest 7 cm in diameter) consistent with metastases.

Bronchoscopy for brush samples and washings revealed malignant cells with scant cytoplasm and nuclear moulding consistent with small cell bronchogenic carcinoma.

The patient commenced treatment with metyrapone and cisplatin with etoposide as palliative chemotherapy.

QUESTIONS

1. What is the most likely cause of this patient's presentation?
2. What is your explanation of the arterial blood gas findings?
3. What are the possible causes of hypokalaemia in this patient; and through what mechanisms?
4. What is the genetic mechanism behind ectopic ACTH production?
5. What characteristics are typical of paraneoplastic malignancies?
6. If this was multiple endocrine adenomatosis, which other tumours might be present?

ANSWERS

1. Cushing's type syndrome due to ectopic ACTH production by a bronchogenic small cell carcinoma. (Note that the term 'Cushing syndrome' relates to clinical hyper-cortisolaemia from whatever cause, but 'Cushing's disease' is when the syndrome is due to excess pituitary ACTH production.)

2. The $PaCO_2$ increases by 0.8 kPa for every increase in HCO_{3-} of 10 mmol/L above 24 mmol/L. Usually the pCO_2 would be expected to be about 7.38 kPa in the presence of simple metabolic alkalosis. In this patient, the $PaCO_2$ is inappropriately low for the bicarbonate of 49.8 mmol/L reported on gas analysis.

3. There are many possible causes of hypokalaemia in this man. He is taking diuretics likely to be associated with hypokalaemia. Prolonged diarrhoea may cause hypoka-laemia through gut losses (but his history of diarrhoea is only 10 days) and finally the osmotic effects of his poorly controlled diabetes leads to potassium loss in the urine. However, the greatest influence will be his Cushing syndrome due to ectopic ACTH secretion. The ECG ST depression is likely to be secondary to his hypoka-laemia. ACTH is produced via the proteolytic conversion of its precursor proopio-melanocortin (POMC). The POMC promoter is methylated and silenced in most tissues, except the pituitary gland. Small cell lung cancer cells are capable of the activation of POMC leading to transcription and translation of POMC protein and hence ACTH release.

4. Paraneoplastic disorders are malignancies of neuroendocrine cells with the associated secretion of peptides, such as hormones. General characteristics of ectopic hormone secretion include:

   a. The hormone is secreted from a site not classically associated with its production or secretion.
   b. The hormone is present in venous effluent from tumour.
   c. mRNA coding for hormone is demonstrable in the tumour tissue.
   d. Genes responsible for hormone production are transcribed via the 'usual' promoter region.
   e. The synthesized/secreted hormone does not always undergo appropriate post-translational processing (often with unusual fragments being released).
   f. The hormones are present in neoplastic tissue at greater concentrations than neighbouring tissue.
   g. The hormone synthesis/secretion greatly exceeds physiological/pathophysiological levels of 'normal' endocrine tissue.
   h. The ectopic hormone secretion is generally autonomous (no negative feedback/or increased secretion post-stimulation by secretogues).
   i. Ectopic hormones can be co-secreted – thus, more than one hormone.
   j. Treatment of the neoplasia is associated with remission of ectopic hormone secretion.

5. Multiple endocrine adenomatosis type 1 involves two or more endocrine glands. In order of diminishing frequency, they are parathyroid adenoma or hyperplasia;

pancreatic islet cell, e.g. gastrinoma, insulinoma, glucagonoma, VIPoma and PPoma; anterior pituitary, e.g. prolactinoma; and adrenal cortex.

6. Cushing's is associated with multiple endocrine neoplasia (MEN) type 1. Medullary cell carcinoma of the thyroid, phaeochromocytoma and parathyroid tumours are associated with MEN type 2.

CASE 15: ELDERLY MAN WITH DYSURIA

History and examination

A 67-year-old man presents to his GP with dysuria and frequency. He had recently undertaken a strict diet in response to the finding of mild hypertension and hypercholesterolaemia which was also treated with simvastatin and lisinopril. Rectal examination revealed a hard nodule in his prostate. On receiving a report indicating an elevated PSA (prostate-specific antigen) and low % free PSA, he was referred to the urologist. Prostatic biopsy revealed malignancy with Gleason scores of 3 + 4. He chose to be treated with radiotherapy. Later that year he presented with complaints of diarrhoea and blood in his stools. Endoscopy demonstrated diverticular disease. However, because of his cachectic state, a computed tomography (CT) scan of his abdomen was arranged which showed bilateral adrenal nodules. At this time, postural hypotension was noted and he complained of feeling weak and dizzy, but this was ascribed to his cachectic state and anti-hypertensive medication. His bloods were as below (sample taken at home).

		Reference range
Sodium	130 mmol/L	135–146 mmol/L
Potassium	5.4 mmol/L	3.2–5.1 mmol/L
Urea	17.4 mmol/L	1.7–8.3 mmol/L
Creatinine	192 µmol/L	62–106 µmol/L
Prostate-specific antigen (PSA)	0.26 µg/L	<5 µg/L
Calcium (adjusted)	2.63 mmol/L	2.15–2.55 mmol/L
Magnesium (adjusted)	0.71 mmol/L	0.65–1.05 mmol/L
Total protein	73 g/L	66–87 g/L
Albumin	39 g/L	34–48 g/L
Alkaline phosphatase	51 U/L	40–129 U/L
Bilirubin	13 µmol/L	<21 µmol/L
Alanine aminotransferase	19 U/L	<41 U/L
Cortisol (random)	112 nmol/L	*

*Cortisol levels vary according to time of test (morning level 171–536 nmol/L, afternoon 64–327 nmol/L).

He was referred to an endocrinologist who arranged a short synacthen test and additional endocrine tests.

Short synacthen test	Time (min)	Cortisol (nmol/L)	Time (min)	Cortisol (nmol/L)
**	0	98	30	123

**Adrenal insufficiency is excluded if there is a rise in the 30-minute cortisol over the 0-minute cortisol >200 nmol/L and the 30-minute cortisol is >550 nmol/L.

		Reference range
Adrenal cortex antibody	Negative	
Adrenocorticothrophic hormone (ACTH) (9 a.m.)	85 ng/L	<50 ng/L
Aldosterone (supine)	<60 pmol/L	100–450 pmol/L

Replacement therapy with hydrocortisone 10mg a.m. and 5 mg p.m. plus fludrocortisone 150 µg daily was commenced.

In view of his CT findings, magnetic resonance imaging (MRI) was arranged which confirmed indeterminate lesions in both adrenal glands and, on the basis of these findings, laparoscopic adrenalectomy was undertaken with additional hydrocortisone cover. Histology showed no evidence of malignancy but evidence of previous adrenal haemorrhage.

QUESTIONS

1. What is the significance of the urea and electrolyte values in this patient?
2. What interpretation do you place on the results of the short synacthen test?
3. What conditions cause a lack of cortisol (Addison's disease)?
4. What is the significance of the ACTH result?
5. What is the significance of the aldosterone result?
6. What is the cause of pigmentation often associated with Addison's disease?
7. What other abnormalities may be associated with Addison's disease?
8. Why is cortisol replacement often prescribed as two doses per day with the lower dose being in the evening?
9. What may be the cause of the hypercalcaemia?

ANSWERS

1. These results indicate significant renal impairment as may be found in an
    Addisonian crisis associated with the inability to retain sodium as found in this
    condition. The hyponatraemia and hyperkalaemia are also typical of Addison's. The
    absence of glucorticoids and mineralocorticoids (cortisol and aldosterone) severely
    impairs the retention of sodium by the kidneys and its exchange for potassium.
    Aldosterone is also responsible for promoting the excretion of potassium by the
    kidneys when concentrations rise in conditions associated with cellular damage.

2. There is an inadequate response to synacthen. Adrenal insufficiency is excluded if
    there is a rise in the 30-minute cortisol over the 0-minute cortisol of >200 nmol/L
    and the 30-minute cortisol is >550 nmol/L.

3. A lack of cortisol may be due to pituitary causes or local adrenal disease. Addison's
    disease is due to the destruction of the cortex of the adrenal glands. While by far
    the most common cause is autoimmune destruction of the adrenals, other processes
    such as secondary malignant deposits, amyloidosis, sarcoidosis, fungal infec-
    tions, HIV and tuberculosis may also destroy the adrenal cortex. When destruction
    of the adrenals is due to local haemorrhage due to meningococcal septicaemia
    (Waterhouse–Friderichsen syndrome), the onset of symptoms may be very rapid.
    Haemorrhagic damage to the adrenals is also a complication of warfarin anticoagu-
    lation. However, with an autoimmune cause, the onset of symptoms is usually more
    insidious. It should be remembered that certain drugs, such as ketoconazole and
    methadone, may inhibit glucocorticoid production.

4. The elevated ACTH result indicates normal pituitary function. The lack of feedback
    by cortisol to inhibit ACTH production leads to raised ACTH concentrations in the
    circulation.

5. The low aldosterone concentration indicates that mineralocorticoid production is
    markedly affected by the disease process in the adrenal cortex. The clinical signifi-
    cance is that the patient will need mineralocorticoid replacement with fludrocorti-
    sone as well as cortisol.

6. The pigmentation in Addison's disease may be general but is classically seen on the
    buccal membranes in the mouth. It is associated with high circulating concentra-
    tions of ACTH or related peptides.

7. Autoimmune Addison's disease may be associated with the presence of vitiligo. In
    addition, Addison's is part of the polyglandular autoimmune syndromes: type I with
    hypoparathyroidism and mucocutaneous candidiasis (an autosomal recessive disor-
    der) and type 2 linked with type I diabetes and autoimmune thyroid disease (either
    Grave's disease or Hashimoto's thyroiditis).

8. The reason for giving hydrocortisone (cortisol) in divided doses is the rapid uptake
    and elimination of the drug. The lower evening dose is given to more closely emu-

late the normal diurnal rhythm of cortisol which falls to low levels at about 2 a.m. in the morning. Loss of this diurnal rhythm has been associated with a greater propensity to the side effects of hydrocortisone therapy.

9. There is an association between Addison's and hypercalcaemia, although the mechanism is far from clear. The hypercalcaemia resolves on treatment with glucocorticoids. Hypercalcaemia has also been noted following cessation of glucocorticoid therapy.

CASE 16: MIDDLE-AGED WOMAN WITH TIREDNESS

History

A 51-year-old female presented with tiredness, lethargy and night sweats. On direct questioning, she indicated her periods were irregular with none in the past three months. Gonadotrophin levels were requested.

Investigations

		Reference range
Luteinizing hormone (LH)	33.5 IU/L	2.4–13 follicular phase
Follicle-stimulating hormone (FSH)	38.9 IU/L	3.5–13 follicular phase

On the basis of symptom scoring, she commenced hormone replacement therapy, but symptoms persisted with unintended weight loss of about 4 kg and report of palpitations. On the basis of her thyroid function tests shown below (initial), she commenced on carbimazole at a dose of 20 mg, but as symptoms persisted the dose was increased to 40 mg daily. Repeat thyroid function tests on carbimazole are as below.

However, due to persistent dyspnoea and palpitations, it was agreed to treat with radioactive iodine. Six months after this treatment, her thyroid function tests were as shown in the table below. She then commenced thyroxine replacement therapy with her dose rising to 125 µg/day.

	Initial	On carbi-mazole	Post^{131}I	On T4	Reference range
Thyroid-stimulating hormone (TSH)	<0.1 mU/L	0.2 mU/L	18.7 mU/L	8.7 mU/L	0.3–4.2 mU/L
Free thyroxine (fT4)	32.1 pmol/L	25.8 pmol/L	9.2 pmol/L	16.7 pmol/L	12–22 pmol/L
Free tri-iodothyronine (fT3)	8.4 pmol/L	5.7 pmol/L		4.9 pmol/L	3.1–6.8 pmol/L
Thyroid per-oxidase (TPO) antibody			358 kU/L		<35 kU/L

However, her TSH on this dose remained elevated. On follow up, her TSH varied between 3.7 and 9.8 mU/L on this dose leading to concerns about dosing.

QUESTIONS

1. Are the levels of LH and FSH diagnostic of menopause?
2. Which conditions might be associated with the initial set of thyroid function tests and through what mechanisms?
3. What is the significance of the raised TPO level following radioiodine treatment?
4. What are the possible causes of the variation in TSH level on her thyroxine replacement dose of 125 µg/day?

ANSWERS

1. The definition of menopause is the absence of menstrual activity for two years. Hence, although the LH and FSH levels are consistent with menopause, they cannot be considered diagnostic. Similarly, the indications for hormone replacement should be based on symptom scoring rather than LH and FSH levels.

2. The initial pattern of thyroid function tests is typical of the hyperthyroid pattern of Grave's disease. This condition is due to the generation of TSH receptor antibodies which mimic the action of TSH thus stimulating thyroid hormone production by the thyroid. There are three types of antibody involved: (1) thyroid-stimulating immunoglobulins acting as LATS (long-acting thyroid stimulants); (2) thyroid growth immunoglobulins binding directly to the TSH-receptor and which have been implicated in the growth of thyroid follicles; (3) thyrotropin-binding inhibiting immunoglobulins which inhibit the normal interaction of TSH with its receptor. The elevated fT4 and fT3 levels feed back to the pituitary and hypothalamus switching off the production and release of thyrotropin-releasing hormone (TRH) and hence TSH levels are suppressed. This is the most common cause of hyperthyroidism.

   Thyroiditis due to viral infection leads to increased release of thyroid hormones which in turn suppress TSH secretion. The pattern is therefore identical to Grave's disease, but may be differentiated clinically by tenderness of the thyroid on palpation and the, usually, transient nature of this condition. Thyroiditis is not uncommon post-partum.

   Hashimoto's thyroiditis may be linked with elevated thyroxine levels in its early stages although it progresses to hypothyroidism.

   A pituitary TSH adenoma causes thyrotoxicosis, although this is very rare, the excessive thyroxine production is driven by TSH which is therefore elevated. The suppressed TSH excludes this possibility in this patient.

   Amiodarone is an iodine-rich compound with a similar structure to thyroxine. It may induce a number of effects including both hypothyroidism and hyperthyroidism.

   Thyroid adenomas may be either non-functional cold adenomas or functional adenomas producing either T4 or T3. The thyroid hormones produced suppress TSH levels.

   Interferon is associated with a number of thyroid problems: hypothyroidism, Grave's disease and destructive thyroiditis. Pretreatment assessment of thyroid status and monitoring during treatment is required.

   Ingestion of thyroxine tablets either surreptitiously or excessive therapeutic dosage will also cause a hyperthyroid pattern of test results. If animal thyroxine is taken, the fT3 may be elevated more than the fT4 indicating the high amounts of T3 in some animal thyroid glands.

3. TPO antibodies at high titre are found in patients with Hashimoto's thyroiditis (95 per cent), primary myxoedema (90 per cent) and Grave's disease (18 per cent). Slightly elevated TPO antibody concentrations may occur in goitre, thyroid carcinoma and in other organ-specific autoimmune diseases, e.g. pernicious anaemia. Antibodies may be predictive of future thyroid disease so the raised value following radioiodine therapy indicates a very high probability that she will develop overt hypothyroidism. As the TSH was higher than 10 mU/L, she commenced thyroxine replacement, in line with current UK guidelines.

4. There are a number of reasons for the variation in TSH results: first, inconsistent or irregular taking of the thyroxine and, second, the effects of the timing of medication and relationship to meals. The most consistent TSH levels are seen in patients who take their thyroxine 1 hour before breakfast.

CASE 17: MIDDLE-AGED MAN WITH SHORTNESS OF BREATH

History

A 52-year-old man complains of increasing shortness of breath over the previous week. He tells his GP that he has had a non-productive cough for the past few days. He has been recently started on ramipril for persistent but mild hypertension.

Pulse 78 per minute regular, blood pressure (BP) 152/88 mmHg, jugular venous pressure (JVP) just visible at 45°, heart sounds normal. He has pitting ankle oedema, more on the right than left. Chest examination reveals no evidence of consolidation, but a few basal crepitations.

Investigations

		Reference range
Haemoglobin	15.1 g/dL	13.5–18.0 g/dL
White cell count	12.9×10^9/L	$4.0–11.0 \times 10^9$/L
Neutrophils	8.7×10^9/L	$2.0–7.5 \times 10^9$/L
Platelets	274×10^9/L	$150–450 \times 10^9$/L
Sodium	132 mmol/L	135–146 mmol/L
Potassium	3.9 mmol/L	3.2–5.1 mmol/L
Urea	5.1 mmol/L	1.7–8.3 mmol/L
Creatinine	77 µmol/L	62–106 µmol/L
Total protein	73 g/L	66–87 g/L
Albumin	44 g/L	34/48 g/L
Globulin	29 g/L	18–36 g/L
Bilirubin	35 µmol/L	<21 µmol/L
Alanine aminotransferase (ALT)	37 U/L	<41 U/L
Alkaline phosphatase (ALP)	110 U/L	40–129 U/L
NT pro brain natriuretic peptide (BNP)	3478 ng/L	Intervention level >400 ng/L
C-reactive protein (CRP)	20.3 mg/L	<5 mg/L
Troponin T	37.6 ng/L	<14 ng/L
D-dimer	389 µg/L	<224 µg/L

QUESTIONS

1. Which medical conditions or treatments may be associated with elevated troponin T concentrations?
2. Why are troponin T assays good markers of myocardial infarction?
3. If the raised bilirubin was due to a pulmonary embolus, what abnormalities would you expect to see in his liver function tests (LFT)?
4. What conditions may cause an elevated serum D-dimer concentration?
5. How do you assess the probability of pulmonary embolus?

ANSWERS

1. Elevated troponin T may occur in congestive heart failure, cisplatin treatment, end-stage renal failure, myocarditis, NSTEMI (non-ST elevation myocardial infarction), polymyositis, pulmonary embolus and severe infections.

    Despite the use of troponins for the diagnosis of myocardial infarction (MI), they are really markers of any process that damages cardiac muscle whether that be from ischaemia, trauma, infection, 'strain' on the heart or toxic effects. About 30 per cent of marathon runners have an elevated troponin at the end of the race!

2. Troponin assays are good markers of myocardial infarction because serum concentrations rise within 4 hours of myocardial damage, the coefficient of variation of modern assays is about 10 per cent at the cut-off level 14 ng/L, and the clinical sensitivity for patients with MI is about 90 per cent. Troponin T has greater specificity than creatine kinase (CK) measurements and troponin T has a greater predictive value for MI than CKMB (myocardial creatine kinase).

    If troponin T at presentation and also at 6 hours is <14 ng/L then a myocardial infarction is excluded. If the troponin T doubles during this time, then this is clinically significant indicating myocardial damage.

    Use of biochemical markers for diagnosis of an acute coronary syndrome:

    a. Take a blood sample for troponin T on initial assessment in hospital.
    b. Take a second blood sample for troponin T 10–12 hours after the onset of symptoms.
    c. Take into account the clinical presentation, the time from onset of symptoms and the resting 12-lead electrocardiogram (ECG) findings when interpreting troponin measurements.

    Newer more sensitive troponin assays may offer advantages over previous assays in terms of diagnostic accuracy, and may allow exclusion of myocardial infarction earlier than the 12-hour time-frame.

    While some laboratories measure troponin T, others assay troponin I. These are different molecules but have the same clinical use and significance.

3. If the raised bilirubin was due to a pulmonary embolus you would expect the bilirubin to be mostly unconjugated and accompanied by a raised aspartate transaminase (AST) and a raised LDH (lactate dehydrogenase). The alanine aminotransferase (ALT) and alkaline phosphatase (ALP) would be likely to be normal.

    Unconjugated hyperbilirubinaemia accompanied by high serum levels of AST and LDH is commonly associated with pulmonary embolus. All three analytes are linked to the breakdown of red cells in the blood clot that is causing the embolus. Raised ALT and ALP will only occur if there is sufficient right heart failure to affect liver function.

4. D-dimer is a fibrin degradation product and is released when a blood clot is degraded by fibrinolysis. Concentrations in plasma may therefore be elevated whenever there has been a clotting process followed by fibrinolysis. Thus, elevated D-dimer is associated with disseminated intravascular coagulation; following surgery and trauma; aortic dissection; in inflammatory conditions, including rheumatoid arthritis, malignancy, liver disease; and in pregnancy. D-dimer results must therefore be considered in the clinical context and the clinical likelihood of deep vein thrombosis or pulmonary embolus.

It should be noted that the clinical sensitivity and specificity of point-of-care tests is not as good as when using laboratory assays.

The clinical specificity of laboratory analyses of D-dimer is 93–95 per cent, but the sensitivity is only 50 per cent, indicating the need to consider results only in the light of clinical suspicion.

False-negative results may occur if samples are taken before fibrinolysis has occurred.

5. The British Thoracic Society guidelines on the use of D-dimer set out a simple process to assess the risk of pulmonary embolus. If the initial chest radiograph is inconclusive, a repeat posteroanterior film is suggested. In addition a simple scoring system is advised assuming there is a reasonable possibility of pulmonary embolus.

- If a pulmonary embolus is more likely than any alternative: score +1
- If there a major risk factor for venous thromboembolism (VTE) (see below): score +1
- The probability from total score: 2 = high, 1 = intermediate, 0 = low.

Major risk factors are recent immobility/major surgery/leg fracture, previous deep vein thrombosis/pulmonary embolism, obstetric, metastatic cancer. It does not include minor risks, such as oestrogens, travel, known thrombophilia, obesity and minor surgery.

CASE 18: ELDERLY WOMAN ADMITTED FOLLOWING A FALL

History

A woman, aged 78 years, was found by her daughter at home on the floor, apparently unconscious. She was admitted to hospital by ambulance. In A&E, she appeared disorientated and apathetic. Her skin appeared pale and her pulse was 65 beats per minute, blood pressure (BP) 125/65 mmHg and respiratory rate 17 per minute. Her rectal temperature was 34.3°C, but she was not obviously shivering. On general examination, there was no evidence of trauma, her chest was clear and there were no neurological localizing signs, although her reflexes appeared rather slow. Electrocardiogram (ECG) showed a bradycardia with low amplitude.

Passive rewarming was commenced together with an infusion of warmed saline.

Investigations

	Initial result	Repeat	Reference range
Haemogolobin (Hb)	15.2 g/dL	13.2 g/L	11.5–16.5 g/dL
WBC (white blood cells)	11.2 × 10⁹/L	10.7 × 10⁹/L	4.0–11.0 × 10⁹/L
Haematocrit (Hc)	0.48 L/L	0.43 L/L	0.37–0.47 L/L
Sodium	140 mmol/L	142 mmol/L	135–146 mmol/L
Potassium	4.5 mmol/L	5.3 mmol/L	3.2–5.1 mmol/L
Urea	10.6 mmol/L	10.2 mmol/L	1.7–8.3 mmol/L
Creatinine	132 µmol/L	126 µmol/L	44–80 µmol/L
Bilirubin	18 µmol/L	17 µmol/L	<21 µmol/L
Total protein	90 g/L	84 g/L	66–87 g/L
Albumin	50 g/L	42 g/L	34–48 g/L
Alanine aminotransferase (ALT)	63 U/L	72 U/L	<31 U/L
Alkaline phosphatase (ALP)	98 U/L	85 U/L	35–104 U/L
Creatine kinase (CK)	1865 U/L	2673 U/L	30–145 U/L
Free thyroxine (fT4)	6.2 pmol/L		12–22 pmol/L
Thyroid-stimulating hormone (TSH)	98 mU/L		0.3–4.2 mU/L
Glucose	8.3 mmol/L	6.7 mmol/L	
Cholesterol	8.5 mmol/L		<5 mmol/L
Triglyceride	2.8 mmol/L		0.8–1.7 mmol/L
Lactate		3.8 mmol/L	0.5–2.2 mmol/L

Arterial blood gases at normal body temperature were within reference ranges.

As her temperature started to rise she started shivering, became more aware and responsive. When she was alert, thyroxine replacement was started at a dose of 25 µg/day.

Ten months later, she was well established on thyroxine replacement, but her GP was concerned at the variation in TSH levels when she had been on the same dose for four months.

	Established on T4	4 months later	Reference range
Free thyroxine (fT4)	20.7 pmol/L	21.2 pmol/L	12–22 pmol/L
TSH	3.9 mU/L	10.9 mU/L	0.3–4.2 mU/L

QUESTIONS

1. Which of the initial results indicate volume depletion?
2. What is the mechanism of volume depletion?
3. Is hyperglycaemia associated with hypothermia and if so what is the mechanism of the hyperglycaemia?
4. What is the cause of the elevated lactate level?
5. What are the possible causes of the raised CK level?
6. What is the most likely cause of her hypothyroidism and what test might indicate this cause?
7. Is this primary or secondary thyroid failure? Give an explanation of your answer.
8. What is the target in thyroxine replacement?
9. Why was she commenced on thyroxine at a dose of 25 µg per day?
10. What are the possible causes of the variation in TSH levels found in this patient?

ANSWERS

1. Volume depletion is indicated by the raised total protein and albumin together with her elevated urea and creatinine. Because she is anaemic, her Hb and Hct do not reflect her volume depletion.

2. There is a saline diuresis in response to hypothermia, due to decreased ADH (anti-diuretic hormone) secretion and renal dysfunction, leading to hypovolaemia and the need for saline replacement. However, there needs to be caution with respect to potassium and phosphate as these will change both on reperfusion (increasing serum concentrations) and the redistribution across cell membranes (decreasing serum concentrations) which follows this.

3. Hyperglycaemia is associated with rapid-onset hypothermia and is due to the increased release of glucagon and catecholamines (stress response) causing increased glycogenolysis and gluconeogenesis. However, if hypothermia is of slow onset, glucose stores may be depleted and hypoglycaemia ensues.

4. As part of the vascular shut down associated with hypothermia, there is increased conversion of glucose to lactate, but no further metabolism due to lack of oxygen. On reperfusion, lactate which has accumulated in muscle is washed out and plasma lactate levels rise, although rarely to a level requiring intervention.

5. CK levels are raised in hypothyroidism because the rate of metabolism/clearance is reduced due to lack of thyroxine. However, the elevation in this patient is much higher than normally found in even severe hypothyroidism. There are two other possibilities: first, the effect of hypothermia causing muscle damage and, second, the effect of lying on the floor semiconscious for a long period of time. ALT levels are also raised in accidental hypothermia.

6. This is the pattern of primary thyroid failure as indicated by the elevated TSH level. This demonstrates that the normal feedback loop to the pituitary is functional.

7. The most likely cause is an autoimmune process which may be shown by elevated TPO (thyroid peroxidase) antibody levels.

8. Returning the TSH to within the reference range is the target. However, some patients remain symptomatic when their fT4 is relatively low, but the TSH is in the reference range. For this reason, some patients are treated to give a slightly low TSH but with a normal fT4 and fT3. Suppression of TSH in treating hypothyroid-ism generates a risk of promoting osteopenia and is not recommended. However, suppression of TSH is required in the treatment of patients following surgery for thyroid carcinoma.

9. Low doses of thyroxine are utilized in the elderly or those with known ischemic heart disease to reduce the risk of precipitating unstable angina or myocardial infarction in someone with such profound hypothyroidism.

10. First, there is the need to check that the patient is taking the medication consistently and that the TSH variation is not due to erratic compliance with therapy. There is evidence that TSH levels are more consistent when thyroxine replacement is taken an hour before breakfast and least consistent when taken in the evening. One theoretical possibility is the time of sampling as there is a diurnal variation in TSH levels. This is of little consequence when TSH levels are normal, but does give significant differences when values are slightly elevated.

CASE 19: ELDERLY MAN WITH NOCTURIA

History

A male aged 68 years presented to his GP with dysuria. On direct questioning, he admitted to nocturia twice nightly and some urgency of micturition. On rectal examination, the prostate was enlarged and the patient complained of discomfort during this examination. The GP arranged for a midstream specimen of urine (MSU) and blood tests, including prostate-specific antigen (PSA) which were taken the following morning.

Investigations

Investigation revealed:

Midstream specimen of urine, no growth

Full blood count (FBC), slight increase in neutrophils.

	Initial findings	6-week follow-up findings	Reference range
Sodium	142 mmol/L	138 mmol/L	135–146 mmol/L
Potassium	4.2 mmol/L	3.9 mmol/L	3.2–5.1 mmol/L
Creatinine	112 µmol/L	95 µmol/L	62–106 µmol/L
Urea	9.2 mmol/L	8.5 mmol/L	1.7–8.3 mmol/L
Estimated glomerular filtration rate (e-GFR)	>60 mL/min/1.73m^2	>60 mL/min/1.73m^2	>60 L/min/1.73m^2
Total PSA	10 µg/L	6 µg/L	<4 µg/L
Free PSA	15%	18%	<15%
C-reactive protein (CRP)		22 mg/L	<5 mg/L

The following week he was admitted via A&E with fever and rectal pain. Blood cultures were positive and a diagnosis of prostatitis was made. Intravenous antibiotics were infused over a 2-week period followed by oral therapy.

He was discharged from hospital and 6 weeks after admission his blood tests were repeated as above.

QUESTIONS

1. What is the half-life of circulating PSA?
2. Was the first PSA a true reflection of his cancer risk? Explain your reasoning.
3. Was his second PSA a true reflection of his cancer risk? Explain your reasoning.

4. Which circumstances may cause the serum PSA to be elevated?
5. What percentage of free PSA indicates a high probability of malignancy?
6. What is the reason for the age-related reference range for PSA?
7. What are the potential clinical uses of tumour markers?
8. What are the limitations to the use of tumour markers?

ANSWERS

1. The circulating half-life of PSA is 2.2–3.2 days, although the half-life of free PSA is much shorter – possibly less than 0.5 days. Following radical prostatectomy, serum PSA values should become undetectable by 3 weeks post-surgery.

2. The blood sample for PSA was taken the day after rectal examination. Although normal rectal examination is usually not associated with any significant increase in PSA levels, it is good practice to take a blood sample for PSA before undertaking a rectal examination of the prostate or waiting for a week after examination. In this patient, it seems likely that he had prostatitis at the time of examination and for this reason the PSA cannot be taken as a reliable indicator of malignancy.

3. This is more problematic. Because of the half-life of PSA, a serum level cannot guarantee to be unaffected by any manipulation or infection of the prostate for 2–3 weeks after the event. The unresolved question is how long following prostatitis do prostatic cells stop being damaged and tissue repair processes completed. The persistence of an elevated CRP value indicates an on-going inflammatory process. If the results were normal (both total and percentage free PSA) at 6 weeks then cancer can be excluded.

4. Prostatitis, sexual intercourse, digital rectal examination, riding a bicycle and urinary retention may all cause elevated serum PSA concentrations. The duration of increase following digital rectal examination, ejaculation and riding a bicycle is short term.

5. The percentage of free PSA (fPSA) indicates a high probability of malignancy when it is less than 15 per cent. Free PSA as a percentage of total PSA is a better marker of malignancy than total PSA. Although prostate cancer tissue has a PSA level about ten times greater than that of either normal or hyperplasic tissue, the clinical specificity and sensitivity of serum PSA as a test for the presence of cancer is poor. The majority of serum PSA is bound to either alpha-2-macroglobulin or alpha-1-antichymotrypsin. The ratio of free PSA to total PSA is inversely related to the likelihood of prostate cancer. Depending on age, digital rectal examination and total PSA, a patient with a free:total PSA ratio of less than 0.15 (free PSA <15 per cent of total) should generally be referred for further investigation. The higher the ratio the more likely it is to be due to benign prostatic hypertrophy, however there is considerable overlap and clinical considerations should take precedence over fPSA when making a diagnosis. The percentage free PSA in patients with slightly elevated total serum PSA has a higher sensitivity and specificity than total PSA.

6. The volume of the prostate increases with age and therefore the amount of PSA it produces. Hence, the reference range for PSA increases with age.

7. Caution is indicated in considering the value of measuring tumour markers, although there are many potential uses including:

   a. Assistance in diagnosis: There needs to be a significant pre-test probability of a given malignancy for the use of tumour markers in the diagnosis of malignancy.

A strong family history, as well as individual clinical presentations and findings will provide a probability.

b. Staging: The level of elevation may assist in determining spread of malignancy.

c. Determining prognosis: Markers may be an indication of tumour aggressiveness.

d. Guidance for intervention/predicting response to treatment: HER-2-positive breast cancer is more likely to respond to herceptin.

e. Monitoring response to therapy: When tumour markers are elevated before initiating treatment, then a reduction in concentration following surgery, radiotherapy or chemotherapy indicates a reduction in tumour mass.

f. Determining recurrence after treatment: When a tumour marker has fallen after treatment, but then rises again, this is an indication of local or more widespread recurrence.

8. Indiscriminate use of tumour markers indicates that the limitations of these assays have not been considered. They include:

a. Lack of specificity for malignancy: No tumour marker is 100 per cent diagnostic for malignancy. Many other disorders and even physiological variations (e.g. serum CA 125 increases with benign ovarian cysts and with menstruation) are associated with elevated serum concentrations.

b. Lack of organ specificity: With the possible exception of PSA, tumour markers are not organ specific.

c. Serum markers are not efficient at detecting early disease: In general, tumour markers are more likely to be elevated with disseminated malignancy. The positive predictive value of serum carcinoembryonic antigen (CEA) in colon cancer is greater in Duke C and D than in stages A and B.

d. Lack of sensitivity: With the possible exception of hCG (human choronic gonadotrophin) in choriocarcinoma, no tumour marker is positive in all cases diagnosed.

e. Determining cause of malignancy: Blanket use of tumour markers when attempting to ascertain the source of malignancy is not an effective use of resources.

CASE 20: MAN WITH SEVERE HEADACHES

History

A 34-year-old man complained of severe headaches which had become more frequent and intense over the past six months. He described the headaches as 'thumping' and has noticed a rapid heart rate during some headaches. He also indicated that he is feeling very anxious following an unpleasant divorce. His GP found his blood pressure to be 180/105 mmHg and commenced treatment with an ACE (angiotensin converting enzyme) inhibitor. Fundoscopy was normal. When the ACE inhibitor failed to control his blood pressure (BP), his treatment was changed to an angiotensin receptor blocker. However, this too failed to control his BP and so the GP referred him to the hospital hypertension clinic where a range of tests were undertaken, with the 24-hour urine being collected when anti-hypertensive agents had been stopped for 3 days.

		Reference range
Sodium	141 mmol/L	135–146 mmol/L
Potassium	3.2 mmol/L	3.2–5.1 mmol/L
Urea	8.5 mmol/L	1.7–8.3 mmol/L
Creatinine	121 µmol/L	62–106 µmol/L
Calcium (adjusted)	2.61 mmol/L	2.15–2.55 mmol/L
Phosphate	0.95 mmol/L	0.87–1.45 mmol/L
Alkaline phosphatase (ALP)	102 U/L	35–104 U/L
Glucose (fasting)	5.4 mmol/L	<6.0 mmol/L
24-h urine normetanephrine	6.1 µmol/24 h	<3.3 µmol/24 h
24-h urine metanephrine	1.9 µmol/24 h	<1.2 µmol/24 h
24-h urine methoxytyramine	2.7 µmol/24 h	<2.5 µmol/24 h

Fasting plasma glucose from a sample taken during a severe headache was 8.5 mmol/L.

A repeat 24-hour urine and blood test was arranged – the 24-hour urine was started at the onset of a headache:

		Reference range
24-h urine normetanephrine	16.5 µmol/24 h	<3.3 µmol/24 h
24-h urine metanephrine	4.9 µmol/24 h	<1.2 µmol/24 h
24-h urine methoxytyramine	3.5 µmol/24 h	<2.5 µmol/24 h
Chromogranin A	195 pmol/L	<60 pmol/L

On the basis of these results, a radioisotope MIBG (iodine-131-meta-iodobenzylguanidine) scan was undertaken.

QUESTIONS

1. What is the most likely diagnosis?
2. Why was it considered necessary to repeat the urine collection for metanephrines?
3. Which conditions may cause an elevation of metanephrine excretion?
4. Which drugs should be stopped, if clinically safe, before collecting a 24-h urine for metanephrine assay?
5. What is the significance of the chromogranin A finding?
6. What is the explanation for the elevated glucose of 8.5 mmol/L?
7. What might be the significance of the serum calcium level and how might this be followed up?
8. What is the purpose of MIBG imaging?

ANSWERS

1. The most likely diagnosis is phaeochromocytoma based on the second collection, although severe emotional stress is a possible cause for the first set of results.

2. Metanephrine values of between 1–4 × ULN (upper limit of normal) are not diagnostic, but require further investigation as they may be associated with other conditions and drug therapy. There is an advantage in collecting a 24-h urine as soon as an 'attack' is noted by the patient, however the effect is more marked if using catecholamine measurements rather than metanephrines.

3. There are a considerable number of conditions which may cause an elevated excretion of metanephrines. They are associated with a stress response which is mediated in part by secretion of adrenal medullary hormones. They include acute psychological stress, hypoglycaemia, obstructive sleep apnoea, vigorous exercise, conditions linked to clinical shock, such as myocardial infarction, severe injury, pulmonary embolus, and use of recreational drugs, such as cocaine. Excessive caffeine intake and nicotine may also influence results.

4. A number of therapeutic drugs are associated with a physiological increase in metanephrine concentrations. In addition, there are drugs which cause analytical interference, but this is very dependent on the method of analysis used by the laboratory. It is preferable to stop these drugs for at least 4 days before starting a urine collection and longer for calcium-channel blockers. Drugs to consider stopping before collecting a specimen for metanephrines include drugs used to control hypertension, e.g. beta-blockers (propranolol), alpha-blockers (doxazosin), calcium-channel blockers (felodipine), drugs inhibiting noradrenaline reuptake (amitriptyline, clozapine), amphetamine-related drugs (ritalin) and dopaminergic drugs (methyldopa). Avoidance of caffeine, nicotine and vitamin C supplementation may also be advised.

   Metanephrine excretion may be reported as total metanephrines or as different fractions, namely metanephrine and normetanephrine. Fractionated metanephrines (as in these results) have a sensitivity of up to 97 per cent and a specificity of about 70 per cent, which makes the assay reliable for detection of phaeochromocytoma but with a rather high false-positive rate – hence the value of repeat estimations, especially following 'an attack'.

   Methoxytyramine is a breakdown product of dopamine and is therefore only raised in dopamine-secreting tumours.

   Please note that laboratory tests for phaeochromocytoma may be based on measurement of catecholamines or their metabolites, the metanephrines. Further tests may be undertaken on urine or plasma. The interference of drugs is different for catecholamine assays than metadrenalines and may also be specific to the analytical method used. It is therefore essential to discuss the question of interference with the assaying laboratory.

5. Adrenal medullary tissue is derived from chromaffin cells which secrete chromogranin A. Although the use of the test is largely associated with investigation of gastrointestinal disorders, its elevation is associated with phaeochromocytoma and is used as a second-line investigation. Recent studies have shown a good sensitivity and specificity. Chromogranin levels are claimed to be proportional to tumour mass. Chromogranin A is used in the diagnosis and monitoring of carcinoid syndrome, although elevated levels may also be found in association with pancreatic cancer and prostate cancer. Liver failure, renal failure and inflammatory bowel disease have also been associated with elevated concentrations.

    Proton pump inhibitor drugs should be stopped before measurement of chromogranin A as these drugs increase secretion.

6. Increased catecholamine secretion, especially as found during 'an attack', will mobilize glycogen stores and increase the rate of gluconeogenesis while inhibiting insulin release. The net effect is an elevation of blood glucose.

7. The raised serum calcium indicates the possibility of hyperparathyroidism and that the phaeochromocytoma is part of MEN2 (multiple endocrine neoplasia type 2). MEN2 comprises medullary cell carcinoma of the thyroid, phaeochromocytoma and parathyroid adenoma or carcinoma. When found in association with Marfanoid characteristics and mucosal adenomas, it is termed Sipple's syndrome or MEN2A. MEN2 is due to a mutation in the pro-oncogene RET and the presence of this mutation may be used to assess the risk in family members.

8. MIBG imaging is important not so much as a diagnostic test, but as a localization test. Up to 10 per cent of tumours are found to be bilateral (more in familial cases) and 10–15 per cent are extra-adrenal.

CASE 21: ELDERLY CONFUSED WOMAN

History

An 82-year-old woman is transferred to A&E in a confused state and unable to cope at home. She lives at home with her husband, aged 86 years, who reports that his wife has been increasingly unwell over the previous 10 days. Her symptoms are non-specific. She has not been eating well because of nausea, has been relatively immobile and now seems unaware of her circumstances and is unable to dress herself.

She appeared dehydrated but was apyrexial. Her pulse was 65 beats per minute, blood pressure (BP) 145/75 mmHg, no ankle oedema and jugular venous pressure (JVP) normal; a few crepitations are found at both bases. No abdominal tenderness is found and there are no focal neurological signs. Previous history from the GP indicates that she has been on thyroxine replacement for many years and that her atrial fibrillation has been well controlled on digoxin and a thiazide diuretic. In addition, she had been treated for breast cancer seven years previously.

Investigations

Admission blood tests showed:

		Reference range
Haemoglobin	12.2 g/dL	11.5–16.5 g/dL
White cell count	10.6×10^9/L	$4.0–11.0 \times 10^9$/L
Neutrophils	5.5×10^9/L	$2.0–7.5 \times 10^9$/L
Platelets	244×10^9/L	$150–450 \times 10^9$/L
Sodium	138 mmol/L	135–146 mmol/L
Potassium	3.2 mmol/L	3.2–5.1 mmol/L
Urea	12.1 mmol/L	1.7–8.3 mmol/L
Creatinine	148 µmol/L	44-80 µmol/L
e-GFR	31 mL/min/1.73m^2	>60 mL/min/1.73m^2
Total protein	80 g/L	66–87 g/L
Albumin	45 g/L	34–48 g/L
Bilirubin	17 µmol/L	<21 µmol/L
Alanine aminotransferase (ALT)	55 U/L	<41 U/L
Alkaline phosphatase (ALP)	195 U/L	35–104 U/L
fT4 (free thyroxine)	12.3 pmol/L	12–22 pmol/L
Tyroid-stimulating hormone (TSH)	19.4 mU/L	0.3–4.2 mU/L

Checking on the laboratory computer, the only previous electrolyes were undertaken by her GP five years previously and showed:

Sodium	140 mmol/L	135–146 mmol/L
Potassium	3.3 mmol/L	3.2–5.1 mmol/L
Urea	6.5 mmol/L	1.7–8.2 mmol/L
Creatinine	79 μmol/L	44–80 μmol/L
e-GFR	64 mL/min/1.73m^2	>60 mL/min/1.73m^2

Rehydration is started initially with dextrose saline. Repeat blood tests the following day revealed:

Sodium	136 mmol/L	135–145 mmol/L
Potassium	3.2 mmol/L	3.2–5.1 mmol/L
Urea	12.6 mmol/L	1.7–8.2 mmol/L
Creatinine	138 μmol/L	44–80 μmol/L
e-GFR	34 mL/min/1.73m^2	>60 mL/min/1.73m^2
Total protein	75 g/L	66–87 g/L
Albumin	40 g/L	34–48 g/l
Bilirubin	16 μmol/L	<21 μmol/L
ALT	53 U/L	<41 U/L
AST	55 U/L	<32 U/L
Alkaline phosphatase	202 U/L	35–104 U/L
Gamma-glutamyl transferase (GGT)	38 U/L	6–42 U/L
Calcium	2.32 mmol/L	2.15–2.55 mmol/L
Adjusted calcium	2.32 mmol/L	2.15–2.55 mmol/L
Phosphate	1.51 mmol/L	0.87–1.45 mmol/L
Digoxin (time after dose not stated)	3.2 μg/L	1–2 μg/L 8–12 h after dose

A section of her electrocardiogram (ECG) rhythm strip is shown in Figure 21.1.

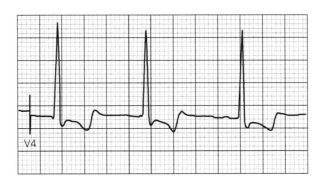

Figure 21.1

In view of her blood results and confusional state, she was treated with Digibind®. Repeat digoxin assay showed little change in her digoxin levels.

QUESTIONS

1. What abnormality is highlighted in the ECG trace and what is its significance?
2. Why is relationship to dose important when interpreting the results of digoxin measurements?
3. What metabolic conditions enhance digoxin toxicity?
4. What is the mechanism for digoxin metabolism and excretion? Why is this pertinent to this case?
5. Why did her serum digoxin concentration not fall when treated with Digibind?
6. What conditions may account for her elevated alkaline phosphatase concentration?

ANSWERS

1. The ECG demonstrates the 'reversed tick' phenomenon with ST segment depression – this is a feature of digoxin therapy, not a sign of toxicity. Any arrhythmia can occur with digoxin toxicity, including paroxysmal atrial tachycardia with atrioventricular block, ventricular ectopics and bigeminy and severe bradycardia.

2. As with most drugs there is a rise in serum concentration following ingestion followed by an uptake by tissues to create a steady-state equilibrium. For digoxin, it takes about 6 hours to reach a steady state. In practice, pre-dose sampling is often more convenient. Routine measurement is unnecessary.

3. Digoxin toxicity is enhanced by hypokalaemia, hypercalcaemia, diuretics (e.g. furosemide), hypomagnesaemia and hypothyroidism. The clinical manifestations of digoxin toxicity include anorexia, nausea/vomiting, visual disturbance (blurred vision – xanthopsia), diarrhoea and arrhythmias.

    The effects of digoxin appear to be due to inhibition of the sodium and potassium ATPase mechanism. The net effect is to increase intracellular calcium concentration and decrease intracellular potassium concentration. Hence hypokalaemia and hypercalcaemia will enhance the actions of digoxin and hence there is an increased risk of toxicity. In hypothyroidism, it is thought the volume of distribution of digoxin is decreased and hence there is a risk of toxicity. Her thyroid function tests show compensated hypothyroidism and this may be a reflection of variable compliance over the preceding months or may be due to a too low dose of thyroxine, causing a compensatory rise in TSH. These should be checked again in two months. Digoxin reduces conductivity at the atrioventricular node and is used commonly to reduce the ventricular rate in atrial fibrillation; it is also a positive inotrope.

4. While up to 20 per cent of digoxin is metabolized in the liver and stomach, the main route for elimination is the kidney. Any reduction in glomerular filtration rate (GFR) is likely to lead to increased circulating concentrations of digoxin. In this case, the significant reduction in renal function was almost certainly the cause for the accumulation of digoxin and the toxicity was enhanced by her borderline hypokalaemia associated with thiazide diuretic treatment. For this reason, monitoring of renal function is essential in patients taking digoxin – especially the elderly.

5. Hypokalaemia and hypomagnesaemia contribute to digoxin toxicity. Bradyarrhythmias are treated with atropine, ventricular arrhythmias are treated by magnesium infusion (8–10 mmol bolus) even in the presence of a normal serum magnesium. Bradyarrhythmias not responding to atropine, or life-threatening ventricular arrhythmias, can be treated with digoxin-specific antibody fragments (Digibind). Temporary pacing may be needed in some cases.

    Treatment with Digibind® captures digoxin in the circulation making it unavailable for uptake by tissues. In addition, it removes digoxin from tissues as it changes the concentration of free digoxin in the blood and hence the dynamic equilibrium between tissues and serum. However, digoxin bound to Digibind® may still be measured in some immunosassays for digoxin. Hence serum digoxin measurements following Digibind® treatment cannot be relied on as an assessment of the efficacy of treatment. The effect is very assay dependent.

6. Alkaline phosphatase is prevalent in bone, liver and placenta with some also found in the intestine. Some tumours are associated with the production of a placenta-like alkaline phosphatase. There are physiological increases in alkaline phosphatase in blood associated with bone growth in children and adolescents and increases from the placenta in pregnancy. In this particular case, the possibility of secondary neoplasia associated with her previous breast cancer is possible, while at her age Paget's disease is also a possibility.

The different tissue-specific isoenzymes of alkaline phosphatase may be separated by electrophoresis and quantified by staining and densitometry.

In primary biliary cirrhosis and gall stone obstruction, there would be a significant elevation of GGT in addition to alkaline phosphatase – there is induction of both enzymes linked to biliary obstruction.

In alcoholic cirrhosis, the AST is usually elevated more than the ALT and in addition the GGT would usually be elevated.

The elevation of alkaline phosphatase without GGT indicates the possible sources as bone, placenta or intestine. In this case, either Paget's disease of bone or secondaries from her breast cancer are possible causes. Paget's disease causes an isolated raised ALP and is a common cause of an isolated raised ALP in the elderly and is often asymptomatic in such patients.

CASE 22: MIDDLE-AGED WOMAN FEELING TIRED

History

A 50-year-old woman complained to her GP of feeling tired all the time and itching. There was no history of fever, night sweats or weight loss. She had been treated for breast cancer five years previously and was believed to be in remission. In addition, a diagnosis of hypothyroidism had been made two years previously and recent thyroid function tests indicated adequate replacement therapy.

Examination

On examination, she appeared mildly jaundiced and small xanthelasma were noted on her upper eye lids. There was no history of abdominal pain, although she admitted to mild discomfort in her right upper quadrant.

Liver function tests were undertaken and on the basis of the findings she was referred for specialist advice.

	GP tests	Specialist tests	Reference range
Bilirubin	48 μmol/L	51 μmol/L	<21 μmol/L
Alanine aminotransferase (ALT)	48 U/L	55 U/L	<31 U/L
Alkaline phosphatase (ALP)	395 U/L	367 U/L	35–104 U/L
Gamma-glutamyl transferase (GGT)		168 U/L	6–42 U/L
Total protein	72 g/L	74 g/L	66–87 g/L
Albumin	35 g/L	33 g/L	34–48 g/L
IgG		13.7 g/L	6–16 g/L
IgA		3.1 g/L	0.8–4.0 g/L
IgM		5.2 g/L	0.5–2.0 g/L
Total cholesterol		8.2 mmol/L	<5.0 mmol/L
Triglyceride		2.2 mmol/L	0.8–1.7 mmol/L
High-density lipoprotein (HDL) cholesterol		1.8 mmol/L	>1.2 mmol/L
Low-density lipoprotein (LDL) cholesterol		5.4 mmol/L	<3.0 mmol/L
Total cholesterol:HDL ratio		4.6	
25 OH Vitamin D		37 nmol/L	50–120 nmol/L
International normalized ratio (INR)		1.4	0.8–1.2

	GP tests	Specialist tests	Reference range
Anti-nuclear antibody (ANA)		Negative	
Anti-smooth muscle antibody		Negative	
Anti-mitochondrial antibody		Positive	
M2-type mitochondrial antibody		Positive	
Anti-gastric parietal antibody		Masked	
Anti-liver/kidney microsomal antibody		Negative	

Viral studies were negative as were tests for haemachromatosis, Wilson's disease and alpha-1 anti-trypsin deficiency.

QUESTIONS

1. Describe the pattern of liver function tests.
2. What are the possible causes of this pattern?
3. Provide an explanation of her immunoglobulin results.
4. What is the cardiovascular risk linked to her lipid findings?
5. Explain the immunology findings.
6. What autoimmune conditions may be associated with primary biliary cirrhosis?
7. What bone disorders are associated with primary biliary cirrhosis and how are they treated?
8. What is the main form of treatment of primary biliary cirrhosis?

ANSWERS

1. The pattern of liver function tests indicates biliary obstruction or cholestasis. The biochemical results pattern indicates the type of liver disorder.

Liver disorder	Bilirubin	Albumin	ALT	ALP	GGT
Acute viral hepatitis	++	N	++	+	+
Acute alcoholic hepatitis	+	N	+	+	++
Chronic viral hepatitis	+ or N	– or N	+	+ or N	+
Cirrhosis	+ or N	–	+	+	+
Gilbert's syndrome	+	N	N	N	N
Primary biliary cirrhosis	++	N or –	+	++	++
Primary sclerosing cholangitis	+	N or –	+	++	++
Secondary neoplasia	+ or N	N	+	++	++

The pattern of cholestasis found in this patient may be due to primary biliary cirrhosis (PBC), primary sclerosing cholangitis (PSC) or tumours in the liver secondary to her breast cancer. The other possibility is gall stone obstruction of the biliary tract, although there is no history of biliary colic. Both secondary neoplasia and gall stone disease may be excluded by ultrasound.

2. A cholestatic pattern of liver tests may be due to (a) extrahepatic causes (due to obstruction of the flow of bile through the biliary tract) and (b) intrahepatic causes (due to impaired secretion of bile from hepatocytes).

   a. Extrahepatic: biliary stones, inflammation of the biliary tract, external obstruction by malignant tumours (usually carcinoma of the head of the pancreas) and biliary atresia (rare).
   b. Intrahepatic: viral hepatitis, drugs (e.g. chlorpromazine), toxins (e.g. alcohol), cholangitis, autoimmune disorder (PBC and PSC), cystic fibrosis.

3. Her immunoglobulins show a significantly raised IgM concentration as found in haemachromatosis.

Immunoglobulin class	Key associated disorders
IgG	Autoimmune disorders, e.g. systemic lupus erythematosis, chronic active hepatitis
IgA	Intestinal disorders, e.g. Crohn's disease
	Respiratory tract disorders, e.g. bronchiectasis, tuberculosis
IgM	Primary biliary cirrhosis, haemoprotazoal infections, e.g. malaria, intrauterine infections (at birth), viral hepatitis, some acute viral infections

Immunoglobulin class	Key associated disorders
IgG, IgA, IgM	Chronic bacterial infections, sarcoidosis, acquired immuno-deficiency syndrome
IgE	Allergic disorders, e.g. extrinsic asthma, atopic conditions, anaphylaxis; response to parasitic infections, e.g. toxocaris, echinococcosis, ascariasis; allergic states secondary to immunodeficiency/suppression

4. Her lipid abnormalities are linked to the presence of xanthelasma. She has an elevated total and LDL cholesterol which are risk factors for cardiovascular disease. However, her HDL is 1.8 mmol/L and a level which will provide considerable protection through reverse cholesterol transport. Her total cholesterol:HDL ratio is 4.6 which at her age as a non-diabetic, normotensive, non-smoker places her in a low risk category (see cardiovascular risk tables in the British National Formulary).

5. The diagnostic test of PBC is the presence of M2-type mitochondrial antibodies which is usually normal in PSC.

   Mitochondrial antibodies are directed to pyruvate dehydogenase complexes and have a close association with primary biliary cirrhosis.

   Smooth muscle antibodies are frequently non-specific or transiently detected. However, they may be associated with type I autoimmune hepatitis. These patients may also have a positive ANA.

   Liver, kidney microsomal (LKM) antibodies are directed against cytochrome P450 proteins and are particularly associated with type 2 autoimmune hepatitis (AIH). This form of AIH presents more commonly in children.

6. Autoimmune conditions associated with PBC include sicca syndrome, Raynaud's phenomenon, rheumatoid arthritis, and hypothyroidism including Hashimoto's thyroiditis.

7. Despite the requirement of bile salts for the absorption of fat and fat-soluble vitamins, osteoporosis is much more common than osteomalacia in patients with PBC; affecting about 30 per cent of patients. It is more common with long-term PBC, a greater degree of jaundice and other general factors, such as post-menopause. Because of this, high-prevalence DEXA (Dual-Energy X-ray Absorptiometry) screening for osteopenia is part of routine follow up. Treatment is with calcium and vitamin D supplements.

8. The mainstay of treatment of PBC is ursodeoxycholic acid. Its actions are multifactorial, but the main route is through promotion of bile salt excretion. It reduces itching and also leads to a reduction in the size of xanthelasmata.

CASE 23: WOMAN WITH IRREGULAR PERIODS

History

A 38-year-old woman complained to her GP that she was having irregular and infrequent periods. She also reluctantly admitted that she was growing rather coarse hair on her arms. The GP noticed her body mass index (BMI) was 31 and on undertaking a stick urine test noted glycosuria. He arranged for tests on suspicion of polycystic ovary syndrome (PCOS) and a glucose tolerance test.

		Reference range
Luteinizing hormone (LH)	5.6 IU/L	2.4–13 IU/L (follicular)
Follicle-stimulating hormone (FSH)	6.1 IU/L	3.5–13 IU/L (follicular)
Oestradiol	374 pmol/L	46–607 pmol/L (follicular)
Testosterone	0.73 nmol/L	0.29–1.67 nmol/L
Sex hormone binding globulin (SHBG)	104 nmol/L	24.6–122 nmol/L
Free testosterone	6 pmol/L	3–33 pmol/L
Prolactin	289 mIU/L	102–496 mIU/L
OGTT, glucose at 0 min (oral glucose tolerance test)	6.8 mmol/L	<6.1 mmol/L, non-diabetic
		6.1–7.0 mmol/L, impaired fasting glycaemia
		>7.0 mmol/L, diabetes
OGTT, glucose at 120 min	10.4 mmol/L	<7.8 mmol/L, non-diabetic
		7.8–11.1 mmol/L, impaired glucose tolerance
		>11.1 mmol/L, diabetes

The patient returned to the surgery to receive the results of the tests and brought a photograph from seven years previously. She indicated that her husband thought her facial features had changed and this was apparent from comparison between her current appearance and the photograph. The GP referred her to the endocrinologist who arranged a glucose tolerance test (GTT) with growth hormone (GH) measurements, an insulin-like growth factor (IGF) assay and other pituitary tests.

		Reference range
IGF-1 (insulin-like growth factor)	85 pmol/L	13–50 pmol/L
Free thyroxine fT4	14.2 pmol/L	12–22 pmol/L
Free tri-iodothyonine fT3	4.8 pmol/L	3.1–6.8 pmol/L
Thyroid-stimulating hormone (TSH)	3.7 mIU/L	0.3–4.2 mIU/L

		Reference range
Cortisol	189 nmol/L	171–536 nmol/L (7–10 a.m.)
Prolactin	376 mIU/L	102–496 mIU/L

Growth hormone suppression test:

Time (min)	Glucose (mmol/L)	GH (μg/L)
0	7.1	18
30	8.2	17
60	9.9	17
90	12.1	16
120	11.9	19

Magnetic resonance imaging (MRI) confirmed the presence of a pituitary tumour. She elected to be treated by radiotherapy. Following pituitary ablation, she required replacement therapy with thyroxine (150 μg/day) and hydrocortisone (10 mg a.m. and 5 mg p.m.).

QUESTIONS

1. Is the pattern of sex hormones indicative of PCOS?
2. What are the findings from the first glucose tolerance test?
3. What are the findings from the second glucose tolerance test?
4. How do you interpret the GH results in the second glucose tolerance test?
5. What other conditions may lead to an impaired GH response to oral glucose?
6. What is the advantage of IGF-1 assays in the diagnosis and monitoring of acromegaly?
7. Why did she need thyroxine and cortisol following radiotherapy?

ANSWERS

1. The pattern of sex hormone results is not suggestive of polycystic ovary syndrome. The key finding in PCOS is an elevated free testosterone concentration even if the total testosterone is normal. This increase in free testosterone is partly due to low concentrations of sex hormone binding globulin (SHBG). Serum concentrations of another androgen, androstenedione, are also raised. In addition, the typical pattern includes an LH value greater than FSH. Prolactin levels are commonly elevated, but usually only to about 600 mIU/L. PCOS is associated with insulin resistance and hence impaired fasting glycaemia and impaired glucose tolerance as found in this patient.

   Only about 2–3 per cent of testosterone is found in the free and active form, the rest being bound mostly to SHBG. Hence, variations in SHBG can generate significant changes in total testosterone. SHBG levels are increased by oestrogens, hyperthyroidism and liver disease and decreased in hypothyroidism, obesity, malnutrition and androgens.

2. The first glucose tolerance test indicates both impaired fasting glycaemia and impaired glucose tolerance. This is commonly associated with obesity and heralds the probability of progression to diabetes and hence is an indication for initial advice on diet and exercise.

3. The second glucose tolerance test shows overt diabetes. Growth hormone antagonizes insulin-mediated uptake of glucose. In addition, it promotes lipolysis increasing the circulating concentrations of non-esterified fatty acids. These cause an accumulation of diacylglycerol in cells which generates the serine phosphorylation of the insulin receptor system rendering it ineffective in promoting the function of glucose transporters on the cell membrane.

4. The normal growth hormone response to an oral glucose load is suppression to below 1 µg/L. The failure to suppress is typical of acromegaly. Some 8 per cent of people with acromegaly do not have very high fasting growth hormone levels, but they still fail to suppress following a glucose load.

5. Other conditions where there is a failure of suppression of growth hormone in response to glucose include chronic renal failure, liver failure, active hepatitis, anorexia nervosa, malnutrition, hyperthyroidism and poorly controlled diabetes. In addition, an atypical response may be found in adolescence.

6. Growth hormone measurements show a diurnal variation, but in addition secretion is pulsatile. Elevated values are associated with exercise, stress, sleep and fasting. IGF-1 mediates many of the actions of growth hormone and is produced in tissues, especially liver, in response to growth hormone. As the concentrations of IGF-1 are more stable than growth hormone during the day they provide a better tool for both the diagnosis and monitoring of acromegaly as almost all patients with acromegaly have elevated IGF-1. However, serum IGF-1 concentrations fall with age and hence an apparently 'normal' value may be high in the elderly. Following

treatment of acromegaly, whether by surgery, drugs or radiotherapy, IGF-1 is used to monitor for the possible recurrence of the tumour.

7. Radiotherapy is likely to damage other cells in the pituitary in addition to those in the adenoma and hence the secretion of TSH, adrenocorticotropic hormone (ACTH), LH and FSH may be impaired. This patient required both thyroxine and cortisol replacement. She did not require mineralocorticoid treatment as the renin-angiotensin-aldosterone system is unaffected by pituitary damage.

CASE 24: MAN WITH PAINFUL KNEES

History

A 40-year-old male lorry driver presented to the orthopaedic clinic complaining of painful knees, particularly on rotation, climbing stairs and kneeling. His knees often locked on bending. On examination, there was swelling around both knees with tenderness over the medial joint spaces and limited flexion. Radiology revealed bilateral degenerative changes with ossified loose bodies in the joint space.

While awaiting a magnetic resonance image (MRI) of his knees, the patient was admitted to A&E having 'collapsed' at home. He complained of nocturia, frequency of micturition, polydipsia, lethargy, nausea, vomiting and an unintended weight loss of 12 kg over the past four months. His urine was strongly positive for glucose and ketones.

He was discharged on oral hypoglycaemic agents. His diabetes remained difficult to control at least in part because of high food intake and drinking 'more than moderate' amounts of beer. His liver function tests (LFT) were repeated.

Investigations

	Initial	Repeat	Reference range
Glucose	30.8 mmol/L		
Bilirubin	17 µmol/L	10 µmol/L	<21 µmol/L
Alanine aminotransferase (ALT)	124 U/L	227 U/L	<41 U/L
Aspartate transaminase (AST)		480 U/L	<41 U/L
Alkaline phosphatase (ALP)	222 U/L	206 U/L	40–129 U/L
Gamma-glutamyl transferase (GGT)	70 U/L	90 U/L	10–71 U/L
Triglyceride		5.1 mmol/L	0.8–1.7 mmol/L
Cholesterol		8.2 mmol/L	<5 mmol/L
Iron		40.2 µmol/L	8.1–28.6 µmol/L
Transferrin		1.8 g/L	2.0–3.6 g/L
Transferrin saturation		87%	5–50%
Ferritin		1267 µg/L	30–400 µg/L
C-reactive protein (CRP)		<5 mg/L	<5 mg/L

In view of the pattern of LFTs, abdominal ultrasound was undertaken revealing a distended gall bladder, but no gallstones and a normal bile duct. Liver autoantibody and viral studies were all negative.

The patient was referred to an endocrinologist who noted a hypogonadal appearance. On questioning, he revealed that he only shaved every 3–4 days. He had smooth skin, sparse body hair and small, soft testes. He admitted an alcohol intake of 40 pints of beer per week. Sex hormone tests were undertaken.

		Reference range
Follicle-stimulating hormone (FSH)	0.7 IU/L	1.5–12.0 IU/L
Luteinizing hormone (LH)	0.9 IU/L	1.7–8.6 IU/L
Testosterone	1.66 nmol/L	8.64–29.0 nmol/L

Thyroid function tests, cortisol and prolactin were all within reference ranges. Insulin stress test indicated adequate growth hormone and cortisol responses to hypoglycaemia. The need to reduce his alcohol intake was stressed. The diagnosis of hereditary haemachromatosis was suspected.

Genetic tests showed he was homozygous for the CYS282TYR variant of this disorder.

Repeated venesection therapy failed to lower his ferritin and he was commenced on testosterone supplements for his hypogonadism and insulin to control his hyperglycaemia.

QUESTIONS

1. Describe the pattern of LFTs seen in this patient?
2. What are the possible causes of his hyperlipidaemia?
3. Is transferrin saturation superior to ferritin in the diagnosis of haemachromatosis? If so, why?
4. What conditions may be associated with an elevated serum ferritin?
5. Which organs may be affected by haemachromatosis and with what effect?
6. What is the significance of the ALT and AST values?
7. What are the possible causes of hypogonadism in type 2 diabetes mellitus (T2DM)?

ANSWERS

1. There are both elements of obstruction, as shown by the raised alkaline phosphatase and GGT, and hepatocellular damage, as shown by the elevated ALT and AST. He has underlying hereditary haemochromatosis (HC) which is an autosomal recessive condition and this patient is one of the 90 per cent of Caucasian individuals with HC who are homozygous for the Cys 282 Tyr (C282Y) variant of the HFE gene.

2. Poor diabetic control, obesity and alcohol excess are largely associated with excessive calorie intake or an inability to deal with a calorie intake through normal processes. When glucose and alcohol cannot be used for energy purposes they are converted to triglyceride in the liver and exported as very-low-density lipoprotein (VLDL) giving elevated serum triglyceride concentrations.

3. As ferritin may be increased in any liver condition where there is hepatocellular damage, a high saturation of transferrin is a better marker of iron overload. A high saturation may be found in haemachromatosis, haemosiderosis, haemolytic anaemia, sideroblastic anaemia and iron poisoning.

4. Ferritin is an acute-phase reactant protein and hence rises in association with infections. For this reason, many laboratories measure CRP when ferritin is requested in order that this possibility is considered by the requesting clinician.

    Obesity is associated with high ferritin as is non-alcoholic fatty liver disease. Both are associated with insulin resistance and a chronic inflammatory state, which may provide an explanation of the high ferritin found in these conditions.

    Hypothyroidism is associated with a low rather than a high ferritin and high serum concentrations are found with thyrotoxicosis. This is thought to be due to the direct effects of thyroid hormones on ferritin production.

    The major intervention in haemachromatosis is venesection as this is the most direct route of reducing iron stores. There are no physiological processes for iron excretion.

    Iron overload conditions are linked with porphyria cutanea tarda. Depletion of iron stores, e.g. by venesection, lead to improvement in the symptoms of porphyria and therefore the presence of porphyria is an indication for venesection.

5. The most commonly involved organs in haemochromatosis are the liver, pancreas, joints, skin, heart, testicles, thyroid and pituitary.

    In the liver, the effects of excessive iron deposition include cirrhosis and liver cancer. The liver is typically the first organ to be affected. Up to 95 per cent of symptomatic patients have liver involvement. Skin involvement from iron deposits in the skin lead to skin discolouration and a bronze appearance. Skin deposition is present in up to 90 per cent of symptomatic patients. Pancreatic effects of iron deposition affects mostly the beta cells leading to glucose intolerance and eventually overt diabetes. This may be seen in more than half of the patients with haemochromatosis. Joint pain (arthralgia) and arthritis are also common (25–50 percent of patients) in haemochromatosis due to local deposition (as in this patient). Haemochromatosis can sometimes involve the heart, causing heart failure or heart rhythm disturbances. Erectile dysfunction may be seen in haemochromatosis due to either testicular or pituitary involvement. Hypothyroidism may result because of haemochromatosis affecting the thyroid gland.

One of the possible late manifestations of hereditary haemochromatosis is referred to as 'bronze diabetes'. This condition occurs when the disease involves the skin (bronze appearance) and the pancreas (diabetes).

6. The AST:ALT ratio has been used to differentiate alcoholic from non-alcoholic liver disease with ratios greater than 2 indicating alcoholic disease. In obesity and diabetes, the AST:ALT ratio is usually less than 1. In addition, AST:ALT ratios are used when contemplating the need for liver biopsy.

7. Hypogonadism is a largely unrecognized complication of T2DM, although cross-sectional studies have indicated that hypogonadotrophic hypogonadism may be present in a third of men with T2DM. This relationship appears to be independent of HbA1c levels, but is inversely correlated with BMI. Those with hypogonadotrophic hypogonadism are more likely to have other features of metabolic syndrome, including a raised CRP.

    Testosterone replacement therapy has been linked to an improvement in insulin sensitivity.

SECTION 2: RADIOLOGY

Case 25: Woman with abdominal pain

Case 26: Woman with cough and weight loss

Case 27: Middle-aged woman with difficulty in
swallowing

Case 28: Young man with chest pain

Case 29: Young woman with loss of vision

Case 30: Middle-aged man with shortness of breath

Case 31: Elderly woman with weight loss

Case 32: Elderly woman with shortness of breath

Case 33: Elderly woman with diabetes

Case 34: Middle-aged woman with a cough

Case 35: Man with a bloody cough

Case 36: Middle-aged man with a cough

Case 37: Elderly man with headache

Case 38: Elderly man with pain in the hip

Case 39: Woman with headache and vomiting

Case 40: Elderly woman with epigastric pain

Case 41: Elderly man with shortness of breath

Case 42: Woman with abdominal pain

Case 43: Middle-aged woman with swelling in hands and feet

Case 44: Middle-aged man with confusion

Case 45: Elderly woman with upper limb weakness

Case 46: Nasogastric feeding on the stroke unit

CASE 25: WOMAN WITH ABDOMINAL PAIN

History

A 21-year-old female student is sent to A&E by the out-of-hours GP. She describes 4 days of abdominal pain and diarrhoea. The abdominal pain is generalized, but worse in the right iliac fossa. It does not radiate and is relieved by lying still. She is having up to ten episodes of diarrhoea a day, which sometimes contains blood. She is not vomiting and has had a reduced appetite for 1 week. She reports weight loss of about 5 kg over the last year without dieting. She also reports intermittent episodes of diarrhoea and abdominal pain over the last two years which her GP has treated as irritable bowel syndrome (IBS). In the last two months, she also reports intermittent abdominal distension and 'squeezing' pain, sometimes associated with vomiting. Her past medical history includes IBS, asthma and anxiety. Regular medicines are peppermint oil capsules, mebeverine, citalopram 10 mg per day and a salbutamol inhaler. She has no allergies, smokes 5–10 cigarettes a day and drinks 10 units of alcohol at weekends.

Examination

On examination she looks unwell. She is flushed, dehydrated and in obvious discomfort. She has a temperature of 38°C, blood pressure (BP) is 95/60 mmHg, heart rate is 110 beats per minute regular, respiratory rate is 16 per minute, oxygen saturations 98 per cent on air. Heart sounds are normal. Auscultation of the chest is clear. Palpation of the abdomen reveals diffuse tenderness, particularly in the right iliac fossa. There is guarding in the right iliac fossa and a sense of fullness to palpation in the same area. Bowel sounds are quiet but present. Digital rectal examination reveals brown stool. There is no rash.

Investigations

		Reference range
Haemoglobin	10.5 g/dL	11.5–16.5 g/dL
Mean cell volume	82.0 fL	76–100 fL
Platelets	440 × 10⁹/L	150–450 × 10⁹/L
White cell count	15 × 10⁹/L	4–11 × 10⁹/L
Neutrophils	11.5 × 10⁹/L	2–7.5 × 10⁹/L
Sodium	135 mmol/L	135–146 mmol/L
Potassium	3.3 mmol/L (3.2–5.1)	3.2–5.1 mmol/L
Urea	10.1 mmol/L (1.7–8.3)	1.7–8.3 mmol/L
Creatinine	90 μmol/L	44–80 μmol/L
Corrected calcium	2.10 mmol/L	2.15–2.55 mmol/L
Albumin	28 g/L	34–48 g/L
C-reactive protein (CRP)	101 mg/L	<5 mg/L
Erythrocyte sedimentation rate (ESR)	80 mm/h	0–15 mm/h

Beta HCG (human chorionic gonadotrophin) is not raised. Urgent imaging is requested.

QUESTIONS

1. What is the clinical suspicion here?
2. How might this influence the choice of imaging modality?
3. What do the images show in Figures 25.1 and 25.2?
4. What are the differential diagnoses for the appearances on imaging?

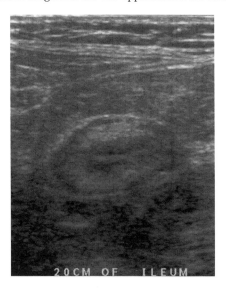

Figure 25.1

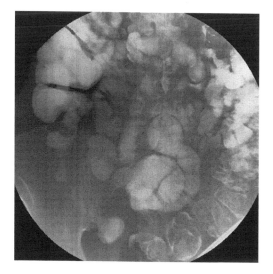

Figure 25.2

ANSWERS

1. The clinical suspicion is that of inflammatory bowel disease, either Crohn's disease or ulcerative colitis. The differential diagnoses in this case would include appendicitis, intra-abdominal infection or possible ovarian pathology.

2. The patient is young and of child-bearing age (note negative pregnancy test) – any imaging should ideally keep ionizing radiation to a minimum. Abdominal x-rays, computed tomography (CT) and barium/contrast studies all involve an ionizing radiation dose, which can be high with CT and barium studies. In this situation, ultrasound and magnetic resonance imaging (MRI) should both be considered as they do not involve ionizing radiation.

   What imaging could you do?

   a. Abdominal x-ray indicated if any suggestion of ileus/obstruction, megacolon or perforation (where combined with an erect chest film to demonstrate free intra-peritoneal air).
   b. Ultrasound can be useful especially in young/thin patients and children. It is accurate in these groups for appendicitis/terminal ileal disease and also for renal/pelvic cases of pain.
   c. CT – high radiation dose, but excellent for visualization of bowel/retroperitoneum. Used in elderly/complex cases.
   d. MRI – not a first-line modality in the abdomen.
   e. Barium studies (small bowel meal/follow-through) are used for the further investigation of suspected small bowel Crohn's disease.

3. The first image is an ultrasound image of the right iliac fossa (Figure 25.3) showing an abnormal loop of terminal ileum (arrow C). Arrow B points to the bowel lumen. Arrow A shows a thickened bowel wall which is hyperechoic secondary to active inflammation. There is inflammatory change in the perimesenteric fatty tissue around the involved segment which suggests inflammation affecting the full thickness of the bowel wall. The differential diagnosis for this appearance could be:

   a. Inflammation, such as inflammatory bowel disease (most common) or secondary to appendicitis
   b. Vascular – intramural haematoma or ischemia
   c. Radiotherapy related
   d. Infiltrative processes, such an amyloidosis
   e. Neoplastic, such as lymphoma or metastases
   f. Infective, tuberculosis can look identical to Crohn's disease.

   The second image is from a barium follow-through showing the small bowel (Figure 25.4). The patient has ingested barium contrast agent which is used to opacify the bowel. The type of barium study depends on which part of the bowel is being investigated. The small bowel has been imaged here with a barium follow-through. There is no obstruction to the passage of contrast which enters the right colon.

A long irregular stricture is seen in the region of the terminal ileum (Figure 25.4, arrows on stricture). There is associated separation of bowel loops in the right iliac fossa secondary to oedema. The appearances are typical of Crohn's disease.

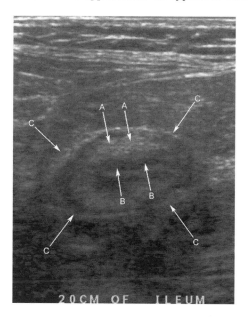

Figure 25.3

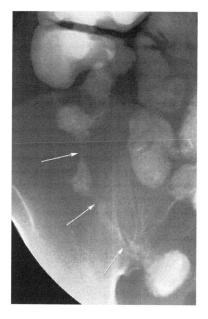

Figure 25.4

4. Conditions causing terminal ileal strictures, such as visualized in this barium study, are:

   a. Crohn's disease
   b. Ischemia
   c. Radiation enteritis
   d. Tumours/malignancy
   e. Carcinoid infiltration
   f. Tuberculosis
   g. 'Backwash ileitis' secondary to ulcerative colitis.

The ultrasound findings are consistent with active Crohn's disease involving the terminal ileum. The barium meal and follow-through shows appearances consistent with a Crohn's stricture of the terminal ileum.

Crohn's disease is a chronic, relapsing inflammatory condition that can affect any part of the gastrointestinal tract from mouth to anus. Patients with small bowel involvement often present with abdominal pain, diarrhoea and weight loss and often there is a mass in the right iliac fossa. Eighty per cent of Crohn's patients have small bowel involvement and the terminal ileum is the most common site.

Other barium study findings in Crohn's disease may be small bowel fold thickening (caused by increase in the volume or fluid of cells in the mucosal or submucosal region) and hyperplasia of lymphoid tissue with or without mucosal erosions (aphthous ulcers). Aphthous ulcers may enlarge and deepen across the bowel wall causing the characteristic 'rose-thorn' ulceration. Late signs include deep fissures or ulcers, pseudopolyps, 'cobblestone' pattern caused by transverse and longitudinal fissures around pseudopolyps, and separation of oedematous bowel loops. Characteristic 'skip lesions' refer to the manner in which lesions occur in multiple sites along the bowel. Strictures are common, especially in the terminal ileum, and are a result of the inflammatory process, and fistulae are also common.

Both Crohn's and ulcerative colitis are associated with extraintestinal manifestations, including:

- Clubbing
- Fatty liver, chronic active hepatitis, sclerosing cholangitis
- Erythema nodosum, pyoderma gangrenosum
- Amyloidosis, ankylosing spondylitis, seronegative arthritis
- Uveitis, episcleritis, iritis.

Different imaging techniques may help to identify complications – barium studies/fistulogram look for fistulae, abscesses or transformation into adenocarcinoma are best seen on CT scan.

Magnetic resonance enterography with gadolinium contrast is an imaging modality that is being increasingly used in Crohn's disease, being useful for assessing the extent of both non-active disease and active disease.

Features which may help differentiate Crohn's disease from ulcerative colitis

	Crohn's disease	Ulcerative colitis
Distribution	Mouth–anus	Colon/ileum (back wash ileitis)
Colon involvement	Right-sided	Left-sided
Ulcers	Deep (rose-thorn)	Superficial (collar stud)
Ileocaeal valve	Thickened	Gaping
Fistulae	Yes	No
Skip lesions	Yes	No
Risk of carcinoma	Slight ↑	Marked ↑
Megacolon	Unusual	More common
Rectum involved	14–50%	95%

There is also an increased risk of small bowel lymphoma and adenocarcinoma in Crohn's disease.

CASE 26: WOMAN WITH COUGH AND WEIGHT LOSS

History

A 60-year-old female presents to her GP with a non-productive cough and weight loss over four months. She complains of generalized aches and pains and more recently she has become constipated. She is a current smoker with a 40 pack-year history, she is a social drinker with no other significant history.

Examination

On examination, her skirt is loose and held up by a belt. Her finger nails are clubbed. She is not cyanosed. Her respiratory rate is 18 per minute and there is reduced air entry in the right upper zone of the chest. Abdominal examination is unremarkable and she is apyrexial and normotensive.

Investigations

Blood tests reveal hypercalcaemia and an elevated parathyroid hormone level. The GP sends her for a chest x-ray and the image is shown in Figure 26.1.

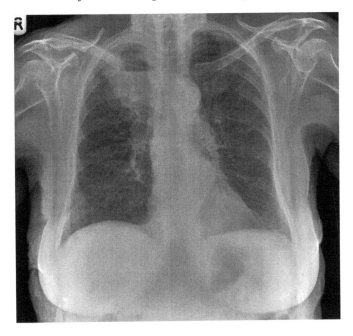

Figure 26.1

QUESTIONS

1. What does the chest x-ray demonstrate?
2. What is the most likely diagnosis?
3. What is the differential diagnosis?
4. What would you do next as the GP?
5. What do the biochemical tests suggest?
6. How would you ensure that a patient is prepared for a computed tomography (CT)-guided lung biopsy?

ANSWERS

1. In the right upper lobe, there is a radiopaque mass measuring 4 cm in diameter. There is an air–fluid level seen behind the medial aspect of the right clavicle. Appearances are consistent with a cavitating lung lesion.

2. The most likely cause in the context of this patient's history is bronchogenic carcinoma, and squamous cell carcinoma (SCC) is the most likely type of lung cancer to cavitate.

3. Causes of cavitating lung lesions can be remembered by the mnemonic 'CAVITY'. Carcinoma, Cystic bronchiectasis, Autoimmune diseases, Vascular disease, Infections and Youth, i.e. congenital causes. Primary or secondary squamous cell carcinomas are the most common causes – remember head, neck and cervix as possible primary sites. Tuberculosis, *Staphylococcus aureus* and *Klebsiella* also cause cavitation, although the patient would be systemically unwell.

4. Urgent respiratory referral is required. If malignancy is suspected, as it is in this case, the respiratory team will request a CT of the chest, abdomen and pelvis for staging purposes and the patient would need to be discussed in a multidisciplinary meeting to make an appropriate management plan.

5. The patient has hypercalcaemia secondary to ectopic secretion of parathyroid hormone from the SCC which is causing constipation and generalized aches and pains. This is known as a paraneoplastic syndrome and is most often seen with SCC of the lung, genitourinary or gynaecological malignancies. Hypercalcaemia may also be related to bone metastases which should be considered and excluded (radionuclide bone scan).

6. Patient preparation includes sufficient explanation of the procedure, with informed, written consent and recent clotting factors with an international normalized ratio (INR) around 1.0. If the patient is on warfarin, it is prudent to discuss with the haematologists. Institutions will have their own protocols which should be checked. In certain cases, warfarin can be stopped temporarily and swapped for daily treatment dose low-molecular-weight heparin (LMWH) injections, omitted the day before the procedure. The INR is monitored until it is approximately 1.0 and the patient is able to have the lung biopsy. Post-biopsy, LMWH and warfarin are restarted until the INR is at a therapeutic level and the LMWH can be stopped. Risks of CT-guided lung biopsy include infection, bleeding and pneumothorax. A chest film 4 hours post-procedure should always be performed to ensure there is no latent pneumothorax (remember to review this, or arrange review and document your findings in the patient's notes).

    The patient was referred to the respiratory physicians and an axial image from the CT of the chest is shown in Figure 26.2. The patient was lying prone at the time of the scan with the head towards the reader. In the right upper lobe, adjacent to the vertebral body, there is a large soft tissue lesion which contains an air – fluid level (arrow A). This corresponds to the mass seen on the chest x-ray. Note vertebral body (arrow B), trachea (arrow C) and a left upper lobe bulla (arrow D). A lung biopsy confirmed squamous cell carcinoma.

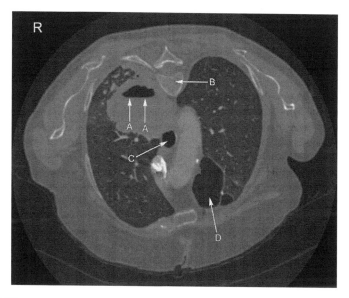

Figure 26.2

Bronchogenic, or lung cancer, is subdivided into small cell lung cancer (SCLC) and non-small cell lung cancer (NSCLC). SCLC is associated with smoking, is usually located centrally within the lung, grows rapidly and metastasizes early. NSCLC includes adenocarcinoma, SCC and undifferentiated large cell carcinoma. Adenocarcinoma is most commonly seen in non-smokers and females, is peripherally located in the lung, grows slowly but may metastasize early. Bronchoalveolar carcinoma is a subtype of adenocarcinoma which may present as a nodule or a focus of consolidation on a chest film. It may develop within an area of scarred lung fibrosis secondary to tuberculosis, bronchiectasis or scleroderma. Persistent consolidation 6–8 weeks after antibiotic therapy should raise the suspicion of cancer and patients require further investigation. SCC is associated with cigarette smoking, may be located centrally or peripherally within the lung and has the slowest growth rate of all the subtypes and is least likely to metastasize distantly. It is, however, the most likely type to cause chest wall invasion. Undifferentiated large cell carcinoma is associated with smoking, is usually large, centrally or peripherally located, grows rapidly and metastasizes early.

Histological confirmation of malignancy and the cell type in conjunction with a staging CT is essential for surgeons, radiotherapists and oncologists to make an appropriate management plan. Biopsy may be performed via bronchoscopy if the lesion is fairly central, or using CT guidance if it is more peripherally located. The TNM (tumour, nodes, metastasis) staging system is used to stage NSCLC and to decide on operability. A staging CT assesses the size of the primary tumour and the extent of invasion into local structures, the presence and size of ipsilateral and contralateral lymph nodes, and the presence of supraclavicular lymph nodes. Spread of cancer to the lymph nodes is suspected when the nodes are enlarged by CT criteria or are round rather than oval in morphology. Finally, metastases within the lungs or pleura, or distant metastases to bone, adrenal glands, brain, and liver, are checked for on the staging CT. TNM staging is revised regularly.

Risk factors for lung cancer include cigarette smoking, male gender, scarred lung fibrosis and exposure to asbestos, uranium and radon gas. Radon gas is a colourless, radioactive gas which is produced by the radioactive decay of uranium in soil and rocks. High levels increase the risk of lung cancer, particularly in smokers and particularly high levels in the UK are found in Cornwall. A relevant occupational and social history is therefore necessary when presenting symptoms suggest bronchogenic carcinoma.

CASE 27: MIDDLE-AGED WOMAN WITH DIFFICULTY IN SWALLOWING

History

A 56-year-old lady presented with a three-month history of difficulty swallowing which is non-progressive. She cannot identify any triggering factors, but notes the dysphagia is to solids more than liquids. She has had a few episodes of vomiting and reflux with reduced appetite and weight. She notes also a one-month history of intermittent bouts of central chest pain worse after food and notes a 2-week history of cough at night, which is non-productive but worsening. She has no other history of note.

Examination

Clinical examination revealed no haemodynamic compromise, respiratory examination revealed scattered coarse crepitations in the base of the right lung, but no evidence of respiratory distress. Cardiovascular, abdominal and neurological examinations were unremarkable. Her weight is currently 64 kg, reduced from 69 kg six months ago.

Investigations

Blood tests showed no evidence of anaemia or infection with normal renal and liver function. Electrocardiogram (ECG) was normal and her chest radiograph showed patchy consolidation at the right base. The patient declined an upper gastrointestinal (GI) endoscopy and underwent a barium swallow for further assessment (see Figure 27.1).

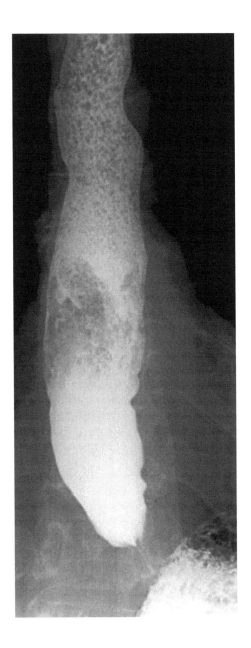

Figure 27.1

QUESTIONS

1. Can you identify the abnormalities seen in Figure 27.1?
2. What is the likely diagnosis in this case?
3. Are there any other investigations that could aid in diagnosis of this condition?
4. How is this condition treated?
5. What are the potential complications?

ANSWERS

1. The main abnormalities are highlighted in Figure 27.2. There is a tight, 'bird beak'-like stricture at the lower oesophageal sphincter (arrow A) with dilatation of the proximal oesophagus containing food debris (arrow B). The stricture is smooth and has no features to suggest it is malignant. Distal to the stricture barium contrast is seen in the stomach suggesting that fluid can traverse the stricture (arrow C).

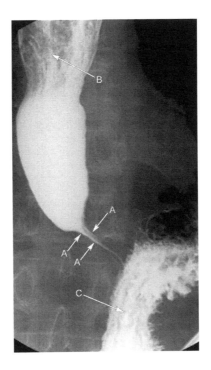

Figure 27.2

2. The most likely diagnosis is achalasia of the oesophagus. This condition is due to dysmotility of the smooth muscle layer of the oesophagus and the lower oesophageal sphincter (LES), due to degeneration of the myenteric plexus. It is characterized by incomplete LES relaxation, increased LES tone and lack of oesophageal peristalsis. This diagnosis is made in the absence of other pathologies such as carcinoma of the oesophagus or fibrosis.

A balance of excitatory transmitters (e.g. acetylcholine and substance P) and inhibitory transmitters (e.g. nitric oxide and vasoactive intestinal peptide, VIP) control the tone and activity of the smooth muscle in this region. The local obstruction with proximal dilatation is similar to Hirschsprung's disease, and in most cases there is an aganglionic segment as in Hirschsprung's disease, but it is acquired rather than congenital and so presents later in life.

The nocturnal cough that this woman described and the right basal consolidation, is most likely a result of aspiration pneumonia due to the reduced or incomplete relaxation of the LES leading to increased regurgitation and inhalation of food products. A condition rather like achalasia can develop as a complication of American trypanosomiasis (Chagas' disease).

3. Barium swallow is useful as achalasia has certain characteristic features and also, as the investigation is dynamic, the hold-up of contrast and failure of sphincter relaxation can be observed in real time. Oesophageal manometry is seen as the reference standard for the diagnosis of achalasia. It may show diagnostic features, such as high resting pressure in the cardiac sphincter, incomplete relaxation on swallowing and absent peristalsis. If manometry is normal but clinical symptoms or radiological evidence suggest achalasia, a condition called pseudoachalasia may be present. Endoscopy (OGD, oesophagogastroduodenoscopy) should be performed to exclude malignancy supplemented by endoscopic ultrasound if available.

4. Treatment options for achalasia include the following:

    a. Endoscopic or fluoroscopic balloon dilatation: where a balloon is inserted into the lower oesophagus via an endoscope or fluoroscopic guidance and it is inflated to stretch the muscle of the oesophagus while leaving the mucosa intact. The success rate is 70–80 per cent with a 5 per cent rate of perforation. If a perforation occurs, emergency surgery is needed to close the perforation and perform a myotomy. However, approximately 50 per cent of patients will require more than one dilatation and roughly one third of patients will develop significant gastro-oesophageal reflux; hence the need for proton pump inhibitors (PPI).
    b. Heller's cardiomyotomy followed by PPI: this operation can be performed laparoscopically where the muscle fibres of the lower oesophagus are divided in a longitudinal direction for about 5 cm, about 1.5 cm above the stomach. The success rate is 85–95 per cent, but 10–15 per cent suffer from reflux symptoms post-operatively, hence the need to use PPI.
    c. Botulinum toxin injection is an alternative to those patients unsuitable for invasive procedures. This is often performed endoscopically where injection of botulinum toxin can be used, but only 30 per cent of patients have satisfactory relief at the end of one year. The injection can also produce an inflammatory reaction that will make surgery difficult.
    d. Calcium-channel blockers and nitrates are useful as they relax the LES. They have been shown to be of limited benefit as they only benefit 10 per cent of patients.

5. Complications of achalasia include:

    a. Untreated achalasia may lead to nocturnal inhalation of food material lodged in the oesophagus and aspiration pneumonia (as seen in the patient in this case).
    b. Carcinoma of oesophagus: Longstanding achalasia increases the risk of oesophageal carcinoma (roughly between 2 and 7 per cent of patients). Presumably potential carcinogens are held in the oesophagus instead of migrating with peristalsis. Malignancy can develop even after successful treatment.

CASE 28: YOUNG MAN WITH CHEST PAIN

History

A 24-year-old gentleman attends A&E complaining of left-sided chest pain which started while he was watching television. The pain came on suddenly, was sharp in nature, did not radiate and was worse on movement and deep breathing. He has felt short of breath since the pain started, but was able to walk into the department. He thinks he had a similar pain before but not as severe and did not seek medical advice previously. He is normally fit and well. He has a family history of ischemic heart disease. There are no allergies and he takes no regular medicines or illicit drugs. He smokes 20 cigarettes a day and drinks alcohol at weekends.

Examination

On examination, he is breathless at rest but able to complete sentences. There is no cyanosis. He is afebrile, blood pressure is 130/85 mmHg, pulse 100 beats per minute regular. Respiratory rate is 24 per minute. Oxygen saturations are 95 per cent on air. Heart sounds are normal. His trachea is central and chest expansion appears reduced on the left with reduced air entry on the left side of the chest and reduced vocal resonance. There are no added sounds.

Investigations

Full blood count, urea and electrolytes, and C-reactive protein are within normal limits. Electrocardiogram shows sinus tachycardia. A chest x-ray is undertaken (see Figure 28.1).

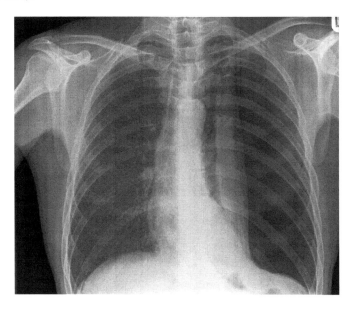

Figure 28.1

QUESTIONS

1. Describe the chest x-ray. What does it show?
2. What is the diagnosis?
3. What causes do you know for this condition?
4. What is the management for this condition?
5. What advice should the patient be given?

ANSWERS

1 and 2.   (Answers 1 and 2). This patient has a large left-sided pneumothorax, seen as lucency (no vessels). This is exerting some mass effect with compression and collapse of the left lung and there is also mediastinal shift to the right, suggesting the pneumothorax is under tension. This is a medical emergency and urgent aspiration/drainage is needed. In patients who are compromised and who have a pneumothorax clinically, then aspiration should be the priority. Patients should not be sent for a chest x-ray as they are in imminent danger of cardiorespiratory arrest.

In this case, although the pneumothorax is large, the patient remains relatively well. This is often the case in younger patients, but when deterioration occurs it can be rapid (increasing air in the pleural space impairs venous return to the heart and causes circulatory collapse).

In Figure 28.2, a chest drain has been inserted (B). Increasingly smaller bore drains are being used in this situation, introduced over a wire passed through a hollow-bore introducer needle (Seldinger technique). This reduces the blunt trauma associated with insertion of larger trocars. The lung edge is well seen (A), as the lung partially reinflates. There is also some surgical emphysema (C).

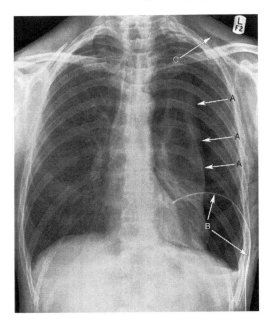

Figure 28.2

3.   Pneumothoraces may be classified as spontaneous or acquired. Acquired pneumothoraces are secondary to trauma or iatrogenic, for example following central line insertion. Spontaneous pneumothoraces may be primary, where there is no evidence

of underlying disease (although apical pleural blebs are common), or secondary to underlying chronic obstructive pulmonary disease, pneumonia, lung cancer, asthma, pulmonary fibrosis or cystic fibrosis. Spontaneous pneumothorax is 2.5 times more common in males, particularly tall, thin male smokers.

4. The aims of management are to allow lung re-expansion and prevent reoccurrence. Treatment is based on estimation of the size of the pneumothorax (difficult, remember the two-dimensional x-ray represents a three-dimensional structure of lungs within the rib cage). The British Thoracic Society guidelines (2010) for management of spontaneous pneumothorax define a small pneumothorax to be less than 2 cm (measuring the interpleural distance at the level of the hilum) and a large pneumothorax to be greater than 2 cm. In clinically stable patients with a small pneumothorax with no underlying lung disease, a period of observation with a repeat chest x-ray at 6–12 hours is appropriate. The resolution rate is approximately 1 per cent per day. If there is no progression, patients can be discharged with follow-up instructions.

    If the pneumothorax is primary and large (more than 2 cm), aspiration of up to 2.5 litres with a 16–18G cannula is recommended. If aspiration fails, a chest drain should be inserted.

    If the pneumothorax is secondary (i.e. there is underlying lung disease, significant smoking history or the patient is over 50 years) and the pneumothorax is more than 2 cm, immediate chest drain is preferred. If it is between 1 and 2 cm and the patient is not breathless, aspiration can be tried, with progression to chest drain if the pneumothorax remains more than 1 cm. If a secondary pneumothorax is small with no breathlessness, the patient can be observed for 24 hours with oxygen therapy (being mindful of any risk of hypercapnic respiratory failure). Finally, any patient with a pneumothorax who is haemodynamically unstable should proceed straight to chest drain. Persistent air leak may require surgical intervention for bullectomy and pleurodesis using a minimal access video-assisted thorascopic (VATS) approach or open thoracotomy approach.

5. There is a suggestion from the history that he may have had a previous pneumothorax. Pneumothoraces can be recurrent, approximately 20 per cent after one previous pneumothorax and 50 per cent after two. As such this man may be considered for pleurodesis. Stopping smoking will also reduce his risk of recurrence. He should be advised not to fly for at least 1 week after the pneumothorax has resolved with complete lung re-expansion (2 weeks after a traumatic pneumothorax).

    A third of pneumothoraces treated by lung re-expansion only will recur. Intervention to prevent recurrence (pleurodesis, bullectomy) is considered after a second pneumothorax or after the first in certain professional contexts (divers, pilots).

CASE 29: YOUNG WOMAN WITH LOSS OF VISION

History

A 27-year-old female presents to A&E with sudden onset of left eye pain and loss of vision. She is under investigation by the neurologists for headaches and an episode of numbness and 'tingling' in her right arm two months previously. Her symptoms are aggravated following a hot bath. She is otherwise fit and well.

Examination

On examination, gait, power and reflexes are normal. On examining her cranial nerves, a light shone into the right eye causes constriction of both the right and left eye. When the light is swung immediately from the right to the left, the pupils appear to dilate on both sides.

Investigations

Blood tests are normal. She is admitted under the medical team and a magnetic resonance imaging (MRI) is arranged, the results of which are shown in Figures 29.1 and 29.2 (Figure 29.1 is an axial FLAIR image through the brain just cranial to the level of the lateral ventricles, while Figure 29.2 is a sagittal T2-weighted image through the cervical cord).

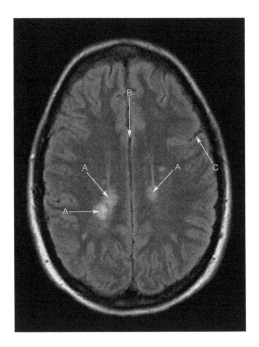

Figure 29.1

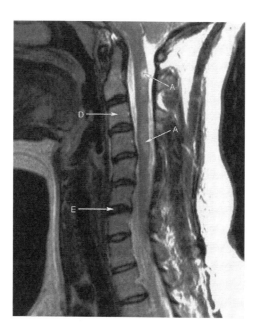

Figure 29.2

QUESTIONS

1. There are arrowed structures on each image. Can you identify the normal anatomy and the abnormality, and name the normal structures labelled?
2. What is the cause of the clinical findings in the eye examination?
3. How is the diagnosis made?
4. What is the course of the disease?
5. What treatments are available?

ANSWERS

1. The abnormalities on the brain MRI are the high signal foci or plaques of demyelination, affecting the white matter of the brain as are seen in multiple sclerosis. These have a periventricular distribution (arrow A). Arrow C shows a left parietal sulcus, arrow B the interhemispheric fissure. Further high signal plaques are seen in the cervical cord (arrow A) on the MRI of the sagittal cervical spine. Arrow D indicates the C3 vertebral body, arrow E the C6/C7 intervertebral disc.

2. The clinical signs from the eye examination demonstrate a relative afferent pupillary defect (RAPD), also known as a 'Marcus-Gunn pupil', and the poor light response in the affected pupil results in pupillary dilatation. A RAPD occurs in optic neuritis which may be a presenting sign of multiple sclerosis (MS).

3. Diagnosis of MS is dependent on lesions being disseminated in time and space, that is, lesions occur at different times in different regions of the brain and spinal cord. MRI of the brain and spinal cord, visual-evoked potentials and lumbar puncture to obtain cerebrospinal fluid (CSF) for analysis for oligoclonal bands may be part of the work up following a thorough central nervous system (CNS) history.

Diagnosing multiple sclerosis
• Comprehensive CNS history
• Relapses disseminated in time and space
• Oligoclonal IgG on CSF analysis
• Plaques in the CNS on MRI (T2-weighted or gadolinium-enhanced)
• McDonald criteria

4. Multiple sclerosis is a disease which can follow a relapsing and remitting pattern, primary progressive, or relapsing progressive pattern. Approximately 80 per cent of patients have the 'relapsing and remitting' type of MS.

5. No cure for multiple sclerosis exists. A multidisciplinary approach to management is essential involving the GP, community nurse, neurologist, radiologist, occupational therapist and physiotherapist. High-dose oral or intravenous corticosteroids are used in the management of acute relapses to reduce their severity. Immunomodulation with interferon may be used for disease modification to reduce the number of relapses. Symptomatic treatment of paraesthesia, constipation, erectile dysfunction and spasticity can be managed with gabapentin, laxatives, Viagra, and baclofen, respectively. Prognosis is very variable ranging from few relapses and no disability to frequent relapses, rapid progressive disability and premature death. Poor prognostic features are the onset of the progressive disease phase, frequent relapses in the first two years after diagnosis, short time between relapses and female sex.

Unusual features in multiple sclerosis

- **Uhthoff's phenomenon.** Reduced visual acuity following exercise or a hot bath.
- **Lhermitte's phenomenon.** 'Electric shock' sensation travelling down the spine and limbs on neck flexion.
- **Pulfrich effect.** Abnormal visual depth perception secondary to differential retinal light stimulation. This effect is exploited with 3D glasses.

Multiple sclerosis is a demyelinating disease of the CNS. Loss of myelin in the white matter of the brain and spinal cord interrupts nerve conduction and causes a motor and/or sensory deficit in the region supplied by that nerve. On T2-weighted MRI of the brain and spinal cord, demyelination is demonstrated as a high signal intensity in the white matter, usually oval in morphology, and measuring a few millimetres to several centimetres in size. Active lesions may enhance following gadolinium administration.

The cause of MS is not clear, although it is thought that genetic and environmental factors, in conjunction with an infection, play a role. MS tends to present in adults between the age of 20 and 40 years and females are affected more than males.

Patients may present with abnormal gait, tremor, paraesthesiae, urinary retention, or visual disturbances which may be secondary to optic neuritis or internuclear ophthalmoplegia. It is essential that a thorough history is taken to address any existing or previous CNS deficit as lesions occur in different sites at different times.

MRI of the brain and spinal cord is the imaging modality of choice and 95 per cent of people with clinically certain multiple sclerosis will have an abnormal MRI brain scan. MRI is also helpful in defining prognosis. After the first attack of demyelination, an abnormal MRI brain scan indicates a high risk of developing multiple sclerosis in the order of 83 per cent risk at ten years. A normal head MRI after a first attack of demyelination reduces the risk of developing multiple sclerosis to 11 per cent.

Signs of optic neuritis include papilloedema, dyschromatopsia (disorder of colour vision), decreased visual acuity and a relative afferent pupillary defect. Internuclear ophthalmoplegia is a sign of impaired conjugate lateral gaze due to demyelination of the medial longitudinal fasciculus (MLF) which is bundles of crossed ascending and descending fibres in the brainstem. The MLF joins the oculomotor nerve in the midbrain on one side with the abducens nerve in the pons on the other side. If there is a lesion in the left MLF then on looking to the left, both eyes will move together normally. On looking to the right, the left eye adducts minimally and there is nystagmus of the right eye. On right lateral gaze, the patient may complain of seeing double. Thus, the MLF lesion is ipsilateral to the eye with impaired adduction.

In transverse myelitis, which is an area of demyelination across the spinal cord at a particular level, patients may present with urinary retention. On examination, a sensory level may be present, below which sensation is impaired, and this level indicates the level of demyelination in the cord.

Oligoclonal bands are immunoglobulins found in serum or CSF. CSF obtained from a lumbar puncture can be sent for electrophoresis or isoelectric focusing to look for oligoclonal IgG. In the context of MS, some oligoclonal bands should be seen uniquely intrathecally (within the CSF) and not in the blood serum. Oligoclonal IgG is present in the CSF of 90 per cent of patients with MS, however, it is also seen in systemic inflammatory conditions, such as lupus, neurosarcoid and CNS infections, such as neurosyphilis.

The differential diagnosis includes acute disseminated encephalomyelitis (ADEM), cerebral vasculitis, cerebrovascular disease, sarcoidosis, Devic's disease, Behçet's disease and CNS lymphoma.

CASE 30: MIDDLE-AGED MAN WITH SHORTNESS OF BREATH

History

A 55-year-old male is referred to the medical assessment unit complaining of increasing shortness of breath over the last few months. He has a long-standing cough productive of white sputum. Over the last 4 days, he feels his breathlessness has deteriorated further. He is now breathless on walking short distances, is coughing up much more sputum than usual and feels generally unwell. He has no chest pain, palpitations or ankle swelling. He has a past medical history of depression. There are no allergies and he takes citalopram 20 mg daily. He has smoked 30 cigarettes a day since the age of 17. He drinks 3 units of alcohol a day. He lives alone and works for the local council.

Examination

He is alert and orientated, and is breathless at rest, but able to complete sentences. He is apyrexial, blood pressure is 140/90 mmHg, pulse 95 bpm regular, respiratory rate is 23 per minute, oxygen saturations are 90 per cent on air. His heart sounds are normal and jugular venous pressure is not raised. Auscultation of the chest reveals diffuse bilateral expiratory wheeze and a prolonged expiratory phase. There is no peripheral oedema.

Investigations

Abnormal blood results include haemoglobin 18.5 g/dL (13.5–18.0 g/dL), white cell count 14×10^9/L ($4–11 \times 10^9$/L) and C-reactive protein (CRP) is 80 mg/L (<5 mg/L). Electrocardiogram reveals normal sinus rhythm.

Arterial blood gas on air shows:

pH	7.33 (7.35–7.45)
PaO_2	7.9 kPa (11.1–14.4 kPa)
$PaCO_2$	6.9 kPa (4.7–6.4 kPa)
HCO_3	30 mmol/L (22–29 mmol/L)
Base excess (BE)	4

Bedside spirometry reveals:

FEV_1	42% predicted
FVC	60% predicted
FEV_1/FVC	52%

A chest x-ray is performed (Figure 30.1).

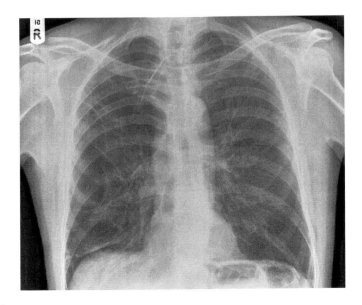

Figure 30.1

QUESTIONS

1. What does the chest x-ray show (Figure 30.1)?
2. What is the likely diagnosis?
3. What is the acute and long-term management of this condition?

ANSWERS

1. The chest x-ray shows a central trachea and a normal mediastinum. The heart is not enlarged. His lungs are hyperinflated with diaphragmatic flattening and, in addition, extensive bullous formation is evident in the right lung (less marked in the left lung). These findings would be consistent with severe chronic obstructive pulmonary disease (COPD) with associated emphysema. No discrete consolidation or mass is seen.

   The development of bullae is common in COPD. Bullae are thin-walled (<1 cm) air spaces as a result of destruction of the alveolar walls. Bullae are seen as thin-walled lucencies, commonly round in shape that compress the normal lung and distort the vasculature that surrounds them. It can be difficult to distinguish an apical bulla from a pneumothorax. The shape of the superior border of the lung may help. If it remains convex from the superior margin to the lateral margin, this is more characteristic of a pneumothorax. An apical bulla will result in a concave shape of the superior margin of the lung. An infected bulla may have an air–fluid level.

   In more advanced disease, the pulmonary arteries may appear large centrally suggesting the development of secondary pulmonary artery hypertension, and cardiomegaly consistent with right heart failure may be seen. In an acute exacerbation, a chest x-ray is useful to look for alternative diagnoses such as lobar pneumonia, pneumothorax and cardiac failure which may mimic an exacerbation (and also to exclude a complicating lung malignancy).

   A subsequent computed tomography (CT) scan of the chest is shown in Figure 30.2 which confirms extensive emphysematous change and the bullous changes (arrowed) seen on chest x-ray.

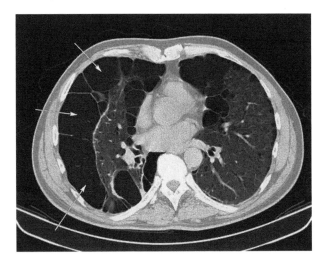

Figure 30.2

2. The chest x-ray and spirometry findings fit with the clinical suspicion of COPD – symptoms of cough, sputum production and dyspnoea in a patient with a long

history of smoking. The history suggests the diagnosis has been present for at least several months and the current presentation represents an acute exacerbation of COPD. His arterial blood gas shows a type 2 respiratory failure which has a chronic (compensated) component but is beginning to decompensate acutely. He has a degree of polycythaemia also secondary to chronic hypoxia.

3. In the acute phase, he should be managed with controlled oxygen therapy due to his risk of worsening hypercapnia maintaining oxygen saturations between 88 and 92 per cent. He should be treated with nebulized bronchodilator therapy (beta-2 agonist and anticholinergic) as required initially and then every 4–6 hours. High-dose prednisolone (40 mg) is recommended for 5–10 days, having evidence for reducing the recovery time by 1–2 days and improving FEV_1. Antibiotics are considered if there is worsening dyspnoea and increased sputum volume and purulence and the choice is based on local protocol.

If there is worsening hypercapnic respiratory failure with acidosis, severe dyspnoea and respiratory distress, non-invasive ventilation is considered. Intubation and ventilation is considered in appropriate patients where there is impending respiratory arrest, impaired conscious level or life-threatening acid-base disturbances despite optimum medical therapy. The overall in-hospital mortality for acute exacerbations of COPD is 8 per cent with an overall one-year survival rate of 77 per cent. This decreases to 65 per cent if an intensive therapy unit (ITU) admission was required.

Once he has recovered from his acute exacerbation, he should have repeat formal lung function testing. This provides a general framework to stage disease and direct treatment (see below).

	Mild	Moderate	Severe
FEV_1	>50% predicted	30–50% predicted	<30% predicted
Treatment	Inhaled short-acting bronchodilator as required	Regular use of short-acting bronchodilator. If control still poor, combination therapy with beta-2-agonist and anti-cholinergic	Inhaled combination of long-acting beta-agonist and corticosteroids. Stop corticosteroids after 4–6 weeks if no improvement. Trial of tiotropium for poor control

A CT of the chest would be indicated if surgical intervention for the bullae was proposed or if initial investigations suggest other pathology. He should be given strong smoking cessation advice and referred for pulmonary rehabilitation. It is recommended that COPD patients receive the influenza vaccine.

The five-year survival of COPD patients ranges from 30 to 60 per cent depending on the severity of the disease based on FEV_1, PO_2 and PCO_2, age and co-morbidities. Low body mass index is an independent risk factor for mortality, particularly in patients with severe COPD. Long-term oxygen therapy improves survival and should be given to patients with respiratory failure (PO_2 <7.3 kPa or SaO_2 <88 per cent) or if the PO_2 is less than 8 kPa with coexistent cardiac failure, polycythaemia or pulmonary hypertension.

CASE 31: ELDERLY WOMAN WITH WEIGHT LOSS

History

A 66-year-old woman is sent to the medical assessment unit by her GP. She feels generally unwell, has lost her appetite and has lost half a stone in weight unintentionally in the last two months. Further enquiry reveals gradually increasing breathlessness and she has constant dull right-sided chest pain. She is a retired teacher, with no other history of note. She has never smoked.

Examination

She is comfortable at rest and is apyrexial, blood pressure 135/90 mmHg, pulse 86 bpm, respiratory rate 17, oxygen saturations are 95 per cent on air.

There is evidence of finger clubbing. Heart sounds are normal. Examination of the chest reveals mildly reduced right-sided expansion and a dull percussion note at the right base. Auscultation of the chest reveals scattered crepitations in the right mid-zone, reduced air entry at the right base and normal air entry on the left side. Her abdomen is soft, non-tender with no organomegaly.

Investigations

		Reference range
Sodium	140 mmol/L	135–146 mmol/L
Potassium	3.6 mmol/L	3.2–5.1 mmol/L
Urea	9.8 mmol/L	1.7–8.3 mmol/L
Creatinine	129 µmol/L	62–106 µmol/L
Erythrocyte sedimentation rate (ESR)	60 mm/h	0–15 mm/h
Haemoglobin (Hb)	9.5 g/dL	11.5–16.5 g/dL
Mean corpuscular volume (MCV)	85.5 fL	76–100 fL
White blood cells (WBC)	6.1×10^9/L	$4.0–11.0 \times 10^9$/L
Neutrophils	2.0×10^9/L	$2.0–7.5 \times 10^9$/L
C-reactive protein (CRP)	96 mg/L	<5 mg/L

A chest x-ray is performed (Figure 31.1).

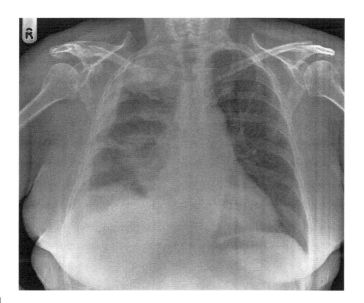

Figure 31.1

QUESTIONS

1. What does the chest x-ray show?
2. What are the differential diagnoses for these appearances?
3. What important part of the history should be enquired about?
4. What is the likely diagnosis?

ANSWERS

1. The chest radiograph demonstrates loss of volume in the right hemithorax. There is lobulated, irregular, pleural thickening in the right hemithorax (arrows, Figure 31.2) extending to the right lung apex, blunting the right costophrenic angle. Some ill-defined airspace opacity is present in the right midzone, possibly inflammatory or mass. No rib destruction is seen, the left lung is clear.

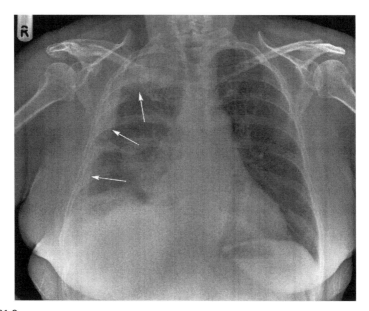

Figure 31.2

2. These features put together (lobular pleural thickening, pleural effusion and volume loss) are highly suspicious for metastatic pleural disease or of mesothelioma. The most common cancers causing metastatic pleural disease are lung and breast, and less commonly haematologic cancers, ovarian and gastrointestinal tumours. Malignant mesothelioma develops in the pleura following exposure to asbestos, and is usually unilateral. Chest x ray or chest computed tomography (CT) scan show diffuse progressive thickening of the pleura on one side. Chest wall invasion or rib destruction may be the only differentiating feature from benign disease, however benign pleural tumours are rare. There may be other evidence of asbestos exposure, such as pleural plaques, pleural or diaphragmatic calcification or pulmonary fibrosis. CT of the thorax may reveal discrete pleural masses, multiloculated effusions and a thick pleural rind in more advanced disease. CT of the thorax also provides staging information in particular relating to bone destruction and mediastinal lymphadenopathy and can be used to guide biopsy of a suspicious lesion for histological diagnosis. Figure 31.3 demonstrates widespread pleural calcification (white arrows) in another patient ('holly leaf' appearance) with a right basal effusion (black arrow).

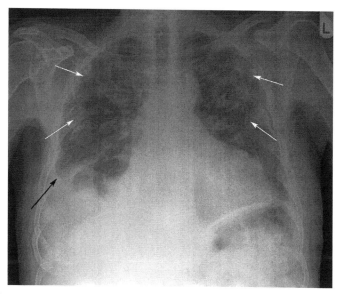

Figure 31.3

3. The important further enquiry in the history is therefore to establish potential exposure to asbestos. It is also important to ask screening questions for other malignancy and undertake the relevant physical examinations. In this case, further enquiry reveals her father was a shipyard worker.

4. Mesothelioma is a tumour of the mesothelial lining of the pleural, pericardial and peritoneal cavities caused by exposure to asbestos (blue asbestos fibres, crocidolite, is the most carcinogenic). It is uncommon with an incidence of eight per 100 000 per year in the UK, affecting men more than women. Asbestos was widely used in the UK until the 1980s. However, there is a long (approximately 40-year) latent period between exposure and presentation, so it has been projected that the incidence is likely to peak in 2020. Any evidence of exposure is relevant, and as in this case people who did not work directly with it are just as much at risk having been exposed to fibres through for example living with or handling work clothes of someone who works directly with asbestos.

The presentation is often insidious with non-specific symptoms initially. The most common symptoms are progressive dyspnoea and non-pleuritic dull chest pain. Systemic features of malignancy include weight loss, night sweats, anorexia and fever. In advanced cases, chest wall mass, hepatomegaly, ascites or cachexia may be present.

Chest x-ray and CT of the thorax is the imaging of choice. Histopathological diagnosis is essential. Samples can be obtained from a pleural aspiration (cytology) or a percutaneous pleural biopsy (histological), however, both have poor sensitivity. If these tests do not yield a diagnosis, surgical biopsy is needed.

Prognosis is related to stage, however, it is generally very poor with a median survival of under a year. In suitable patients, surgery, radiotherapy and chemotherapy are offered, although there is no significant evidence for surgery and mesothelioma is a very radioresistant and chemoresistant tumour. Radiotherapy has a palliative role to treat chest pain and prophylactic for needle aspiration, chest drain or biopsy sites. Video-assisted thoracoscopic (VATS) decortication and pleurodesis can be offered for palliation of symptomatic pleural effusions. There are compensation schemes in place for industry-related asbestos exposure and families should be aware of this.

Other forms of asbestos-related chest disease
Lung fibrosis (asbestosis) lower zone
Pleural plaques (most common form)
Pleural thickening
Pleural calcification
Benign effusion (must exclude malignancy)
Risk of lung carcinoma

CASE 32: ELDERLY WOMAN WITH SHORTNESS OF BREATH

History

A 72-year-old woman attends A&E acutely short of breath. She tells you she has been under investigation for breathlessness and is awaiting a computed tomography (CT) scan of her chest for a 'shadow on the lung' seen on a recent chest radiograph. She has been breathless for several weeks but has become markedly worse over the last 24 hours and is now very breathless at rest and struggling to complete sentences. She reports a recent history of recurrent chest infections and weight loss. Her past medical history includes a myocardial infarction eight years ago, hypercholesterolaemia and hypertension. Current medications are aspirin 75 mg/day, simvastatin 40 mg at night, ramipril 5 mg at night, bisoprolol 2.5 mg/day and bumetanide 1 mg/day. She is an ex-smoker of 20 years, having previously smoked ten cigarettes a day for 25 years.

Examination

On examination, she is breathless at rest and using accessory muscles. Her oxygen saturations are 90 per cent on air, respiratory rate 20 per minute, blood pressure 110/80 mmHg, pulse 95 bpm, regular, temperature 36.5°C. Heart sounds are normal with nil added. On examination of the chest, she has reduced expansion on the left side. Percussion note is dull on the left side of the chest and, on auscultation, there is reduced air entry throughout the left side of the chest. Her abdomen is soft and non-tender and there is no peripheral oedema.

Investigations

She undergoes blood tests, an arterial blood gas and a chest x-ray. The results are shown below. Her electrocardiogram shows no significant acute changes.

		Reference range
Haemoglobin	10.0 g/dL	11.5–16.5 g/dL
Mean cell volume (MCV)	78 fL	76–110 fL
White cell count	13.0×10^9/L	$4.0–11.0 \times 10^9$/L
Neutrophil count	8.5×10^9/L	$2.0–7.5 \times 10^9$/L
Platelet count	161×10^9/L	$150–450 \times 10^9$/L
Urea	11 mmol/L	1.7–8.3 mmol/L
Creatinine	110 µmol/L	44–80 µmol/L
Potassium	3.1 mmol/L	3.2–5.1 mmol/L
Sodium	148 mol/L	135–146 mmol/L

		Reference range
Arterial blood gas		
pH	7.40	7.35–7.45
PaO$_2$	7.0 kPa	11.1–14.4 kPa
PaCO$_2$	5.0 kPa	4.7–6.4 kPa

Anteroposterior (AP) sitting chest x-ray is performed (Figure 32.1).

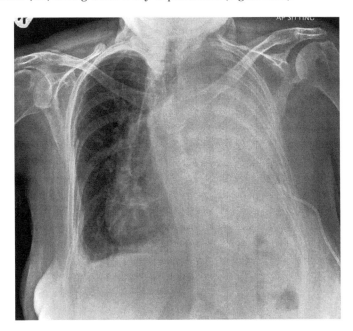

Figure 32.1

QUESTIONS

1. Describe the appearance of this x ray.
2. What is the differential diagnosis for this appearance?
3. What other x-ray features help to confirm the diagnosis?
4. What other investigations are indicated?
5. What is the on-going management?

ANSWERS

1. (Answers 1–3) There is complete opacification of the left hemithorax. This is an AP film and the patient is rotated. Allowing for this, there is evidence of mediastinal shift away from the affected side, suggesting mass effect. There are several causes for this – the most common cause is a large pleural effusion. Other causes for hemithoracic opacity might include a large mass, or possibly extensive acute consolidation (less likely and there is no evidence of consolidation, e.g. air bronchogram on the film).

2. It is important to differentiate an effusion from the other causes of hemithorax opacity which are associated with volume loss, namely mediastinum shifted to the affected side, including lung collapse or previous pneumonectomy/lobectomy (look for evidence of previous surgery, clips at hilum or rib defects). Figure 32.2 is a chest radiograph in a patient with a left lung collapse due to an occluding tumour obstructing the left main bronchus (black arrow); note mediastinal shift to the left.

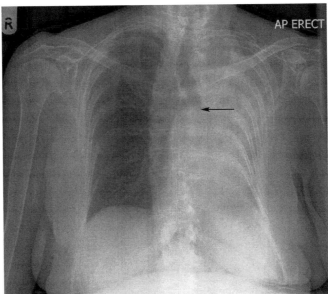

Figure 32.2

3. We know this patient had a possible lesion on a recent chest radiograph – make sure you always try to look at any previous films – this lung opacification is new and secondary to likely effusion. Underlying lung malignancy needs to be excluded in the first instance and there are likely to be several litres of fluid in her chest.

4. A pleural effusion is the accumulation of fluid in the pleural space. It is not a diagnosis, but a manifestation of underlying disease. There are many causes for effusions, but the most common causes are cancer, pneumonia and heart failure. Effusions are classified as transudates or exudates based on their protein content

(less than 25 g/L in transudates and more than 35 g/L for exudates; if the protein concentration is between these two, then Light's criteria are applied). Transudates arise from an imbalance of oncotic and hydrostatic pressures in conditions such as heart failure, liver failure, renal failure or hypoalbuminaemia. Exudate is a result of altered pleural or local capillary permeability in inflammatory or neoplastic conditions, such as malignancy, pneumonia, autoimmune disease, pancreatitis, or secondary to some drugs, such as amiodarone or methotrexate. Effusions may also be haemorrhagic due to trauma, bronchial carcinoma, bleeding disorders, or they may be chylous due to an obstructed thoracic duct. Serum albumin level and serum lactate dehydrogenase (LDH) should be requested to compare with pleural fluid analysis.

5. The patient should be managed using the ABCDE approach (airway, breathing, circulation, disability, and exposure). This patient's effusion is large and causing respiratory compromise, and should therefore be drained. A drain has been placed and position checked on x-ray. Samples of the pleural fluid should also be sent to seek the underlying cause, fluid sent for microbiology, cytology and clinical chemistry including protein, LDH, pH, glucose, and differential cell count. Amylase can also be checked if there is any suggestion of pancreatitis as a cause.

Do remember, as always, if you are unsure at any stage as to the cause of radiological appearances, seek senior advice or speak to a radiologist. If the patient is not *in extremis*, an ultrasound of the chest can help confirm the presence of an effusion and whether it is loculated. The best position for access and also depth of effusion from the skin can also be marked. Ultrasound can be performed in the radiology department or on the ward. Risks of pleural aspiration include infection, bleeding and pneumothorax. Consent the patient appropriately, document all procedural aspects in the patient notes and arrange and review the post-drainage/aspiration chest radiograph. In some institutions, pleural drain insertion is only done under ultrasound guidance by a radiologist to minimize such risks to the patient. When fluid is drained, this patient will need CT of the chest/abdomen to assess the underlying cause.

CASE 33: ELDERLY WOMAN WITH DIABETES

History

A 79-year-old woman is found on the floor at home. Neighbours raised the alarm after they had not seen her for 2 days. She has a past medical history of type 2 diabetes, hypertension, stroke and osteoarthritis. Her regular medicines are aspirin 75 mg/day, dipyridamole 200 mg twice a day, metformin 1 g three times a day, gliclazide 80 mg twice a day, bendroflumethiazide 2.5 mg/day, ramipril 5 mg/day, omeprazole 20 mg/day and simvastatin 20 mg/day. She smoked 15 cigarettes a day until ten years ago. She normally lives alone and independently.

Examination

On examination, she has a Glasgow Coma Scale (GCS) score of 9 (E, 3; V, 2; M, 4). Her blood pressure is 168/100 mmHg, pulse 70 bpm regular. She is afebrile. Respiratory rate is 10 per minute and her saturations are 100 per cent on high-flow oxygen. Heart sounds are normal, auscultation of the lungs reveals a few crackles at the right base. Her abdomen is soft and non-tender. Neurological examination reveals increased left-sided limb tone and hyper-reflexia with a dense left hemiparesis and left-sided facial droop. There is evidence of left-sided neglect. Her left plantar reflex is up-going.

Investigations

		Reference range
Haemoglobin	10.5 g/dL	11.5–16.5 g/dL
Mean cell volume	80.1 fL	76–100 fL
White blood cells	6×10^9/L	$4.0–11.0 \times 10^9$/L
Neutrophils	4×10^9/L	$2.0–7.5 \times 10^9$/L
Platelets	212×10^9/L	$150–450 \times 10^9$/L
Urea	6 mmol/L	1.7–8.3 mmol/L
Creatinine	160 µmol/L	44–80 µmol/L
C-reactive protein	33 mg/L	<5 mg/L
Glucose	4.0 mmol/L	

An urgent computed tomography (CT) of the head is performed (Figure 33.1).

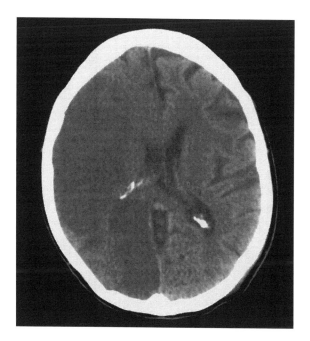

Figure 33.1

QUESTIONS

1. What does the head CT scan show?
2. What is the acute and long-term management of this condition?
3. Are any further investigations indicated at this time?

ANSWERS

1. Figure 33.2 is an axial unenhanced CT section through the brain at the level of the bodies of the lateral ventricles. There is a large, wedge-shaped, area of low attenuation (dark) seen in the right cerebral hemisphere, predominately involving the parietal lobe (arrows A). This involves the distribution of the right middle cerebral artery. There is evidence of associated mass effect with cerebral swelling (note some midline shift to the left, arrow B shows displaced interventricular septum). There is distortion and compression of the body at the right lateral ventricle (arrow C). The appearances are those of an extensive and acute right middle cerebral artery infarction. CT should be performed urgently, especially in patients who may be candidates for thrombolysis; ideally patients should have been admitted, scanned and thrombolysed within 4.5 hours of the event.

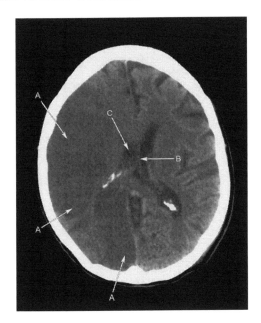

Figure 33.2

CT is the initial imaging modality of choice for the diagnosis of stroke and to differentiate infarct from haemorrhage. Figure 33.3 is a CT scan and demonstrates a large intracerebral haematoma (A) in the left parietal region (in another patient). There is mass effect with surrounding oedema (arrow B). If CT is performed early on, within hours, of the cerebrovascular event, scanning may be normal or changes subtle. In these cases magnetic resonance imaging (MRI) can be valuable (see below). CT will also exclude other mimics of stroke (e.g. tumour, subdural haematoma, abscess), is rapid to complete and is generally well tolerated by patients. CT can also help triage patients who are suitable for thrombolysis – a patient with a large area of infarction, as in this case, would be at high risk of haemorrhage into the infarcted area and would not be considered suitable for thromobolysis.

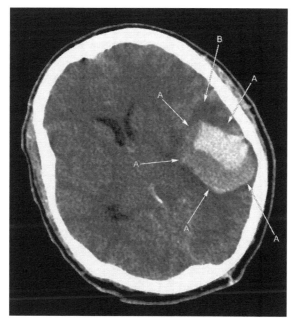

Figure 33.3

2 and 3. The patient should be managed according to the ABCDE approach (airway, breathing, circulation, disability and exposure) and immediate treatable causes of stroke, e.g. hypoglycaemia, excluded.

MRI (to include diffusion weighting) can be helpful in the diagnosis of reversible ischemia, but is not widely available especially out of hours. Carotid ultrasound is used to triage patients who may benefit from carotid endarterectomy after stoke – surgery can benefit patients with severe (>70 per cent) internal carotid artery stenosis who have had either transient ischemic attack or a stroke with good recovery involving the anterior circulation.

Stroke is a sudden-onset neurological deficit of vascular origin lasting more than 24 hours. It is the third most common cause of death in the Western world and a major cause of disability with an incidence of 200 per 100 000 a year affecting males more than females. There are many risk factors including increasing age, hypertension, smoking, hypercholesterolaemia, diabetes mellitus, ischemic heart disease, peripheral vascular disease, atrial fibrillation, coagulopathies, oral contraceptive pill use and vasculitis. Eighty per cent of strokes are ischemic in origin, 10 per cent are a result of primary intracerebral haemorrhage and 10 per cent due to subarachnoid haemorrhage. Specific clinical patterns can arise from infarction of different anatomical territories and are detailed by the Oxford Community Stroke Project classification. Differential diagnosis includes epileptic seizure with Todd's paresis, migraine, cerebral tumours, hypoglycaemia, subdural haematoma, encephalitis, cerebral abscess, cerebral vasculitis and cerebral venous thrombosis.

Haemorrhagic transformation and oedema can lead to clinical deterioration and death. Seizures can occur acutely or later on after the stroke. Approximately 45 per cent of patients will have an element of dysphagia putting them at risk of aspiration. The resulting physical disability of a stroke may predispose patients to deep vein thrombosis, pulmonary embolism and pressure sores. Infection, most commonly aspiration pneumonia, is a common cause of death.

There is now an increasing evidence base for the use of thrombolysis (recombinant tissue plasminogen activator) within 4.5 hours of ischemic stroke to improve outcome in carefully selected patients at specialist centres. Aspirin 300 mg is given as soon as possible after the onset of stroke symptoms if there is no haemorrhage and thrombolysis is not being considered.

The aims of on-going management are to modify existing risk factors and implement secondary prevention measures. Antiplatelet therapy should be commenced with aspirin 300 mg for 2 weeks followed by clopidogrel 75 mg/day. Immediate lowering of blood pressure is usually not recommended as it may increase the risk of cerebral hypoperfusion and possible extension of stroke. Longer-term control of blood pressure (after 14 days) is essential as lowering blood pressure reduces the risk of further stroke. Treatment with an angiotensin-converting enzyme (ACE) inhibitor and a thiazide is recommended. Anticoagulation with warfarin is recommended in patients with atrial fibrillation. If there are no contraindications, warfarin should be started 2 weeks after the stroke to reduce the risk of haemorrhagic transformation. Statin therapy should be instituted as a secondary prevention at 48 hours and smoking cessation advised.

Prognosis depends on age and stroke type. Overall mortality is 19 per cent at one month and 31 per cent at one year. However, the prognosis following haemorrhage is significantly worse, with a high rebleed rate.

CASE 34: MIDDLE-AGED WOMAN WITH A COUGH

History

A 53-year-old female office worker is seen by her GP with a persistent cough which started 4 weeks ago. In the last few days, it has become productive of yellow and green sputum. She has just completed a second course of antibiotics which have not improved her symptoms. She denies breathlessness, but reports feeling notably fatigued in recent weeks, with excessive sweating, particularly at night, which she thought may be related to the menopause. She has never smoked, and has not travelled outside Europe since returning from South Africa with her family as a teenager. She has no other medical history of note.

Examination

She is noticeably thin. She has a temperature of 37.5°C, blood pressure 135/83 mmHg, heart rate 92 beats per minute and regular, oxygen saturation 96 per cent on room air and respiratory rate of 18 per minute. Further examination reveals no lymphadenopathy, there is no clubbing, and the chest is clear.

Investigations

Routine blood tests reveal a normocytic anaemia, but are otherwise normal.

The GP sends her for a chest x-ray (Figure 34.1).

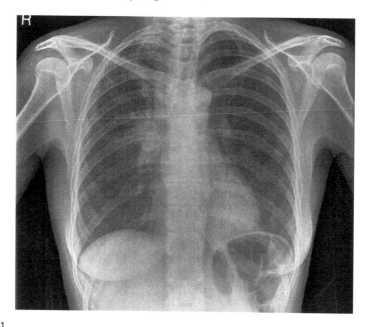

Figure 34.1

QUESTIONS

1. What does the chest x-ray show?
2. What is the likely diagnosis?
3. What else should you consider in this patient?
4. What would you do next as her GP?

ANSWERS

1. The chest radiograph demonstrates a bulky and dense right hilum (arrows A) and increased soft tissue in the right paratracheal region (arrows B) consistent with lymphadenopathy (Figure 34.2). Ill-defined infiltrates are seen within the right upper lobe with perihilar consolidation.

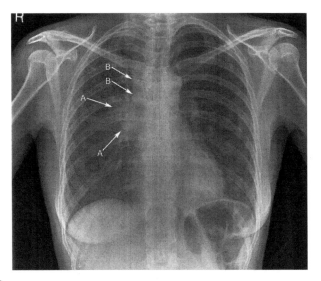

Figure 34.2

2. In the context of this patient's history, symptoms and chest x-ray findings, pulmonary tuberculosis (TB) is the most likely diagnosis. Differential diagnoses include sarcoidosis, and primary lung malignancy. Pulmonary tuberculosis may occur concomitantly with sarcoidosis, particularly if the individual is undergoing steroid treatment. Lymphoma and metastases, particularly from adenocarcinoma of the gastrointestinal tract, breast or ovary, may demonstrate similar radiological signs.

3. Further history-taking may reveal potential risk factors for tuberculosis and direct further clinical tests. These include close contact with an infected individual, living in crowded or poor housing, homelessness, or chronic alcohol or drug misuse. Progression from latent to active disease is caused by defects in cell-mediated immunity, most commonly coinfection with human immunodeficiency virus (HIV). Other factors which can trigger reactivation are advanced age, diabetes, renal failure, malnutrition, malignancy, corticosteroid use and immunosuppressive drugs.

4. A referral to a respiratory physician specializing in tuberculosis should be made for treatment and contact tracing. Notification of a new case of tuberculosis must be made to the Health Protection Agency. Patient education with regard to transmission and the importance of compliance with treatment should be initiated. Multiple sputum samples should be sent for microscopy and culture for acid-fast bacilli, prior to treatment commencing. Treatment should not be delayed while awaiting

results if there is a high clinical suspicion of TB. Full blood count, liver and renal function, colour vision and acuity should be checked prior to commencing treatment.

Tuberculosis is an airborne infectious disease caused by *Mycobacterium tuberculosis*, which shows a predilection for the lungs but may affect any organ in the body. It differs from other bacterial infections in that the inflammatory response involves cell-mediated immunity (hypersensitivity reaction). There has been a resurgence in incidence in tuberculosis in Western countries since the 1980s associated with coinfection with HIV, immigration and the development of multidrug-resistant tuberculosis. Recognition and early treatment of tuberculosis is therefore important.

Primary tuberculosis, which occurs in previously unsensitized individuals, is often asymptomatic and undetectable on physical examination, but is an incidental finding on chest x-ray. In primary infection, *Mycobacterium tuberculosis* is taken up by alveolar macrophages and then replicates, with spread via the lymphatics to the hilar lymph nodes. Cell-mediated immunity leads to granuloma formation, limiting further bacterial replication and disease spread. The site of primary infection is usually in the periphery of the mid-zone of one lung producing an opacity of 1–2 cm. This is the Ghon focus and, together with lymphadenopathy on the side of the lesion, forms the primary complex. In time, the primary complex may become fibrotic, calcified or resolve completely. If the host's immune response is unable to contain replication, active disease occurs (primary progressive tuberculosis). Adenopathy is a feature of primary progressive tuberculosis and is much more common in children. Imaging may offer the only way of diagnosing and evaluating the extent of tuberculosis in infants and children when clinical suspicion is high, i.e. previous exposure and a positive tuberculin test.

Tuberculosis can be acquired in childhood and remain clinically latent for years, with only a small proportion progressing to active disease. Reactivation, or post-primary tuberculosis, occurs one to two years after the initial infection in around 5 per cent of individuals, but can also evolve decades later, usually as a result of an impaired immune response. Most commonly, this is due to coinfection with HIV, but may be due to advanced age, diabetes, renal failure, malignancy, corticosteroid or other immunosuppressive therapy. Once reactivation occurs, unlike in primary tuberculosis whereby the infection is contained by the immune response, progression is inevitable.

In primary tuberculosis, lesions can occur throughout the lungs and tend to favour the bases, however, reactivated TB tends to involve the apical and posterior segments of the upper lobes and superior segments of the lower lobes.

Complications, such as bronchogenic spread, may occur due to erosion of the bronchial walls by caseous tissue, resulting in bronchopneumonia or pulmonary consolidation. If the disease spreads into the pleural cavity, a pleural effusion, or empyema, may form. Haematogenous spread may result in widespread dissemination to extrapulmonary sites and is associated with increased mortality. Early dissemination may appear as miliary tuberculosis on chest x-ray, identified as millet-sized (1–2 mm) nodules throughout the lung fields, with a predilection for the upper lobes. Brain involvement is common in miliary tuberculosis and therefore CT/ MR imaging should be performed even in the absence of neurological signs.

What is the Ghon focus?

The primary site of pulmonary tuberculosis infection – a calcified granuloma in the lower lobe associated with calcified hilar nodes (the Ghon complex).

Symptoms may be insidious and non-specific, but pulmonary tuberculosis most commonly presents with a persistent cough, which becomes productive, with dyspnoea and haemoptysis in more advanced disease. Weight loss, fatigue, night sweats and intermittent fever are also presenting features. Examination may be normal or there may be signs of weight loss, consolidation or pleural effusion, and lymphadenopathy. There may also be evidence of extrapulmonary disease, for example skin changes, cranial nerve or meningeal involvement, and spinal disease (Pott's disease).

As well as a thorough medical history, which may identify previous contacts and risk factors, and physical examination, the diagnosis of active tuberculosis is usually made with positive chest x-ray findings and the presence of acid-fast bacilli (AFB) in at least three sputum samples. Ziehl–Neelsen (ZN) staining provides a quicker test to identify acid-fast bacilli and a positive result implies probable mycobacterium tuberculosis (as the most common acid-fast bacilli). Positive AFB cultures are required to confirm these findings but results can take several weeks. Bronchoscopy may be necessary to obtain bronchoalveolar lavage (BAL) samples if sputum samples are inadequate. In extrapulmonary disease, biopsies may be required. Chest x-ray may show upper lobe infiltrates or cavitation, lymphadenopathy or changes related to previous tuberculosis infection, such as calcification and fibrosis. Histological findings demonstrate a caseous, or necrotic, granuloma (in contrast to the non-caseating granulomas found in sarcoidosis and Wegener's granulomatosis).

What is Simon's focus?

A calcified nodule that forms in the apex of the lung following haematogenous spread from the primary site in primary tuberculosis infection, often, the site of disease reactivation.

The aim of treatment is to cure the disease, prevent transmission and avoid drug resistance. Typically, the treatment course is 6 months, with a four-drug regimen (rifampicin, isoniazid, pyrazinamide and ethambutol) in the first two months and a continuation phase of two drugs in the last four months. Directly observed therapy (DOT) aims to increase compliance with nurse-supervised treatment and observed ingestion of medication.

A repeat chest x-ray should be performed at the end of treatment for pulmonary tuberculosis to confirm resolution of pulmonary disease.

CASE 35: MAN WITH A BLOODY COUGH

History

A 73-year-old man presents to his GP with a 3-day history of haemoptysis. He has had a dry cough for the last 3 weeks. He denies breathlessness or chest pain. On further probing, he reports unintentional weight loss of 10 kg in the last six months, loose stools for several weeks and feels 'bloated'. He has a history of hypertension which is well controlled with amlodipine. He has never smoked and was previously employed as a mechanic.

Examination

On examination, he is cachectic and his finger nails are clubbed. He is afebrile, heart rate 84 per minute, blood pressure (BP) 125/85 mmHg, respiratory rate 16 per minute, oxygen saturations 95 per cent on room air. There is a hard enlarged lymph node in the left supraclavicular region. His chest is clear on auscultation and heart sounds are normal with no peripheral oedema. His abdomen is mildly distended with no palpable masses or organomegaly and bowel sounds are present. Digital rectal examination is unremarkable and urine dipstick is normal.

Investigations

		Reference range
Haemoglobin	11.5 g/dL	13.5–18.0 g/dL
White blood cell count	5.6×10^9/L	$4.0–11.0 \times 10^9$/L
Platelets	256×10^9/L	$150–450 \times 10^9$/L
Mean corpuscular volume (MCV)	70 fL	76–100 fL
Sodium	136 mmol/L	135–146 mmol/L
Potassium	4.1 mmol/L	3.2–5.1 mmol/L
Urea	7.8 mmol/L	1.7–8.3 mmol/L
Creatinine	96 µmol/L	62–106 µmol/L
C-reactive protein (CRP)	22 mg/L	<5 mg/L
Total protein	88 g/L	66–87 g/L
Albumin	26 g/L	34–48 g/L
Bilirubin	4 µmol/L	<21 µmol/L
Alanine aminotransferase (ALT)	86	Up to 41 IU/L
Aspartate aminotransferase (AST)	98	Up to 40 IU/L
Alkaline phosphatase (ALP)	159	40–129 IU/L
International normalized ratio (INR)	1.3	0.8–1.2

A chest x-ray is performed (Figure 35.1).

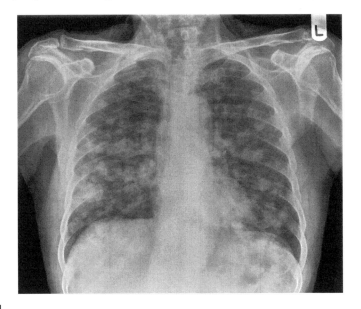

Figure 35.1

QUESTIONS

1. What does the chest x-ray show?
2. What is the differential diagnosis?
3. What do the blood tests suggest?
4. Which further investigations would you request?

ANSWERS

1. There are multiple nodular opacities of varying sizes throughout both lung fields, heart size normal, no overt bone destruction. These nodules are ill-defined, and no cavitation or associated calcification is present.

2. The most likely diagnosis is pulmonary metastases (from a non-lung primary or lung primary). Other differentials would include Wegener's granulomatosis, rheumatoid nodules, fungal infection (e.g. aspergillus), tuberculosis and sarcoidosis. Wegener's granulomatosis, although uncommon, may mimic pulmonary metastases in clinical presentation and radiological findings. It commonly affects the upper airways; renal impairment (haematuria/protein on urine dipstick) is found in 80 per cent of patients at presentation and cytoplasmic anti-neutrophil cytoplasmic antibodies (c-ANCA) are a relatively sensitive test (positive in 90 per cent of Wegener's granulomatosis cases). The most likely diagnosis given the history and examination is pulmonary metastases from a primary in the gastrointestinal tract.

3. The patient has a microcytic anaemia and mildly deranged liver function. In the context of the clinical picture this is likely to suggest occult blood loss from the gastrointestinal tract with metastases to the liver.

4. In light of the chest x-ray findings, computed tomography imaging of the chest, abdomen and pelvis to enable further characterization of the nodules and identify the extent of disease and locate the primary tumour would be appropriate at this stage. Contrast-enhanced computed tomography (CT) scan is generally preferred for radiological staging as it improves the identification of vascular anatomy, particularly of the liver, and may improve visualization of nodal disease.

   Further tests which may be useful include tumour markers, which are non-specific, but may assist in the diagnosis. Carcinoembryonic antigen (CEA) is non-specific for bowel cancer and may be raised in non-malignant disease, such as Crohn's, chronic obstructive pulmonary disease, pancreatitis and in smokers. However, if raised, it can be a useful marker of disease pre- and post-treatment.

   The patient underwent a contrast-enhanced CT of the chest, abdomen and pelvis. An axial lung windowed image of the CT of the chest is shown in Figure 35.2. Throughout both lungs, there are multiple nodular opacities (A) of variable sizes with a pleural lesion also demonstrated on the right. CT of the sigmoid colon revealed a stricture with thickened colonic wall consistent with a possible primary malignancy, and further large ill-defined lesions throughout the liver. Colonoscopy confirmed the diagnosis of sigmoid carcinoma. The oesophagus (B) and descending thoracic aorta (C) are also shown in figure 35.2.

   Malignant tumours commonly metastasize to the lungs via haematogenous or lymphatic spread. Those which commonly metastasize to the lungs are breast, gastrointestinal (GI) tract and renal cell carcinomas, as well as head and neck, soft tissue sarcomas and melanoma. Less common malignancies which may metastasize to the lungs include thyroid and testicular tumours.

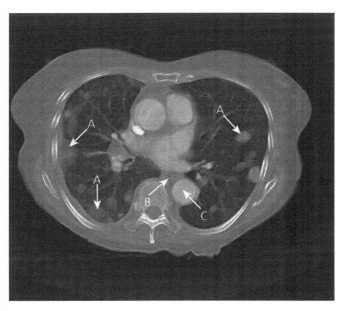

Figure 35.2

Colorectal cancer is the third most common cancer in the UK, around 65 per cent of these are in the left side of the colon. Most cases arise from adenomatous polyps. Ninety-five per cent of colorectal cancers are adenocarcinomas with the remainder being squamous cell carcinoma, carcinoid tumour, sarcoma and lymphoma. The most common sites for metastases are the liver and lymph nodes, but metastatic spread to the lungs, as well as peritoneum, pelvis and adrenals also occurs. Only one third of colorectal cancer is diagnosed in the early stages (Duke's stages A and B).

It is associated with advancing age, with more than 80 per cent of those diagnosed being over the age of 60 years, a high fat and low fibre diet, inflammatory bowel disease (ulcerative colitis) and a hereditary predisposition, the two major forms of which are familial adenomatous polyposis (FAP) and hereditary non-polyposis colon cancer (HNPCC).

The most common presenting symptoms depend on the site of the lesion within the colon and rectum and are often non-specific, but include change of bowel habit, rectal bleeding, tenesmus, abdominal pain and weight loss. Patients with a lesion in the left side of the colon are more likely to present with bowel obstruction, whereas lesions on the right, where the lumen diameter is larger and stool is more fluid, tend to present later as an iron-deficiency anaemia. Severe anaemia may cause symptoms of breathlessness and fatigue. Patients may, however, present with symptoms related to metastatic disease, the most common of which is cough and haemoptysis, but also pneumonia, pleuritic chest pain and dyspnoea.

There are two staging systems used for colorectal cancer in the UK; the TNM (tumour, node, metastasis) system is more commonly used, but staging may also be referred to by Duke's classification. 'T' describes how far the tumour has infiltrated the wall of the intestine and spread to local areas. 'N' is the extent of spread to regional lymph nodes and 'M' is the extent of metastatic spread to other areas of the body.

Colon cancer staging systems: TNM and Duke's

TNM staging system		Duke's staging system		5-year survival rate (%)
Stage	Definition	Stage	Definition	
0	Tis N0 M0		*In situ.* Only involves the mucosa	
I	T1 N0 M0	A	Limited to bowel wall	85–95
	T2 N0 M0			
IIa	T3 N0 M0	B	Extension into serosa or mesenteric fat	60–80
IIb	T4a N0 M0		Extension through wall, but not into nearby tissues	
IIc	T4b N0 M0		Extension through wall, and into nearby tissues	
III	Any T N1 M0	C	Lymph node metastases	30–60
	Any T N2 M0			
IV	Any T any N M1	D	Distant metastases	<10

Management of this patient involves a multidisciplinary team. Histological confirmation of malignancy and cell type is important for further management by the surgical and oncological teams. A colonoscopy and biopsy of the lesion identified in the colon on CT scan would be appropriate. Bronchoscopy with biopsy may also be required if there is doubt regarding the primary or secondary nature of the lung lesions.

Definitive treatment for localized colorectal cancer (Duke's A + B) is surgical resection. Treatment for Duke's C usually involves surgical resection followed by chemotherapy. In patients with advanced disease, chemotherapy may prolong survival. Colonic stenting may be required if a patient presents with acute large bowel obstruction.

The bowel cancer screening programme for 60–75 year olds (variable age inclusion by country) was rolled out in the UK in 2010. The programme involves faecal occult blood testing (FOBt) every two years and subsequent referral for colonoscopy in the event of abnormal results. The aim is earlier diagnosis of colorectal cancer and improved mortality rates.

CASE 36: MIDDLE-AGED MAN WITH A COUGH

History

A 45-year-old Caucasian male has been referred to respiratory outpatients. He has a 3-month history of worsening shortness of breath with an associated non-productive cough, which is more severe at night. He feels generally lethargic and achy, and has also experienced sweats and shivering at night. His weight is steady. He has also noticed some painless swelling of his cheeks. He is married with two children and works as a solicitor. He does not smoke and drinks only socially. There is no other history of note.

Examination

On examination, he looks well and is apyrexial. There is bilateral, firm, symmetrical and non-tender swelling of his parotid glands and there are multiple small, hard nodes in the anterior triangles of his neck. Cardiothoracic examination is unremarkable.

You review his chest x-ray undertaken by his general practitioner (Figure 36.1). Initial blood results including full blood count, area and electrolytes, and liver function tests are unremarkable. There is an increase in serum corrected calcium and also C-reactive protein.

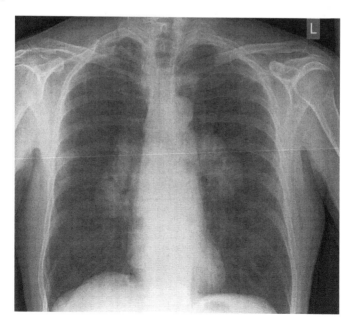

Figure 36.1

QUESTIONS

1. What abnormality is present on the chest radiograph?
2. What is the most likely diagnosis in this patient?
3. How might you confirm the diagnosis?
4. What abnormality might you find on cutaneous examination?
5. How should he be further managed?

ANSWERS

1. The chest radiography demonstrates bilateral hilar lymphadenopathy (BHL) with symmetrical lobulated hilar enlargement. There is no evidence of significant paratracheal lymphadenopathy, although there is some splaying of the carina suggesting subcarinal lymphadenopathy (an enlarged left atrium, e.g. secondary to mitral stenosis can also do this).

2. The most likely diagnosis in the context of the clinical presentation and the chest radiographic findings is that of sarcoidosis. Sarcoidosis is a multisystem granulomatous disease of unknown cause, most common in adults under 50 years of age and more common in women, and African Americans and Scandinavians. Sarcoidosis can involve the parotid glands – the combination of uveitis, parotid enlargement and facial nerve palsy with pyrexia is known as Heerfordt's syndrome (uveoparotid fever). This patient does not report eye symptoms, but formal ophthalmological assessment of all patients presenting with sarcoidosis is essential – posterior uveitis may be asymptomatic and can be sight-threatening.

3. Sarcoidosis can affect any organ and usually a tissue diagnosis is necessary for confirmation. Histologically, non-caseating granulomata are identified. Computed tomography (CT) of the chest is useful to further evaluate thoracic disease and to assess whether interstitial lung involvement is present. This patient underwent CT – an axial post-contrast section through the chest is shown in Figure 36.2 – this confirms hilar lymphadenopathy (arrow B), subcarinal lymphadenopathy (arrow A). Note normal ascending aorta (arrow C) and main right pulmonary artery (arrow D). No lung fibrosis was apparent on lung window settings. CT and clinical examinations will help identify sites suitable for biopsy. Cutaneous scars are often infiltrated by sarcoid granulomata and are readily amenable to biopsy. In this patient, there is

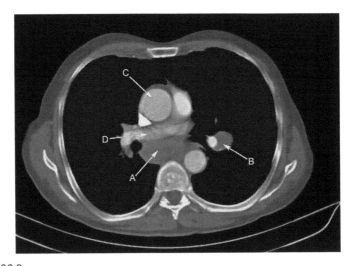

Figure 36.2

likely involvement of the parotid glands and cervical lymph nodes and ultrasound-guided core biopsy can be utilized to obtain a tissue sample from either of these areas. Non-caseating granulomata are a non-specific finding and other conditions, including tuberculosis, lymphoma and fungal infections, can cause granuloma formation and mimic sarcoidosis. Foreign body reactions, beryllium exposure and common variable immunodeficiency are other mimics.

Other investigations include:

a. Immunoglobulin estimation – sarcoidosis is associated with a polyclonal gammopathy.
b. Alkaline phosphatase (normal in this patient; if raised, may suggest hepatic involvement).
c. Serum angiotensin-converting enzyme (ACE). This is secreted by granulomata, but is non-specific. ACE is raised in 60 per cent of patients at the time of diagnosis – the degree of elevation may correlate with granuloma load, there is no prognostic value, however, and the use of this investigation is limited.
d. Lung function tests in the presence of respiratory symptoms (restrictive defect if pulmonary fibrosis present).
e. Electrocardiogram for cardiac arrhythmia or conduction delay which may suggest cardiac involvement.
f. Tuberculin skin test. If positive, tuberculosis needs to be excluded.
g. Serum calcium. Granulomas secrete 1,25 vitamin D and cause hypercalcaemia in 10 per cent of patients (as in this case).
h. Magnetic resonance imaging is indicated for the detection of suspected neurological sarcoidosis and positron emission tomography (PET) imaging is increasingly being used for evaluation and follow up of complex, multisystem disease.

4. Erythema nodosum is a common cutaneous manifestation of sarcoidosis and careful lower limb cutaneous assessment is necessary. Erythema nodosum, arthralgia, malaise and BHL are known as Lofgren's syndrome which has a good prognosis, with spontaneous recovery frequent. Lupus pernio may occur (chronic cases), hypo/hyperpigmentation, skin nodules and scar infiltration are also recognized.

5. Many patients do not need treatment and the disease can regress spontaneously. The main treatment option is oral corticosteroids. There are certain absolute indications for oral steroids:

a. Hypercalcaemia
b. Neurological involvement
c. Cardiac involvement
d. Ocular involvement (if topical steroids have failed).

Steroids can be of benefit to patients with moderate to severe chest symptoms or changes suggestive of interstitial lung disease on imaging.

UK guidelines advocate initial treatment with prednisolone 0.5 mg/kg per day for one month, then reducing the dose over six months to a maintenance dose of 10 mg, or less, per day. Patients should start on an oral bisphosphonate to prevent steroid-induced osteoporosis. Steroid treatment is usually for 12–24 months at least. If steroids fail, then other immunosuppressive agents can be used, e.g. azathioprine, methotrexate, cyclophosphamide, although these are toxic. If these fail, or are not tolerated, treatment with a tumour necrosis factor inhibitor (e.g. infliximab) can be considered and these can be highly effective.

Factors associated with a poor prognosis include:

a. Black patient
b. Patient >40 years of age at onset
c. Chronic uveitis
d. Chronic hypercalcaemia or nephrocalcinosis
e. Neurological or pulmonary disease.

The patient in this case would benefit from steroid treatment (age >40, moderately severe respiratory symptoms and hypercalcaemia).

CASE 37: ELDERLY MAN WITH HEADACHE

History

A 66-year-old man is brought to A&E by his wife with a worsening headache and new onset of vomiting. The headaches started a couple of months ago, are worse in the morning and have not responded to over-the-counter pain relief. His wife reports that her husband has been confused and agitated lately and has been aggressive on occasions, which is completely out of character. Prior to this, he has been fit and well with no history of headache. He stopped smoking five years ago after a 20 pack-year history and rarely drinks alcohol. He does not take any other medications.

Examination

The patient's vital signs are normal. He has clubbing of the fingernails, otherwise general medical examination is normal. Neurologically, the patient is disorientated, scoring 5/10 on the abbreviated mental test, with no signs of meningism. He has a mild dysarthria and an ataxic gait. There is a vertical nystagmus. Fundoscopy reveals blurring of the optic discs with venous engorgement. Cranial nerve examination is normal. Peripheral examination reveals a mild generalized weakness of 3/5, but is otherwise normal.

Investigations

Routine blood tests were normal except for a sodium of 126 mmol/L (135–145 mmol/L) and a C-reactive protein (CRP) of 19 mg/L (reference range <5 mg/L). Blood sugars are normal.

An urgent computed tomography (CT) of the head is requested (Figure 37.1).

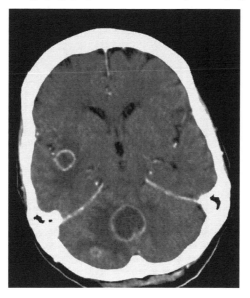

Figure 37.1

QUESTIONS

1. What does the CT show?
2. What is the differential diagnosis?
3. What do the blood tests suggest?
4. Which other signs may be elicited on neurological examination?
5. As the admitting doctor in A&E, what would you do now?

ANSWERS

1. Figure 37.2 shows multiple ring-enhancing lesions (A) with perifocal oedema (B) and mass effect with compression of the fourth ventricle. The largest lesion is in the midline in the cerebellum. There is no midline shift and no generalized oedema and the lateral ventricles are not dilated. Ring enhancement is thick and irregular. The patient is showing signs of raised intracranial pressure (non-resolving headaches, worse in the morning, vomiting, papilloedema), as well as neurological impairment secondary to the location of the lesions. He has a high risk of obstructive hydrocephalus secondary to the posterior fossa pathology and fourth ventricular compression.

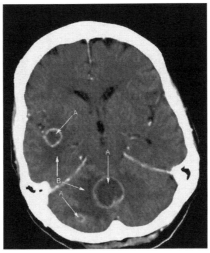

Figure 37.2 An axial post-contrast CT section through the frontal horns of the lateral ventricles and posterior fossa.

2. The differential diagnosis for multiple intracranial ring enhancing lesions is:

   a. Brain metastases – lung, breast, melanoma
   b. Primary brain tumour – especially glioblastoma
   c. Multiple sclerosis
   d. Lymphoma
   e. Cerebral abscess
   f. Atypical infection, e.g. toxoplasmosis.

3. Hyponatraemia in a euvolaemic patient with a suspected malignancy, particularly the brain and lungs, should raise the suspicion of a paraneoplastic syndrome. The syndrome of inappropriate antidiuretic hormone (SIADH) hypersecretion is caused by tumours which secrete ectopic antidiuretic hormone (ADH) leading to free water uptake which results in excessive water in the intravascular space. It is more prevalent in small cell carcinomas. Symptoms associated with hyponatraemia include malaise, nausea, generalized weakness, confusion and anorexia, although onset may be insidious and may be asymptomatic, unless very severe.

4. The large lesion in the midline of the cerebellum may elicit any of those clinical signs associated with cerebellar disease. These can be remembered by the mnemonic DASHING (Dysdiadochokinesis, Ataxia, Slurred speech, Hypotonia, Intention tremor, Nystagmus, Gait (ataxic)).

   Temporal lobe lesions may present with behavioural change but may demonstrate visual defects on examination.

   With multiple brain lesions, a mixed neurological picture may unfold.

5. The CT shows features which are acute and life-threatening, and in keeping with a clinical picture suggestive of raised intracranial pressure (papilloedema, prolonged and progressive headache and vomiting) and he needs an urgent referral to the neurosurgeons. He is likely to be started urgently on high-dose steroids to reduce cerebral oedema (once an infective cause has been excluded). This may allow a ventricular shunt to be avoided – urgent brain radiotherapy may be considered depending on results of further investigations. This would prevent the complications of raised intracranial pressure.

   A chest x-ray (Figure 37.3), and when the patient is considered stable, a CT chest/abdomen/pelvis, may identify a possible primary tumour.

   Less urgently, but to complete the examination, the patient should undergo a rectal examination, full skin examination and, in females, a breast examination. Tumour markers may also assist in the diagnosis, but these are not specific and may be falsely negative. Liver function tests and a bone profile should be included in the initial biochemical tests.

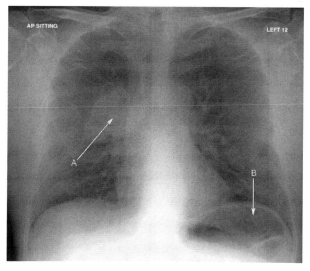

Figure 37.3 Note the right hilar mass (A) consistent with a likely primary lung malignancy and (B) gastric fundus.

Discussion

The differential diagnosis of lesions in the brain is guided by age, the number of lesions, single or multiple, and the features of the lesion. Brain metastases spread haematogenously and the tumour damages the blood–brain barrier, which allows contrast to leak into the brain. Multiple sclerosis, gliomas, infections and infarctions can also damage the blood–brain barrier. In metastatic disease, contrast-enhanced imaging demonstrates a ring-enhanced lesion, irregular and with an often necrotic centre. There is often marked vasogenic oedema surrounding the focal lesion. Primary tumours are usually solitary, but metastases can often present as a single lesion. Abscesses are generally smoother in appearance, well-defined and with a thin, uniform ring of enhancement. Significant perifocal oedema is common in malignant lesions, and on magnetic resonance imaging (MRI) most malignant tumours will be of low signal intensity on T1 - weighted imaging and high on T2 - weighted imaging, with the exception of metastatic melanoma for which the opposite is true (melanin alters the signal). The cerebellum is a common site for brain metastases.

Of all cancers which present with symptoms of brain metastases, lung cancer is the primary malignancy in about three-quarters of cases. Other cancers which commonly metastasize to the brain are breast, melanoma, renal and colon. Lung and melanoma metastases often present as multiple lesions, while renal and colon metastatic lesions are often singular.

While onset is often insidious, with a slowly progressive course, metastatic brain lesions can present acutely due to infarction or haemorrhage.

The management of brain metastases is two-fold. Brain protection and alleviation of life-threatening complications should be initiated on presentation, with longer-term management based on a multidisciplinary approach to determine treatment options. This may be a combination of surgical resection, chemotherapy and radiotherapy, but will be driven by histological confirmation and expected sensitivity to different treatments. In the later stages of disease, palliative treatment to reduce symptoms may be initiated. Immediate management includes the insertion of a shunt by the neurosurgical team which will relieve the raised intracranial pressure which, if left untreated, may eventually restrict blood supply to the brain, flow of cerebrospinal fluid (CSF) and cause herniation. Urgent focal radiotherapy should relieve pressure symptoms by reducing the size of bulky tumours. Dexamethasone may be used acutely to reduce cerebral oedema.

CASE 38: ELDERLY MAN WITH PAIN IN THE HIP

History

A 69-year-old man presents to his GP with pain and stiffness in his left hip. He has had intermittent pain for some months which is getting worse and is particularly painful at night, with no radiation. He has previously been very active, but his walking is now severely restricted. He also has the pain at rest and denies any injury. He has been taking ibuprofen with no relief. He has no other joint pain. He reports being troubled by urinary frequency at night which he has had 'for years' and he recently had an episode of urinary retention and currently has a urinary catheter *in situ*. He is awaiting urology review. He has no constitutional symptoms or weight loss and takes bendroflumethiazide and amlodipine for hypertension.

Examination

On examination of his hip, there is no obvious deformity or skin change, and gait is normal. Palpation of the superior pubic rami reveals mild tenderness. Movement of the left hip is extremely limited in all directions due to pain. Neurovascular examination is unremarkable. The rest of the musculoskeletal examination is normal.

Investigations

Routine blood results showed a haemoglobin of 10.6 g/dL (13.5–18 g/dL), erythrocyte sedimentation rate (ESR) 43 mm/h (0–15 mm/h), C-reactive protein (CRP) 29 mg/L (<5 mg/l) and alkaline phosphatase 704 IU/L (40–129 IU/L).

The GP sends him for an x-ray of the pelvis and left hip (Figure 38.1).

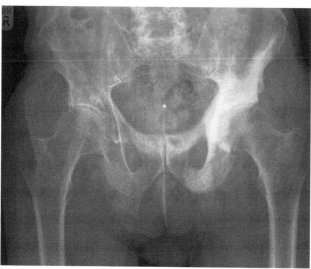

Figure 38.1

QUESTIONS

1. What does the x-ray show?
2. What is the differential diagnosis?
3. What is the most likely diagnosis?
4. Which further tests would you request and which further examination would be appropriate?

ANSWERS

1. The pelvic x-ray shows ill-defined sclerotic lesions affecting a large portion of the left hemi-pelvis, including the acetabulum, ischium and pubic rami, and also the superior pubic ramus on the right (for lesions, see arrows on Figure 38.2). No fracture is seen. Note his urinary catheter.

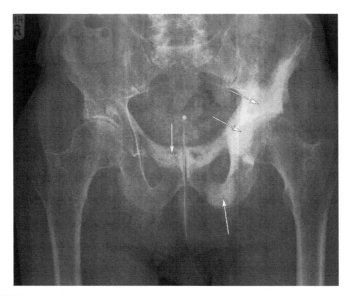

Figure 38.2

2. The differential diagnosis for bony sclerotic lesions can be remembered by the mnemonic 'VINDICATE'.

Vascular	Haemangiomas, infarct
Infection	Chronic osteomyelitis
Neoplasm	Primary osteoma/osteosarcoma, secondary prostate, breast
Drugs	Vitamin D, fluoride
Inflammatory/idiopathic	
Congenital	Osteopoikilosis
Autoimmune	
Trauma	Stress fractures
Endocrine/metabolic	Hyperparathyroid, Paget's disease

In this age group, the most likely differentials to consider are metastatic disease and Paget's disease. Paget's disease is an important radiological differential as it can mimic malignant disease. It has three phases: an osteolytic phase, followed by a mixed phase of osteolytic and osteoblastic activity, then an osteoblastic phase. This causes bone growth and deformity with multiple potentially life-threatening complications. Appearances on x-ray will depend on the phase of disease with a cotton wool appearance during the mixed phase. The three classic features of Paget's disease on plain x-ray are bony enlargement, coarse trabeculae and a thickened cortex. The pelvis is the most common bone affected, followed by the femur. A classic large lytic lesion of the skull seen in Paget's disease is called 'osteoporosis circumscripta'.

3. These sclerotic lesions are not typical of Paget's disease and in a male of this age metastatic prostatic carcinoma is the most likely diagnosis.

4. A bone profile (remember to exclude hypercalcaemia), prostate-specific antigen (PSA) test and digital rectal examination would be appropriate at this stage, with an urgent referral to the urology department and a radionuclide bone scan. In this case, a firm, irregular prostate and raised PSA strongly suggested a prostatic primary.

Metastases and multiple myeloma are the most common malignant bone tumours. Age is an important consideration in the differential diagnosis, as these present most commonly in the over 40 age group. In the over 70s, bone pain is a red flag symptom. The site of bone lesions is another important consideration. Bone lesions most commonly involve the axial skeleton – the skull, spine, pelvis, ribs, proximal humerus and femur are common sites. Those which are distal to the elbows and knees are uncommon, but when they do occur they are often related to a lung primary. Lesions may be focal, multifocal, single or diffuse; skeletal metastases are usually focal, but may be diffuse. Diffuse or multiple focal sclerotic lesions, particularly in the pelvis, suggest either a breast or prostate primary.

Differential diagnosis of lytic bone lesions

Mnemonic 'FOG MACHINES'
- F, fibrous dysplasia
- O, osteoblastoma
- G, giant cell tumour
- M, metastasis/multiple myeloma
- A, aneurysmal bone cyst
- C, chondroblastoma
- H, hyperparathyroidism, haemangioma
- I, infection
- N, non-ossifying fibroma
- E, enchondroma/eosinophilic granuloma
- S, simple bone cyst

Primary tumours which frequently metastasize to the bone are breast, prostate, lung and kidney, but also thyroid, colon and melanoma. Many lesions are asymptomatic, but pain is the primary presentation in those who are symptomatic. It is progressive, often worse at night and is not relieved by rest. Patients may also present with pathological fractures, symptoms of spinal cord compression or hypercalcaemia, or symptoms related to bone marrow infiltration, such as anaemia.

Metastases may also be lytic or mixed lytic/sclerotic. A lytic deposit in the cuboid bone secondary to renal cell carcinoma is shown in Figure 38.3 (arrow).

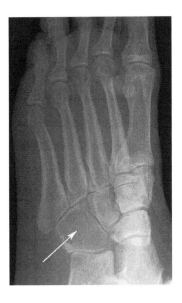

Figure 38.3

CASE 39: WOMAN WITH HEADACHE AND VOMITING

History

A 79-year-old female presents to A&E complaining of acute severe headache with several episodes of vomiting. The headache has been present for 3 hours, the onset being sudden. The pain is worse on moving her head and she describes it as constant and generalized. She has a past medical history of poorly controlled hypertension. She denies any history of trauma.

Examination

She looks unwell, but is conscious and orientated. She is apyrexial, pulse 100 beats per minute, blood pressure 160/105 mmHg. Cardiorespiratory examination is unremarkable and no focal neurological defect is present. Fundal examination is technically difficult as she finds the light uncomfortable.

Investigations

Routine bloods are unremarkable. Electrocardiogram (ECG) confirms sinus rhythm, with no acute changes. An urgent computed tomography (CT) scan of the head is performed (see Figure 39.1). This is an axial section through the brain at the level of the third ventricle.

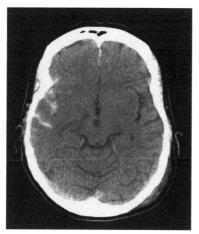

Figure 39.1

QUESTIONS

1. What are the CT findings?
2. What is the diagnosis?
3. Can you think of any other possible diagnosis with this clinical presentation?
4. What other symptoms/signs may this patient have?
5. What is the management of this condition?

ANSWERS

1. On CT (Figure 39.2), there is high density material consistent with blood seen in the sulci and Sylvian tissue (arrow A), in the right temporoparietal region (arrow B) with parafalcine blood also present (arrow C).

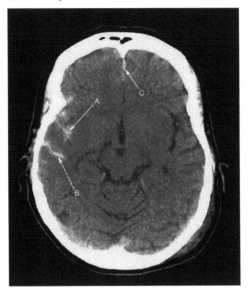

Figure 39.2

2. The appearances are consistent with an acute subarachnoid haemorrhage (SAH).

3. Possible differentials in this clinical scenario include: meningitis, migraine, intracerebral bleed, cerebral venous sinus thrombosis.

4. Commonly patients with SAH present with severe headache (often patients describe the headache as the worst they have ever had and resembling being hit with a bat at the back of the head), vomiting, collapse, seizure and coma. Patients often have meningism – nuchal rigidity, Kernig's sign (pain elicited when the leg is bent at the hip and knee to 90° and then the knee extended), or Brudzinski's sign (involuntary lifting the patient's legs off the couch when lifting the head).

5. There should be urgent referral to the neurosurgeons for further management. Patients may undergo urgent cerebral angiography to identify a possible aneurysmal source and then surgical or radiological (coils) treatment, although this may be delayed depending on the patient's condition.

   Subarachnoid haemorrhage is defined as spontaneous bleeding into the subarachnoid space, which lies between the arachnoid membrane and the pia mater surrounding the brain. It most commonly results from a ruptured cerebral aneurysm, or may result from traumatic head injury.

Headache caused by SAH is sudden, i.e. onset is within seconds to minutes and, due to the meningeal irritation, it is constant. The headache can often radiate towards the occipital region.

CT is the initial imaging modality of choice with high sensitivity for intracranial blood. CT can be negative in 5–10 per cent of cases and also a normal scan does not exclude raised intracranial pressure (look for papilloedema).

Lumbar puncture is indicated where CT is negative and in the absence of raised intracranial pressure, with high accuracy for red cells and also xanthochromia (a breakdown product of haemoglobin). This takes at least 12 hours to appear in the cerebrospinal fluid.

SAH can lead to death or severe disability (neurological or cognitive impairment), even when diagnosed and treated at an early stage. Up to half of all cases of SAH are fatal and 10–15 per cent of patients will die before reaching hospital.

Up to one third of patients have no symptoms, apart from the characteristic headache. Vomiting may be present and approximately 1 in 14 patients present with seizures. Confusion, decreased level of consciousness or coma may be present, as may neck stiffness and other signs of meningism.

In 85 per cent of cases of spontaneous SAH, the cause is rupture of a cerebral aneurysm. The aneurysms tend to be located in the circle of Willis and its branches. While most cases of SAH are due to bleeding from small aneurysms, larger aneurysms, which are less common, are more likely to rupture.

Intracerebral hemorrhage is twice as common as SAH and can be misdiagnosed as the latter. SAH can be initially misdiagnosed as a migraine or tension headache, which can lead to a delay in obtaining a CT scan. Interestingly, some SAH patients may have experienced prior sentinel headache perhaps due to a small warning leak from the offending aneurysm (in around 6 per cent). As surgery is more successful in the least symptomatic patients, it is important to always be suspicious of any patient presenting with sudden headache with neck or back pain.

Management of SAH patients is as follows:

a. Urgent referral of all proven SAH to neurosurgeons.
b. Re-examination/continuous assessment of patients via the central nervous system (CNS), blood pressure (BP) recordings, pupillary examinations with Glasgow Coma Score (GCS) monitoring.
c. Maintenance of cerebral perfusion aiming for systolic above 160 mmHg and the patients should be kept well hydrated.
d. Nimodipine, a calcium-channel blocker that reduces vasospasm and consequent morbidity from cerebral ischaemia, a serious complication of SAH.
e. Endovascular coiling is preferred to surgical clipping.

f. Intravascular stents can be introduced radiologically and balloon remodelling can be used to treat wide-necked aneurysms. Microcatheters can now traverse tortuous vessels to treat previously unreachable lesions.

Cerebral aneurysms can be identified using CT or conventional catheter angiography. To reduce the risk of further bleeding from the same aneurysm, clipping or coiling of the aneurysm is performed. Clipping requires a craniotomy to locate the aneurysm, followed by the placement of clips around the neck of the aneurysm. Coiling is performed endovascularly. When the aneurysm has been located, platinum coils are deployed that cause a blood clot to form in the aneurysm, thus sealing off the aneurysm.

Delay in diagnosis of SAH (for example, by mistaking the sudden headache for migraine) contributes to poor outcome. Other factors associated with poorer outcome include low GCS at the time of presentation, systolic hypertension, a previous diagnosis of SAH, large volume of subarachnoid bleeding or large aneurysms detected on the initial CT scan, and increasing age of the patient.

CASE 40: ELDERLY WOMAN WITH EPIGASTRIC PAIN

History

A 62-year-old woman presents with a 4-week history of mild non-specific band-like epigastric pain radiating to the back. The pain seems to be worse at night with no relieving factors and is dull in nature, but constant. She also complains of weakness of her lower limbs over the last week prior to admission, which has been progressively worsening. The only other relevant history she gives is a bout of diarrhoea and vomiting 2 weeks ago, which settled without treatment. On direct questioning, she denies symptoms of bladder or bowel dysfunction, weight loss, loss of appetite, weakness, pins and needles or numbness of the upper limbs and denies other symptoms of note. She is a non-smoker with minimal alcohol intake and no past medical history.

Examination

She looks well and is apyrexial. Respiratory, cardiovascular and abdominal examinations are unremarkable. Neurological examination of the upper limbs showed power 5/5, with normal tone, reflexes and sensation. Neurological examination of the lower limbs showed power of 3/5 in all the muscle groups of both limbs, with diminished dermatomal sensation in distribution L2–S1 bilaterally. No reflexes at the knees and ankles bilaterally were elicited with down-going plantars. Formal gait examination was difficult to assess given this patient's leg weakness, but other cerebellar function appeared normal. Cranial nerve I–XII examination was unremarkable.

Investigations

This lady's initial bloods showed mildly raised alkaline phosphatase at 180 IU/L (35–104 IU/L) (the rest of the liver function tests were normal) with mild normocytic anaemia, haemoglobin (Hb) 10.5 g/dL (11.5–16.5 g/dL), MCV 80 fL (76–100 fL) with normal renal function and inflammatory markers. A magnetic resonance image (MRI) examination of the spine was performed. A sagittal T2-weighted section through the upper thoracic region is shown in Figure 40.1 with an axial T2-weighted image at the T7 level shown in Figure 40.2.

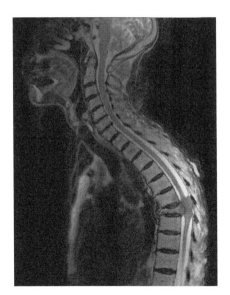

Figure 40.1

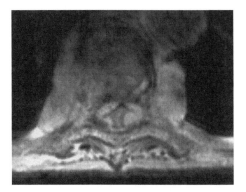

Figure 40.2

QUESTIONS

1. Identify the abnormalities seen in the Figures 40.1 and 40.2.
2. What is the diagnosis?
3. What further investigations should be performed?
4. What is the differential diagnosis?
5. How should she be managed?

ANSWERS

1. A magnified view from Figure 40.1 is repeated on this page as Figure 40.3 and Figure 40.2 is repeated as Figure 40.4, annotations included.

   A = cord compressed between collapsed T7 vertebral body and tumour within the posterior canal.
   B = cord below the level of compression at T7. Note linear high signal within the cord which represents dilation of the central canal distal to the obstruction.
   C = cord above the level of obstruction. Note high signal cerebrospinal fluid (CSF) around the cord.
   D = tumour, which encroaches upon and largely effaces the spinal canal. Note paravertebral mass also.
   E = the compressed cord. No CSF can be seen around the cord.

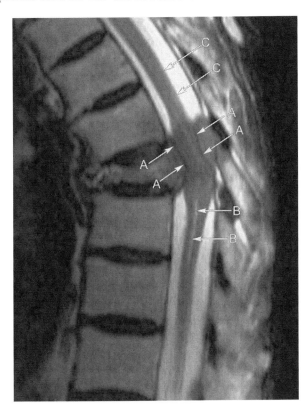

Figure 40.3

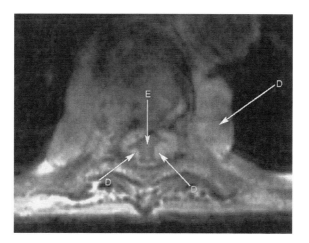

Figure 40.4

2. This patient has acute severe cord compression, likely secondary to malignancy. This is a medical emergency and she needs urgent treatment.

3. Other investigations will be needed (bloods, chest radiograph, body computed tomography (CT), among others), but these must not interfere with the urgent treatment of her compressed cord (see below).

4. This patient has a collapsed and infiltrated T7 vertebral body, with a paravertebral mass. These appearances are not those of either uncomplicated osteoporotic collapse or a discitis, and malignancy is likely. She does not have a disc prolapse. Primary bone tumours are unusual and either metastasis or myeloma is most likely. The hunt for a primary can wait until the acute cord compression has been treated.

5. She needs urgent discussion with neurosurgery and also oncology. In a patient with a known or suspected malignancy, high-dose oral steroids should be started immediately to reduce swelling and urgent radiotherapy may suffice. In other patients who are operatively fit with no known diagnosis, urgent surgical decompression is indicated assuming the patient is fit, and biopsies can also be obtained at that time.

It cannot be over-stressed how important it is to image (MRI) these patients urgently, i.e. within an hour or two, and get them to the surgical unit or radiotherapy as soon as possible thereafter. Do not send a form for an MRI down to radiology marked 'urgent' and expect it to be done – you must discuss the case in person. Plain films and radioisotope bone scans are of no real use in this situation. MRI is excellent at delineating spine, cord and disc anatomy. If MRI is contraindicated (e.g. pacemaker, claustrophobia), then spinal CT can be used but is less effective.

In everyday practice, breast, lung, renal, prostate carcinoma or myeloma are the most common causes of metastatic cord compression. Full staging and further treatment can be undertaken once the cord situation has been resolved and a diagnosis made. Do remember to carefully assess bladder and anal sphincter function at the time of presentation; these are affected particularly in cauda equina syndrome. The aim must be to diagnose and treat before irreversible neurological damage occurs.

CASE 41: ELDERLY MAN WITH SHORTNESS OF BREATH

History

A 76-year-old man presents with a 2-week history of worsening shortness of breath on exertion and a 1-week history of a non-productive cough. He also notes that he has been having difficulty sleeping, often waking with fits of coughing and gasping for breath. His breathing difficulty has been present for the past six months initially on walking upstairs only, but for the past 2 weeks on walking flat surfaces for shorter distances. He has also noted some swelling of his ankles. He denies any other symptoms on direct questioning, in particular no chest pain or haemoptysis. He is currently on no medication. He has had a myocardial infarction in the past, but no other medical history of note.

Examination

The patient appeared dyspnoeic at rest, normotensive, pulse 100 bpm regular and mildly clammy. Clinical examination revealed raised jugular venous pressure at 7 cm, normal heart sounds, scattered wheeze throughout the chest with fine crepitations in both lung bases. He had bilaterally pitting oedema to the mid-shins. Abdominal and neurological examinations were unremarkable.

Investigations

Blood tests results showed mildly raised urea of 9 mmol/L (1.7–8.3 mmol/L) with the other biochemical and haematological parameters including blood glucose being normal. Troponin-T was not raised.

Electrocardiogram (ECG) showed sinus tachycardia with old ischemic changes in the anterior leads, unchanged when compared to previous ECGs.

A chest x-ray on admission is seen in Figure 41.1.

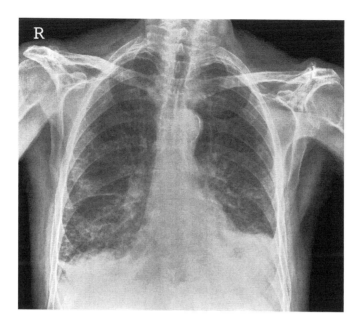

Figure 41.1

QUESTIONS

1. What are the chest x-ray abnormalities?
2. What is the most likely diagnosis?
3. What other chest radiographic features may be observed in this condition?
4. How is this condition treated?

ANSWERS

1. Figure 41.1 demonstrates:

    a. Bilateral basal pleural effusions, larger at the left base
    b. Septal (Kerley B) lines
    c. Fluid in the horizontal fissure
    d. Linear infiltrates in the mid/lower zones bilaterally.

    Note that the heart does not appear enlarged.

2. The appearances would be consistent with acute cardiac failure and pulmonary oedema. In acute heart failure, the heart size may well be normal.

3. In chronic/congestive cardiac failure, cardiomegaly is likely to be observed. Upper lobe blood diversion may also be seen, due to upper lobe redistribution of blood due to increased vascular resistance at the lung bases. This sign is often difficult to identify with confidence. Pulmonary oedema may also appear as more confluent, airspace ('alveolar') opacity often in a perihilar ('bat's wing') distribution. Kerley B (septal) lines are well shown in this case – a magnified image of the right lower zone is included in Figure 41.2, septal lines shown with arrows. Septal lines are due to interstitial oedema in the interlobular lymphatics. They tend to be peripheral, horizontal and subpleural in the lower zones. Pulmonary oedema is the most common cause (others include sarcoidosis, lymphangitis carcinomatosa). Kerley A lines are also described and are line densities radiating from the hilak. Note that alveolar/airspace opacity is a non-specific, but important radiological sign. It indicates consolidation within the airspace. Pulmonary oedema (water), infection (pus), haemorrhage and tumour can all cause this appearance. Clinical history and previous radiographs are essential to help differentiate.

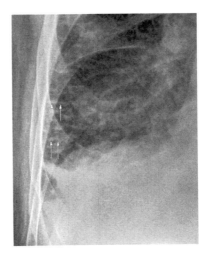

Figure 41.2

4. This patient has acute cardiac failure, with evidence of both left- and right-sided failure. It is important to consider and exclude a causative myocardial infarction.

    Acute cardiac failure is a medical emergency, so immediately:

    - Sit patient upright
    - High flow oxygen by mask
    - Intravenous access (bloods)
    - Furosemide 40–80 mg i.v. slowly
    - Diamorphine 2.5–5 mg i.v. (slowly, morphine is a venodilator and off loads the heart, watch for respiratory depression).

    This patient responded well to initial therapy: a post-treatment radiograph is shown in Figure 41.3. He will need an echocardiogram and cardiology input as to his further management and medication; reduced ventricular function secondary to previous ischaemic heart disease is likely in this case. If patients do not respond to initial therapy, nitrates (venous dilators) can be administered sublingually or by infusion (if systolic blood pressure >90 mmHg) and additional i.v. furosemide can be administered. If the blood pressure starts to drop, this may be due to cardiogenic shock and the patient needs urgent intensive care unit (ICU) referral and inotropic support (prognosis is poor).

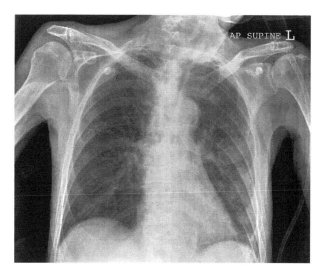

Figure 41.3

CASE 42: WOMAN WITH ABDOMINAL PAIN

History

A 32-year-old woman presents to A&E with abdominal pain, bloody diarrhoea and fever. She reports having had cramping abdominal pain, watery diarrhoea and nausea 2 weeks previously. She had visited the GP after 3 days who took stool samples and prescribed imodium, buscopan and dioralyte. The diarrhoea continued and she now has 8–10 bowel movements per day. She has not consumed food or fluids in over 24 hours. She was previously well, has not travelled abroad recently, has not been in contact with anyone who was sick and was not aware of any family history of illness. She is an ex-smoker of 5 pack-years. She has no drug allergies. She works for a theatre company.

Examination

On examination, she looks unwell. She is alert and orientated in time and place. She has a temperature of 38.0°C, heart rate 110 bpm regular, blood pressure 95/62 mmHg, oxygen saturations 98 per cent on room air and respiratory rate 18 per minute. She has dry mucous membranes. Her abdomen is distended with generalized tenderness, no rebound or voluntary guarding, tympanic with quiet bowel sounds. Per rectum examination reveals bloody stool and mucous, but no masses. There are no skin changes or rashes. Urine dipstick normal.

Investigations

		Reference range
Haemoglobin	9.9 g/dL	11.5–16.5 g/dL
White cell count	14.8×10^9/L	$4.1–11.0 \times 10^9$/L
Platelets	626×10^9/L	$150–450 \times 10^9$/L
Mean cell volume	68 fL	76–100 fL
Sodium	131 mmol/L	135–146 mmol/L
Potassium	2.9 mmol/L	3.2–5.1 mmol/L
Urea	10.4 mmol/L	1.7–8.3 mmol/L
Creatinine	80 µmol/L	44–80 µmol/L
Alanine aminotransferase (ALT)	22 IU/L	Up to 31 IU/L
Aspartate aminotransferase (APT)	24 IU/L	Up to 32 IU/L
Alkaline phosphatase (ALP)	174 IU/L	35–104 IU/L
Bilirubin	4 µmol/L	Up to 21 µmol/L
Albumin	32 g/L	34–48 g/L
Total protein	85 g/L	66–87 g/L
International normalized ratio (INR)	1.2	0.8–1.2

		Reference range
C-reactive protein (CRP)	136 mg/L	<5 mg/L
Erythrocyte sedimentation rate (ESR)	32 mm/h	0–15 mm/hr

An arterial blood gas is performed:

pH 7.54 (7.35–7.45) HCO_{3^-} 34
PO_2 12.5 kPa (11.1–14.4 kPa)   Base excess (BE) 7.8
PCO_2 4.5 kPa (4.7–6.4 kPa)   Lactate 1.7

An erect chest x-ray revealed no abnormalities, and the abdominal x-ray is shown in Figure 42.1.

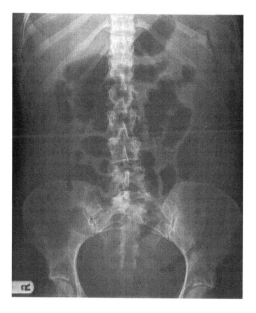

Figure 42.1

QUESTIONS

1. What does the abdominal x-ray show?
2. Why was an erect chest x-ray performed?
3. What is the most likely diagnosis?
4. What do the blood tests and clinical observations suggest in light of the x-ray findings?
5. What would be your immediate management of this patient?

ANSWERS

1. The abdominal x-ray shows an oedematous thick-walled left colon extending from the splenic flexure into the pelvis, demonstrating 'thumb-printing' (arrows A in Figure 42.2) which is visible in the left upper quadrant and is a result of mucosal and submucosal oedema. Gas is visible in the stomach (arrow B) and throughout the colon. Transverse colon is shown by arrows C. There is a loss of normal haustral pattern. Some mildly prominent small bowel loops are present in the central abdomen.

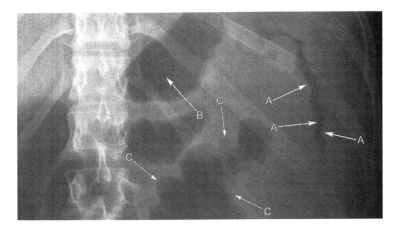

Figure 42.2

2. An erect chest x-ray has been obtained to exclude an associated perforation. A good quality chest film performed erect can detect as little as 1 cc of free intraperitoneal air.

3. The most likely diagnosis is toxic colitis based on clinical features and radiological evidence. The underlying cause may be inflammatory bowel disease (most likely), infective, drug-induced or ischaemic colitis. Although the history is not suggestive of an infective cause, investigations should aim to rule this out. Ischaemic colitis would be unusual in this age group. It is usually sudden in onset, and there is usually a history of atherosclerotic disease, hypoperfusion or vasculitis, and associated pain is severe and cramping with bright red rectal bleeding being a prominent feature. Toxic colitis can rapidly progress to toxic megacolon as the damaged bowel wall impairs the contractile ability of the large bowel with gas building up in the colon. A colonic diameter of >6 cm indicates toxic megacolon which is at risk of perforation.

4. Anaemia, raised inflammatory markers and white cell count, thrombocytosis, electrolyte abnormalities, fever, tachycardia and hypotension, with a metabolic alkalosis suggest a severe toxic colitis. Hypoalbuminaemia is another important marker of poor prognosis. The extent of metabolic alkalosis is related to the severity of the disease.

5. This patient should be managed on the high-dependency unit (HDU). Urgent referral to the gastroenterologists is required and review by the colorectal surgeons
   is recommended for joint management. Three stool specimens should be sent for
   microscopy and culture and *Clostridium difficile* toxin, along with blood cultures.
   Intravenous fluid resuscitation should be initiated immediately while correcting
   electrolyte abnormalities, blood transfusion if necessary, and the patient should be
   catheterized for fluid management. The patient should be made nil by mouth and
   a nasogastric tube inserted to assist with deflation of the bowel. Prompt initiation of i.v. corticosteroids is required. With no previous diagnosis of inflammatory
   bowel disease, a possible infective cause of colitis and with potential development
   to toxic megacolon and perforation, i.v. antibiotics would be appropriate. Repeat
   abdominal x-rays should be requested to monitor progress. If the patient is on any
   opioids, antidiarrhoeals and anticholinergics, these should be stopped immediately.
   Sigmoidoscopy or proctoscopy may be required in this case if the cause of colitis
   is uncertain, as the rectal mucosa can be visualized and biopsies taken. Steroid
   enemas can also be administered.

Discussion

Toxic colitis is a life-threatening condition. There are a number of causes of colonic
inflammation, but the majority occur in individuals with inflammatory bowel disease,
particularly ulcerative colitis. Around 30 per cent of new cases of inflammatory bowel
disease will present with toxic colitis and around 1 per cent of patients with inflammatory bowel disease will have toxic megacolon at some stage. Toxic megacolon is
defined as segmental or total colonic distension >6 cm in the presence of acute colitis
and systemic toxicity.

The management of severe acute colitis is dependent on early recognition and prompt
treatment. Diagnosis is based on clinical features and radiological findings, with plain
abdominal x-ray being the imaging modality of choice for both initial management
and monitoring of progress, which may be required every 12–24 hours. This is one
of the few life-threatening conditions which can be confidently diagnosed on plain
x-ray. CT may be useful where radiological features are equivocal or complications
are suspected, but is rarely indicated in the initial management of severe acute colitis. Barium enema is contraindicated in toxic colitis and megacolon due to the risk of
perforation.

Patients are generally systemically unwell with abdominal tenderness and distension.
Severity of disease is defined by Truelove and Witt's Classification of Severity of Acute
Colitis:

Activity	Mild	Moderate	Severe
Number of bloody stools per day	<4	4–6	>6
Temperature (°C)	Afebrile	Intermediate	>37.8
Heart rate (beats per minute)	Normal	Intermediate	>90

Activity	Mild	Moderate	Severe
Haemoglobin (g/dL)	>11	10.5–11	<10.5
Erythrocyte sedimentation rate (mm/h)	<20	20–30	>30

A number of factors may precipitate the onset of toxic colitis:

- Drugs that slow gastric motility, such as opioids, anticholinergics (e.g. buscopan), and antidiarrhoeals (e.g. loperamide), non-steroidal anti-inflammatory drugs (NSAIDs), chemotherapy and barium enemas.
- Infection with organisms, such as *Salmonella*, *Shigella*, *Entamoeba histolytica*, *Campylobacter*, *Escherischia coli* and *Clostridium difficile* (pseudomembranous colitis), which may either cause toxic colitis *de novo* or precipitate colitis in patients with inflammatory bowel disease. Cytomegalovirus (CMV) causes colitis in patients with immunodeficiency.
- Hypokalaemia/hypomagnesaemia
- Patients who abruptly discontinue treatment with 5-aminosalicylic acid (5-ASA) or corticosteroids may also induce toxic colitis.

Features of acute colitis on plain x-ray:

- Wall thickening due to mucosal oedema
- Loss of haustra
- Mucosal islands (oedematous mucosa surrounded by deep ulceration)
- Thumbprinting due to submucosal oedematous infiltration
- Dilated large bowel loops, more commonly of ascending and transverse colon
- Multiple loops of dilated small bowel, worrying sign of imminent perforation.

The management of toxic colitis is initially medical unless there is free air, localized or diffuse peritonitis, distension of the colon >10 cm, major haemorrhage or uncontrolled sepsis, all of which are indications for emergency laparotomy. The patient should be under the joint care of gastroenterologists and colorectal surgeons as one-third of patients will require surgical treatment. A 5-day course of i.v. corticosteroids is the mainstay of treatment with i.v. ciclosporin as adjuvant therapy if patients are not responding to steroids. Regular monitoring and correction of electrolytes is important as hypokalaemia may worsen with corticosteroid therapy.

All patients should receive prophylactic heparin treatment as the risk of venous thromboembolism in acute colitis is high. Improvement, based on clinical observation, blood tests and repeat plain abdominal x-ray, should be seen within 3 days, otherwise discussion regarding surgical treatment options should be initiated.

The indications for surgical intervention include:

- Failure to improve with medical therapy (usually by 48–72 hours)
- Progressive toxicity or dilatation
- Perforation
- Uncontrolled bleeding.

Surgical intervention is life-saving at this point and involves either a total or sub-total colectomy with ileostomy.

The main types of colitis	
Inflammatory	Ulcerative colitis
	Crohn's disease
Vascular	Ischaemic colitis
Infectious	Pseudomembranous colitis (C. *difficile*)
	Salmonella, Shigella, Campylobacter, E. coli
	Entamoeba histolytica
Viral	Cytomegalovirus

CASE 43: MIDDLE-AGED WOMAN WITH SWELLING IN HANDS AND FEET

History

A 45-year-old woman presents to her GP complaining of stiffness and swelling in both hands and feet each morning, which improves during the day. She has had similar problems with her knees in the past. She feels quite tired and a bit down, and is struggling with daily activities such as making a cup of tea.

Examination

On examination, there is diffuse swelling over the metacarpophalangeal (MCP) joints bilaterally and the proximal interphalangeal joints (PIPJ) in her hands. The joints are warm and swollen. There is also swelling related to the lateral aspect of the right foot, in the region of the fourth and fifth metatarsophalangeal (MTP) joints.

Investigations

Blood test results demonstrate a raised erythrocyte sedimentation rate (ESR), elevated C-reactive protein (CRP) and rheumatoid factor and the presence of anticyclic citrullinated peptide antibodies. The patient was sent for x-rays of her hands and feet. The right foot x-ray is shown in Figure 43.1.

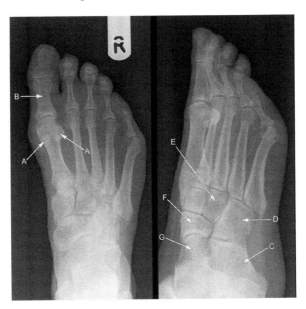

Figure 43.1

QUESTIONS

1. Which views have been taken of the foot?
2. Name the normal anatomy (A–G) and the abnormality on the foot x-ray?
3. Which other joints might you expect to be involved?
4. What x-ray findings would you expect with osteoarthritis?
5. How would you manage this patient?

ANSWERS

1. The image on the left is an AP (anteroposterior) view of the foot and the image on the right is an oblique view.

2. Normal anatomy:

   A. Sesamoid bones
   B. Proximal phalanx big toe
   C. Calcaneus
   D. Cuboid
   E. Lateral cuneiform
   F. Navicular
   G. Talus.

   The abnormality is seen in the head of the fifth metatarsal. There is periarticular erosion of the bone in this region with decreased bone density (osteopenia) around the joint, joint space loss and soft tissue swelling. The erosions are annotated in a magnified view (Figure 43.2). These features are radiological hallmarks of rheumatoid arthritis (RhA).

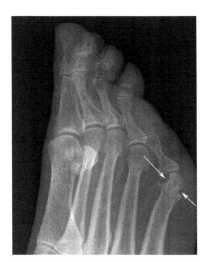

Figure 43.2

3. The small joints of the hands and feet are typically involved in RhA. Problems with hand grip can be secondary to swelling or pain, or may be due to extensor tenosynovitis. Other joints which may be involved are the wrist, shoulders, elbows, cervical spine, hips and knees. Finger deformities in RhA include a swan neck deformity (flexion at the PIPJ and hyperextension at the distal interphalangeal joint (DIPJ)) and Boutonnière's deformity (hyperextension at the DIPJ and flexion at the PIPJ). Ulnar deviation may also occur.

4. The hallmarks of osteoarthritis are joint space loss, subchondral cysts and sclerosis and osteophyte formation. The carpus and distal interphalangeal joints tend to be more involved.

5. A full history should be taken to assess for other joint involvement. Adequate pain relief is essential and non-steroidal anti-inflammatory drugs (NSAIDs) are the initial mainstay. The patient should have appropriate blood tests and x-rays and be referred to a rheumatologist for specialist management. The main aims of management are to reduce symptoms and improve prognosis with modification of the disease. Patients should be screened for depression as patients with rheumatoid arthritis are twice as likely to suffer from depression as the general population.

Rheumatoid arthritis (RhA) versus osteoarthritis (OA)

RhA	OA
Less common than OA	Most common arthritis
Inflammatory autoimmune disease	Also known as degenerative joint disease
Primarily affects synovium → synovial hypertrophy and pannus	Primarily affects cartilage 'wear and tear' → reactive bony hypertrophy (osteophytes)
Classically a symmetrical polyarthritis	Asymmetrical monoarthritis in large joints
Hot, swollen, red joint	Bony swelling in the hands
Early morning stiffness lasts at least 1 hour	Early morning stiffness lasts less than 1 hour
Gentle movements may relieve symptoms	Movement aggravates symptoms, pain relieved by rest, stiffness recurs following rest
Ulnar deviation, Boutonnière's deformity, swan neck deformity	Bouchard's nodes (PIP joint) and Heberden's nodes (DIP joints)
Extra-articular features	No extra-articular features

Discussion

Rheumatoid arthritis is a chronic multisystem inflammatory disease which affects synovial joints, as well as tendons and bursae causing an erosive arthritis leading to joint destruction with deformity and subluxation, and significant disability. It affects women more frequently than men in the fourth decade, but in the sixth decade men and women are equally affected.

A genetic predisposition and an environmental trigger are thought to cause rheumatoid arthritis and it is considered an autoimmune disease. The inflammatory process attacks the joints causing synovial thickening and pannus – the formation of abnormal granulation tissue – which produces enzymes that destroy cartilage and eventually leads to bone erosion. As well as joint involvement, tenosynovitis of the hands and bursitis may occur. Acute flare ups occur over a background of progressive joint destruction.

The radiological hallmarks of musculoskeletal RhA are soft tissue swelling, joint space loss, peri-articular osteopenia and bone erosions. Bone erosions tend to occur later in the disease process with subluxation and carpal destruction. In the wrist, the distal ulnar subluxes dorsally and the carpal bones sublux volarly (towards the palm). The fingers demonstrate ulnar deviation as they sublux transversely towards the ulna. In the neck, atlanto-axial subluxation occurs and the C2 body migrates superiorly. Erosion of the odontoid peg (C2) also occurs.

There are several extra-articular features of RhA. These may present as part of a syndrome, such as Caplan syndrome or Felty syndrome. Caplan syndrome is seropositive RhA with lung nodules in the upper lobes and periphery of the lung which may cavitate. There may be associated pulmonary fibrosis and a pleural effusion (usually unilateral). Felty syndrome is RhA associated with splenomegaly, neutropenia and lymphadenopathy. Other extra-articular manifestations include eye disease (e.g. keratoconjunctivitis sicca), pericardial effusion, vasculitis, peripheral sensory neuropathy, carpal tunnel syndrome, elbow nodules and periungal erythema. Atherosclerosis is accelerated by the production of cytokines.

Pharmacological management includes NSAIDs for pain management, steroids to treat acute flare-ups, disease-modifying agents (DMARDs) to induce remission, and biologic agents (anti-TNFα) to inhibit cytokine production when the disease remains active despite the use of two DMARDs. Side effects of NSAIDs include gastrointestinal irritation and bleeding, renal failure and fluid retention. Disease-modifying agents have various side effects which include myelosupression, hepatotoxicity, pneumonitis and proteinuria. Blood test monitoring is required. The use of biologic agents increases the risk of infections, such as tuberculosis, and skin reactions. Monitoring is with blood tests and chest x-rays.

Patients with rheumatoid arthritis require individual tailored care with multidisciplinary input, including physiotherapy, to encourage regular exercise and occupational therapy for aids and splints. Frequent contact with the GP is important as rheumatoid arthritis can result in significant disability.

The differential diagnosis of RhA includes acute viral polyarthritis, e.g. parvovirus B19, rubella, or hepatitis B virus, however, these usually last fewer than 6 weeks. Systemic lupus erythematosis is a differential, although erosions are not a feature. Psoriatic arthropathy also affects the small joints of the hands, but is a seronegative spondyloarthropathy. Pseudogout may be chronic, but is usually a monoarthritis.

Diagnosing rheumatoid arthritis – the American College of Rheumatology revised criteria (four criteria are required)

Morning stiffness >1 hour before improvement
Swelling of ≥3 joints for >6 weeks
Swelling of the proximal interphalangeal, metacarpophalangeal or wrist joints
Symmetrical swelling
Characteristic x-ray changes
Subcutaneous rheumatoid nodules
Rheumatoid factor positive

CASE 44: MIDDLE-AGED MAN WITH CONFUSION

History

A 56-year-old male builder is brought into A&E by his wife. Over the past week, he has been complaining of increasing headache and over the past 24 hours he has become mildly confused, and she has also noticed some weakness in his left arm and leg. The only other history of note is that while standing up at work he hit his head hard on a steel gilder, although this was 3 weeks previously and he had suffered no immediate effects. He has two children and is a non-smoker; he is on no medication currently apart from paracetamol for his headache.

Examination

On examination, his observations are stable and he is apyrexial. Cardiorespiratory and abdominal examination is unremarkable. He is mildly disorientated in time and place, but knows his name. Neurologically, he has reduced power 4/5 in his left arm and leg, with brisk reflexes and mildly increased tone. There is nothing else of note. Initial routine blood results are unremarkable as is his electrocardiogram (ECG).

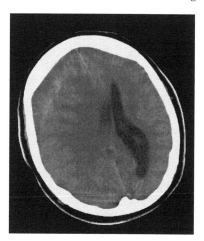

Figure 44.1

QUESTIONS

1. What are the current recommendations for cranial computed tomography (CT) scan post-trauma in adults?
2. What is the differential diagnosis for this presentation?
3. What does the CT image in Figure 44.1 demonstrate? This is an axial section at the level of the bodies of the lateral ventricles (unenhanced).
4. Would you consider any other forms of imaging?
5. How should he be further managed?

ANSWERS

1. The current indications for cranial CT post-injury to be performed within 1 hour of request:

   a. Glasgow Coma Score (GCS) <13
   b. GCS <15, 2 hours or more after injury
   c. Depressed/base of skull fracture
   d. More than one episode of vomiting (adult) (>3 episodes of vomiting in a child)
   e. Seizure
   f. Coagulopathy
   g. Focal neurological defect.

   This case is complicated in that the trauma was several weeks previously. However, this is a (relatively) young patient with altered conscious level and focal neurology and urgent cranial imaging is needed. There is a history of previous trauma and in this context CT is the initial imaging modality of choice to detect possible intracranial blood.

2. Differential diagnosis includes:

   a. Cerebrovascular accident (thrombotic or haemorrhagic)
   b. Subdural, possible extradural haematoma
   c. Cerebral abscess (less likely, he is afebrile with a normal white cell count)
   d. Metabolic causes (e.g. hypoglycaemia, less likely).

3. The CT image (see Figure 44.2) shows a right-sided extracerebral collection of fluid. Note that the inner margin of this (overlying the brain) is concave (arrows B), suggesting this is subdural in location. The collection itself is relatively hypodense to

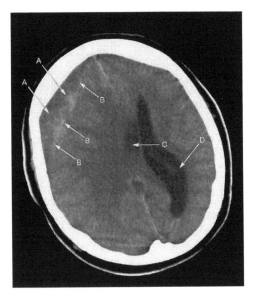

Figure 44.2

brain, but is inhomogeneous containing areas of hyerintensity (arrows A). With the history of trauma and the appearances of the collection, this is likely to represent a subacute subdural haematoma, containing areas of fresh (white) haemorrhage. There is considerable associated mass effect with adjacent cerebral swelling and sulcal effacement, compression of the body of the right lateral ventricle (arrow C), midline shift to the left and some dilation of the body of the contralateral left lateral ventricle (arrow D).

4. Magnetic resonance imaging (MRI) can be helpful in some cases where CT is equivocal – no further imaging is needed in this case.

5. He needs urgent referral to neurosurgery and decompression of his haematoma.

On CT, acute subdural/extradural blood appears bright/hyperdense. As this matures, by 7–10 days, it becomes relatively isodense to brain. This is when CT can be difficult to interpret, especially in cases where subdurals are bilateral and symmetrical, where the scan can appear normal at first glance. MRI is helpful if there is doubt, as blood at this stage contains methaemoglobin, which is bright on TI-weighted MRI and usually obvious. As blood matures further and the subdural becomes chronic (haemosiderin formation), the collection becomes hypodense/dark. The situation is complicated in some cases where repeated small venous rebleeds cause a mixture of different aged blood (as in this case).

Differentiation from extradural haematoma is usually feasible both clinically and on CT. Extradural haematomas arise due to collections of blood between the dura and the skull and often arise following temporal/parietal bone fractures with arterial injury (middle meningeal artery). They are high pressure and cause rapid changes in intracranial pressure, often after a lucid interval post-injury. Subdural haematomas arise due to blood between the dura and arachnoid and are often secondary to sheering injury with damage to bridging veins. Bleeding is at lower pressure and the haematoma may accumulate gradually with presentation subacute or chronic. Subdural blood can travel along the inside of the skull with a typically concave inner margin, stopping only at dural reflections, such as the falx cerebri and the tentorium cerebelli. Extradural haematoma has a typically biconvex, lentiform configuration and cannot pass beyond sutural lines.

Figure 44.3 is an axial CT section through the posterior fossa following occipital head injury showing the bioconvex appearance of an extradural haematoma in the posterior fossa (arrows A).

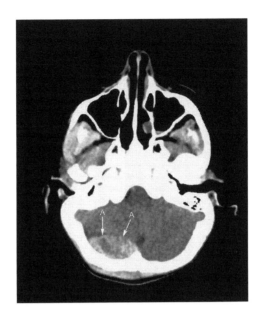

Figure 44.3

CASE 45: ELDERLY WOMAN WITH UPPER LIMB WEAKNESS

History

A 78-year-old female presents with pain and weakness of the right upper limb, drooping of her right eye first noted one month ago and a 2-week history of change and hoarsening in her voice. She describes some weight loss, general malaise and intermittent night sweats. She is a life-long smoker with moderate alcohol intake and suffers from diabetes, which is diet controlled.

Examination

The patient is haemodynamically stable and afebrile; cardiovascular and abdominal examinations are unremarkable. Respiratory examination reveals finger clubbing, reduced air entry bilaterally with no added sounds and dullness to percussion at the right apex. Neurological examination reveals reduced power of the muscles in the right upper limb at 3/5, with reduced sensation to light touch; tone and reflexes are normal. The left upper limb and lower limb neurological examination is unremarkable.

Investigations

		Reference range
Full blood count		
Haemoglobin	9.8 g/dL	11.5–16.4 g/dL
White cell count	7.3 × 10⁹/L	4.0–11.0 × 10⁹/L
Neutrophils	6.5 × 10⁹/L	2.0–7.5 × 10⁹/L
Platelets	322 × 10⁹/L	150–450 × 10⁹/L
Mean corpuscular volume (MCV)	85 fL	76–96 fl
Renal function		
Sodium	149 mmol/L	135–145 mmol/L
Potassium	4.5 mmol/L	3.5–5.0 mmol/L
Urea	6.1 mmol/L	3.0–6.5 mmol/L
Creatinine	120 µmol/L	60–125 µmol/L
Liver function		
Bilirubin	23 µmol/l	3–17 µmol/l
Alkaline phosphatase (ALP)	325 IU/L	100–300 IU/L
Alanine aminotransferase (ALT)	30 IU/L	5–35 IU/L
Aspartate transaminase (AST)	23 IU/L	5–35 IU/L
Total protein	86 g/L	63–80 g/L
Albumin	33 g/L	32–50 g/L

		Reference range
Other inflammatory markers		
Erythrocyte sedimentation rate (ESR)	90 mmol/L	<5.0 mmol/L
C-reactive protein (CRP)	22 mg/L	<5 mg/L

A chest x-ray was undertaken (Figure 45.1).

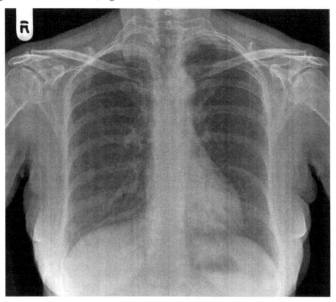

Figure 45.1

QUESTIONS

1. What abnormalities can you see in Figure 45.1?
2. What is the most likely diagnosis?
3. What might you find on cranial nerve examination?
4. What further investigations are needed to confirm the diagnosis?
5. How is this condition treated?

ANSWERS

1. The chest x-ray shows an opacity at the right lung apex (arrows C) seen on a magnified view of the right apex included in Figure 45.2. Here the associated destruction of the posterior right upper second rib can be clearly seen (arrows A). The corresponding normal second rib is annotated for comparison (arrows B). There is no mediastinal lymphadenopathy.

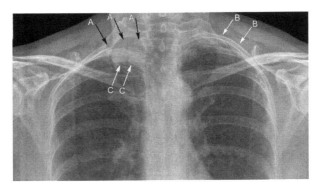

Figure 45.2

2. This patient has a superior sulcus (Pancoast) lung carcinoma.

3. Pancoast tumours can present in a number of ways due to local/chest wall infiltration:
   a. Horner syndrome, due to disruption of the sympathetic plexus as it dips down below the thoracic inlet – this comprises ptosis, miosis and anhydrosis on the affected side. There are other causes of Horner syndrome where the sympathetic plexus is involved in the neck or at the skull base (e.g. trauma, tumour) and, depending on the level that damage occurs, sweating over the face may be spared.
   b. Pain/loss of function due to brachial plexus infiltration (look for small muscle hand wasting).
   c. Pain due to chest wall/rib invasion.
   d. Hoarse voice due to infiltration of the recurrent laryngeal nerve.

4. This patient will need a staging CT thorax/abdomen, this can also be used to guide needle biopsy. Magnetic resonance imaging (MRI) is very helpful in some cases to better delineate the apical mass and soft tissue/nerve root infiltration. MRI is also useful if there is suggestion of spinal infiltration/cord compression.

5. Unfortunately, by their nature these tumours are usually inoperable by the time they present due to chest wall/mediastinal invasion. Treatment as such is often palliative, revolving around chemoradiotherapy, depending on histology. Lesions are often squamous cell carcinomas or adenocarcinomas (arising in old areas of scarring).

CASE 46: NASOGASTRIC FEEDING ON THE STROKE UNIT

History

At 11 p.m., you are asked to review a 75-year-old female patient on the stroke unit. The nursing staff have passed a nasogastric tube which was technically difficult and would like to start feeding the patient. A post-procedural chest radiograph has been undertaken.

The chest radiograph is shown in Figure 46.1.

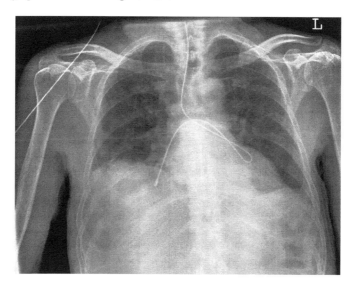

Figure 46.1

QUESTIONS

1. What does the x-ray show?
2. How will you advise the nursing staff?
3. What are the important principles around nasogastric tube placement that you should remember?

ANSWERS

1. The chest x-ray (Figure 46.2) shows the nasogastric tube passing down the trachea (A), coiling in the left main bronchus (B) and then passing over the carina with the tip lying in the right lower lobe bronchus (C).

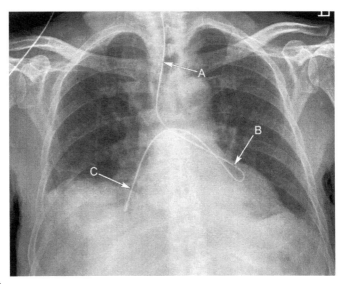

Figure 46.2

2. The nursing staff must not feed the patient and need to remove the nasogastric tube. This needs to be reinserted. However, it is reasonable (and fair on the patient) that this is reattempted the next morning (unless feeding is urgent, this is unusual). A normally positioned nasogastric tube is shown in another patient (Figure 46.3) with the tip well beneath the left hemidiaphragam (arrow).

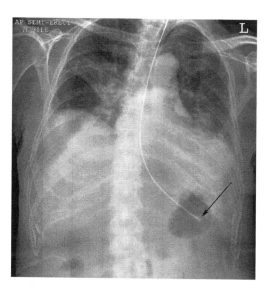

Figure 46.3

3. Nasogastric tube insertions are generally performed on the ward by nursing staff, but junior doctors may be called in difficult cases or where a chest x-ray has been performed following tube insertion to confirm position. Unfortunately, nasogastric tube insertion is associated with morbidity and mortality usually due to malpositioning in a bronchus and written guidance on insertion should always be available.

4. Generally, if the nurses have struggled to insert a tube or if the litmus test for stomach contents is negative on aspiration of the tube, then a chest x-ray will be requested to confirm tube position. This is where difficulties can arise. Ideally, tube insertion should be done during the day when senior medical and nursing staff are available (also radiologists in the department). They can advise and assist with tube insertion and radiograph interpretation. Errors arise at night when junior staff try to assess tube position and make a mistake. Assessment can be difficult and errors can be catastrophic with feeding occurring into the lung. If you are unsure about an x-ray appearance and are put on the spot late at night, it may be best to advise a delay in any feeding until the morning when senior help is readily available, or seek senior help at the time. Always document all discussions and decisions in the patient record and sign/date/time all entries, document any discussions with colleagues also. Also check carefully you are looking at the correct x-ray in the correct patient. Mistakes have occurred in patients who have had multiple x-rays with the nasogastric tube position assessed on a previous film and incorrect advice then given.

SECTION 3: HAEMATOLOGY

Case 47: Elderly woman with constipation

Case 48: Young woman with profound fatigue

Case 49: Middle-aged man with lethargy

Case 50: Teenager with chest pain

Case 51: Elderly woman with light-headedness

Case 52: Elderly woman with anaemia

Case 53: Middle-aged woman with anaemia

Case 54: Confused elderly woman

Case 55: Elderly woman with bruising

Case 56: Elderly man with hip pain

Case 57: Teenager with unexplained bruises

Case 58: Teenager with panic attacks

Case 59: Elderly man with nose bleeds

Case 60: Teenager with a swollen knee

Case 61: Woman with a heavy period

Case 62: Young woman with leg pain and swelling

Case 63: Elderly woman with fever and lethargy

Case 64: Woman with emergency hip repair

Case 65: Middle-aged woman with right-sided weakness

Case 66: Middle-aged man with increasing tiredness

Case 67: Elderly man with abnormal blood test results

Case 68: Middle-aged man with cellulitis

CASE 47: ELDERLY WOMAN WITH CONSTIPATION

History

A 72-year-old woman presented to the surgical assessment unit (SAU) with abdominal pain, distension, and constipation for the past week. She reports having not felt well for the past few months, with progressive tiredness and shortness of breath when walking up the hill to her local shops. She has become anorexic, has been unable to open her bowels for the past week and has been suffering from worsening constipation for a couple of months, despite taking senna and lactulose prescribed by her GP. Over the past couple of days, her abdomen has become distended and painful.

She has a past medical history including stable angina, asthma, a previous laparoscopic cholecystectomy for cholecystitis and a right hip replacement for arthritis. She has no known allergies, and apart from the laxatives, takes anti-hypertensives, aspirin and salbutamol (as needed). She drinks no alcohol, but has smoked 15–20 cigarettes a day for the past 56 years. There is no family history of note. She currently lives alone in a ground-floor flat with no carers, and is independent in activities of daily living.

Examination

Examination of the cardiorespiratory system revealed occasional scattered expiratory wheezes and hyper-expanded lungs. Her abdomen was distended and tender to palpation, but soft, with no palpable masses or hepatosplenomegaly. Shifting dullness was absent, as was rebound tenderness.

Investigations

		Reference range
Haemoglobin	9.8 g/dL	11.5–16.0 g/dL
White cell count	7.2×10^9/L	$4.0–11.0 \times 10^9$/L
Neutrophils	4.4×10^9/L	$2.0–7.5 \times 10^9$/L (40–75%)
Lymphocytes	0.9×10^9/L	$1.5–4.0 \times 10^9$/L (20–45%)
Mean corpuscular volume (MCV)	71 fL	76–96 fL
Mean corpuscular haemoglobin (MCH)	23 pg	27–33 pg
Haematocrit	0.35	0.37–0.47
Platelets	355×10^9/L	$150–400 \times 10^9$/L
Sodium	136 mmol/L	135–146 mmol/L
Potassium	3.9 mmol/L	3.5–5.0 mmol/L
Urea	7.2 mmol/L	2.5–6.7 mmol/L
Creatinine	120 µmol/L	79–118 µmol/L

		Reference range
Corrected calcium	2.58 mmol/L	2.12–2.65 mmol/L
Phosphate	0.99 mmol/L	0.8–1.42 mmol/L
Bilirubin	12 μmol/L	3–17 μmol/L
Alkaline phosphatase (ALP)	122 U/L	39–130 U/L
Alanine aminotransferase (ALT)	37 U/L	5–40 U/L
Total protein	63 g/L	60–80 g/L
Albumin	33 g/L	35–50 g/L
C-reactive protein (CRP)	9 mg/L	<10 mg/L

Her abdominal x-ray is shown in Figure 47.1.

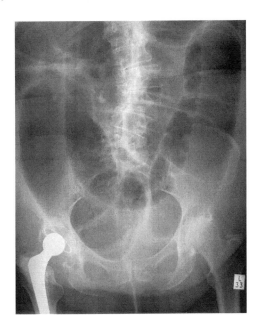

Figure 47.1

QUESTIONS

1. What is the likely cause of this woman's constipation?
2. What other biochemical investigations would help in this case?
3. What is the next investigation needed prior to treatment?

ANSWERS

1–3. This lady has an acute large bowel obstruction, most likely secondary to a primary colonic malignancy. The large bowel is dilated into the left pelvis suggesting a low obstructing lesion, note absence of gas in the rectum. The tumour will have been slowly increasing in size, causing her progressive problems with constipation, until the tumour size caused complete bowel obstruction: the cause of her acute presentation. Her microcytic anaemia would suggest that she is suffering from iron deficiency anaemia, which often occurs secondary to a lower gastrointestinal malignancy. Blood loss can be chronic and at a rate too slow for overt black stools (melaena) to be noted by the patient. Assessment of the patient's iron status with a serum ferritin will confirm the iron deficiency, but care must be taken as ferritin can be falsely elevated in acute infection or inflammation.

A staging computed tomography (CT) scan of the chest, abdomen and pelvis will enable better delineation of the site of obstruction, while also assessing for the presence of distant metastases. Assessment of tumours within the pelvis often requires the addition of pelvic magnetic resonance imaging (MRI). Acute management of this patient will be surgical, and will involve nasogastric decompression of the proximal bowel, along with intravenous fluid resuscitation, while plans for surgical intervention are made.

Differential diagnosis

Breathlessness

This lady has asthma with hyper-expanded lungs on examination. Along with her smoking history, she is more likely to be suffering from chronic obstructive pulmonary disease (COPD) than asthma. She also has stable angina which indicates an element of ischaemic heart disease and possible heart failure. Questioning for orthopnoea and paroxysmal nocturnal dyspnoea will help discern this. Finally, her colonic malignancy is likely to be advanced – hence its causing bowel obstruction. It is therefore possible that she has distant metastases, including lung metastases, which may account for her breathlessness. Another point to note is that malignancy is a strong provoker of thrombosis through a number of mechanisms, both with direct effects, such as compression by the tumour of the iliac vessels within the abdomen and pelvis, and also from thrombogenic factors released from tumour cells. Hence, pulmonary embolus must also be considered in the differential.

Microcytic anaemia

The main acquired causes of microcytic anaemia are iron deficiency and acquired sideroblastic anaemia. Other causes of microcytic anaemia are congenital, and can therefore be excluded when a previous full blood count is shown to have a normal MCV.

They include thalassaemia, sickle cell disease, congenital sideroblastic anaemia, and hereditary spherocytosis.

Key points
• A change in bowel habit with microcytic anaemia, particularly from the fifth decade onwards, strongly suggests bowel pathology, and further investigation is warranted. In this case, the symptoms and anaemia were left until the tumour was so large that bowel obstruction occurred, indicating advanced-stage malignancy. Charting a patient's MCV with historic results, if available, can often show the slow progression of microcytosis when chronic low level blood loss is present, and before the MCV is outside the 'normal' range.

CASE 48: YOUNG WOMAN WITH PROFOUND FATIGUE

History

A 22-year-old student presents to her GP with profound fatigue that has been developing over the previous few months. She suffers from hypothyroidism and is on replacement therapy, and wonders if she needs to increase her dose of thyroxine.

She denies any recent coughs or colds, fevers, weight loss or change in bowel habit, and apart from fatigue, has no other symptoms. She has mild asthma which rarely troubles her, and there is a family history of heart disease.

Apart from her thyroxine, she is on no other medication, and has an allergy to penicillin after developing a rash with previous use. She does not smoke, and drinks approximately 18 units of alcohol per week. She denies any recreational drug use, or unprotected intercourse.

The fatigue is now severe enough to interfere with her coursework and she has been finding it hard to concentrate on lectures.

Examination

Cardiovascular, respiratory and abdominal examination was normal with no cardiac murmurs present, and a regular pulse rate of 82 beats per minute. No wheeze was audible and the abdomen was soft and non-tender, with no palpable masses. No lymphadenopathy was palpable. Examination of the oropharynx revealed a normal-sized, slightly erythematous tongue, but no ulcers were noted.

Investigations

		Reference range
Haemoglobin	8.2 g/dL	11.5–16.0 g/dL
White cell count	5.4×10^9/L	$4.0–11.0 \times 10^9$/L
Neutrophils	2.8×10^9/L	$2.0–7.5 \times 10^9$/L (40–75%)
Lymphocytes	1.2×10^9/L	$1.5–4.0 \times 10^9$/L (20–45%)
Mean corpuscular volume (MCV)	112 fL	76–96 fL
Haematocrit	0.29	0.37–0.47
Platelets	155×10^9/L	$150–400 \times 10^9$/L
Sodium	136 mmol/L	135–145 mmol/L
Potassium	3.7 mmol/L	3.2–5.1 mmol/L
Urea	6.2 mmol/L	1.7–8.2 mmol/L
Creatinine	65 µmol/L	79–118 µmol/L

		Reference range
Corrected calcium	2.22 mmol/L	2.12–2.65 mmol/L
Phosphate	0.98 mmol/L	0.42–0.8 mmol/L
Bilirubin	11 mmol/L	3–17 µmol/L
Alkaline phosphatase (ALP)	56 U/L	39–130 U/L
Alanine aminotransferase (ALT)	33 U/L	5–40 U/L
Total protein	74 g/L	60–80 g/L
Albumin	39 g/L	35–50 g/L
C-reactive protein (CRP)	5 mg/L	<5 mg/L
Thyroid stimulating hormone (TSH)	0.6 mU/L	0.5–5.7 mU/L
Free thyroxine	16 pmol/L	9–22 pmol/L

QUESTIONS

1. What is the differential diagnosis?
2. What tests would you like to perform next?
3. How would you manage this patient?

ANSWERS

1. There are a number of possible causes of macrocytic anaemia, which include haematinic deficiencies of folate and vitamin B12, as well as liver disease, alcohol excess, untreated hypothyroidism, myelodysplastic syndromes and a number of prescription medications.

2. Investigations would look to exclude these differentials, with B12/folate, thyroid functions tests, liver function tests and a blood film to confirm macrocytosis and exclude myelodysplastic syndrome. In this particular case, the woman had a serum B12 of 86 µg/L (normal range, 160–925 ng/L) consistent with B12 deficiency. The fatigue, out of proportion to the anaemia, along with the glossitis would fit with this diagnosis.

3. The cause of this woman's B12 deficiency needs to be ascertained. Enquiries into her dietary habits are essential as vegan diets are particularly prone to being low in B12. However, in a young patient with a normal diet, autoimmune disorders need to be investigated – particularly as this patient's hypothyroidism may be autoimmune in nature. Pernicious anaemia is an autoimmune condition with antibodies directed against gastric parietal cells or intrinsic factor itself, which prevents absorption and binding of B12 from the diet. In order to bypass these problems with absorption of B12, parenteral replacement with intramuscular hydroxycobalamin is instituted as set out in the British National Formulary, and continues lifelong. Blood transfusion is not usually required in the treatment of anaemia from B12 deficiency as correction of the deficiency usually reverses this, and the patient can usually tolerate the anaemia until this happens. Furthermore, transfusion is not a risk-free procedure, and should be avoided when possible.

Key points
• Macrocytic anaemia has a number of possible causes, some of which are more common in patients with co-existing autoimmune disorders.
• Treatment of pernicious anaemia involves the administration of parenteral vitamin B12 replacement with hydroxycobalamin.
• Blood transfusion is rarely required, except in the most extreme cases, and should always be discussed with the haematologists first.

CASE 49: MIDDLE-AGED MAN WITH LETHARGY

History

A 43-year-old man is referred to the medical team by A&E after presenting with lethargy and shortness of breath. He was found in a semi-conscious state outside the local fast food restaurant and brought in by ambulance. After a few hours of intravenous fluid resuscitation, he came round and gave doctors there a 2-month history of progressive shortness of breath and tiredness after walking half a mile.

His past medical history included mild osteoarthritis of the hands, appendicectomy, cholecystectomy and hypertension. He denied taking any regular medication and has an allergy to penicillin. He currently lives alone in a bedsit, and smokes 30 roll-ups a day. He admits to drinking a bit more than he should, and on direct questioning admits to drinking ten cans of strong lager a day (7 per cent alcohol).

Examination

The patient appeared dishevelled and unshaven, and was tremulous. His conjunctivae were pale. Cardiorespiratory examination was normal, but abdominal examination revealed mildly enlarged and irregular hepatomegaly. No peripheral oedema was noted, and no other stigmata of chronic liver disease were seen.

Investigations

		Reference range
Haemoglobin	7.5 g/dL	13.5–18.0 g/dL
White cell count	3.6×10^9/L	$4.0–11.0 \times 10^9$/L
Neutrophils	2.2×10^9/L	$2.0–7.5 \times 10^9$/L (40–75%)
Lymphocytes	1.0×10^9/L	$1.5–4.0 \times 10^9$/L (20–45%)
Mean corpuscular volume (MCV)	112 fL	76–96 fL
Haematocrit	0.23	0.40–0.54
Platelets	156×10^9/L	$150–400 \times 10^9$/L
Sodium	130 mmol/L	135–146 mmol/L
Potassium	3.6 mmol/L	3.5–5.0 mmol/L
Urea	1.9 mmol/L	2.5–6.7 mmol/L
Creatinine	80 µmol/L	79–118 µmol/L
Corrected calcium	2.31 mmol/L	2.12–2.65 mmol/L
Phosphate	0.77 mmol/L	0.42–0.8 mmol/L
Bilirubin	22 µmol/L	3–17 µmol/L
Alkaline phosphatase (ALP)	156 U/L	39–130 U/L

		Reference range
Alanine aminotransferase (ALT)	46 U/L	5–40 U/L
Total protein	56 g/L	60–80 g/L
Albumin	30 g/L	35–50 g/L
C-reactive protein (CRP)	8 mg/L	<5 mg/L
Lactate dehydrogenase (LDH)	422 IU/L	70–250 IU/L
International normalized ratio (INR)	1.5	1.0–1.3

QUESTIONS

1. How many units of alcohol per week is he consuming and what is the diagnosis?
2. What investigations would you perform next?
3. How would you manage this patient?

ANSWERS

This man has macrocytic anaemia in the presence of alcohol excess. One litre of lager at 7 per cent contains 7 units of alcohol. Ten cans (500 mL each) of lager is 35 units. His weekly alcohol intake is therefore 245 units. Recommended weekly alcohol limits are 21 units for men and 14 units for women. This is therefore a significant alcohol intake.

Macrocytic anaemia combined with alcohol intake raises the possibility of liver disease causing his macrocytosis, but this would not necessarily cause an anaemia as well. With the majority of this man's daily calorie intake coming from alcohol, his diet is the next main concern, and haematinic deficiency should be investigated. This patient had a folate level of 0.7 µg/L (normal range, 2.5–18 µg/L) with a normal B12 level, which confirmed the suspicion of diet-induced haematinic deficiency secondary to alcohol consumption. It is important in these cases to check for B12 deficiency as co-existent folate and B12 deficiencies are relatively common. In these cases, replacement of B12 should start before folate because replacement of folate can rapidly increase red cell production, further exacerbating any B12 deficiency, and may result in subacute combined degeneration of the spinal cord (SACD).

In view of the irregular hepatomegaly, a liver ultrasound scan should also be performed to investigate the cause of this, although alcoholic cirrhosis is likely here. Full hepatitis screening and a blood film should also be requested, and the patient should be started on folic acid replacement. Despite the anaemia, immediate blood transfusion is not required in this patient as his symptoms only become significant with moderate exertion. He can therefore be treated just with folic acid, and should see a gradual improvement in his haemoglobin levels, and therefore symptoms, without the need to expose the patient to donated red cell infusions, and the risks associated with transfusion.

Differential diagnosis

- Macrocytosis secondary to liver disease/alcohol, with gastrointestinal bleeding secondary to varices – but note the normal urea levels
- Folate or B12 deficiencies
- Hypothyroidism
- Haematological malignancies, although other blood indices are normal

---

Key points

- Taking an alcohol history should include direct questioning as to the volume and strength of alcohol consumed.
- Excess alcohol consumption often results in decreased dietary vitamin and mineral intake.
- In the absence of very symptomatic anaemia, blood transfusion is not usually necessary, and replacement of folic acid should result in a gradual and progressive recovery of blood counts.

CASE 50: TEENAGER WITH CHEST PAIN

History

A 17-year-old male presented to A&E with chest pain and a cough, which had started 2 days previously. He is tachypnoeic and in obvious distress with his chest pain, which is worse on inspiration. He is unaccompanied in the department, and unable to give much history due to his pain, but is asking for pain relief with morphine, having been given this on previous attendances to A&E with similar symptoms.

He is on no regular medication, and denies any allergies. He reports having tried codeine, diclofenac and paracetamol for the chest pain, which helped at first, but is no longer providing benefit. His cough started 2–3 days ago, and has now become productive of green sputum, without blood staining. He denies any previous cardiac problems or asthma. He is unaware of any family history, as he was adopted from an orphanage in his native Nigeria as a child. He is currently taking his A-levels at college. He denies any illicit drug usage, excessive alcohol intake or foreign travel recently. He has had no prolonged immobility or recent operations.

Examination

He is tachypnoeic, but lying very still on the bed, taking rapid shallow breaths. He is sweaty with an elevated temperature of 39°C, and pale conjunctivae. Breath sounds are reduced bilaterally, but absent from the right lung base, and dullness to percussion is present at this site. He is tachycardic, with a regular pulse of 110/min, but no audible murmurs and is normotensive. There are no splinter haemorrhages present. Abdominal examination is unremarkable with a soft, non-tender abdomen, and no organs palpable. Bowel sounds are present and normal.

Investigations

		Reference range
Haemoglobin	7.4 g/dL	13.5–18.0 g/dL
White cell count	14×10^9/L	$4.0–11.0 \times 10^9$/L
Neutrophils	11×10^9/L	$2.0–7.5 \times 10^9$/L (40–75%)
Lymphocytes	2.8×10^9/L	$1.5–4.0 \times 10^9$/L (20–45%)
Mean corpuscular volume (MCV)	66 fL	76–96 fL
Haematocrit	0.220	0.40–0.54
Platelets	420×10^9/L	$150–400 \times 10^9$/L
Sodium	130 mmol/L	135–146 mmol/L
Potassium	4.4 mmol/L	3.5–5.0 mmol/L
Urea	7.2 mmol/L	2.5–6.7 mmol/L
Creatinine	135 µmol/L	79–118 µmol/L

		Reference range
Corrected calcium	2.32 mmol/L	2.12–2.65 mmol/L
Phosphate	0.82 mmol/L	0.42–0.8 mmol/L
Bilirubin	225 μmol/L	3–17 μmol/L
Alkaline phosphatase (ALP)	126 U/L	39–130 U/L
Alanine aminotransferase (ALT)	54 U/L	5–40 U/L
Total protein	66 g/L	60–80 g/L
Albumin	44 g/L	35–50 g/L
C-reactive protein (CRP)	122 mg/L	<5 mg/L
Lactate dehydrogenase (LDH)	455 IU/L	70–250 IU/L

A chest radiograph confirmed right basal consolidation.

QUESTIONS

1. What is the cause of this man's chest pain?
2. What is the initial management of his case?
3. What other information do you require?
4. What is the likely underlying diagnosis?

ANSWERS

1. This young man has presented with signs and symptoms of a community-acquired pneumonia. Examination suggests a right lower zone consolidation, and the plain chest radiograph confirms this. His presenting symptoms are of a productive cough and pleuritic chest pain. The most likely cause for this man's chest pain is therefore inflammation of the pleura secondary to the underlying pneumonia. However, another possible cause of the chest pain, indicated by the blood results, is that of a sickle cell crisis, causing bony pain in the ribs. The full blood count reveals a microcytic anaemia, while the biochemistry shows a raised bilirubin and LDH, consistent with sickle cell disease with active red cell haemolysis. If a reticulocyte count was requested, this would usually be significantly elevated, confirming the high red cell turnover, with new immature red cells (reticulocytes) being produced to compensate for their decreased lifespan. If a past medical history is unavailable from the patient, a blood film should confirm the diagnosis, along with a sickle solubility test. Figure 50.1 shows sickle-shaped cells characteristic of sickle cell disease (see arrow). With the institution of population-based neonatal screening for sickle cell disease in the UK, along with a positive family history, most patients will be able to inform you of their condition. Nevertheless, new diagnoses are occasionally made in older patients.

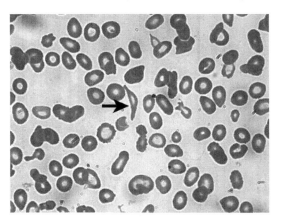

Figure 50.1

2 and 3. With the shallow breathing secondary to chest pain, the resultant hypoventilation will cause progressive hypoxia, which in turn causes increased red cell sickling. This sickling causes further rib pain, the cycle spirals downwards and significant morbidity and mortality can result if not managed appropriately. With these patients, early intervention is required to prevent further red cell sickling, the causes of which include hypoxia, hypothermia, infection and dehydration. Initial treatment should include high-flow oxygen, intravenous fluids, thromboprophylaxis, antibiotics to cover encapsulated organisms as per local guidelines (as sickle cell patients will have autoinfarcted their spleen in childhood, rendering them functionally asplenic), adequate analgesia to facilitate ventilation despite painful ribs and nursing in a high-dependency

area with regular review by doctors and nurses experienced in the care of sickle cell patients. Blood transfusion should not automatically be given and consideration of the individual patient's baseline haemoglobin is essential. Steady-state haemoglobin levels vary between sickle patients, but can be as low as 6 g/dL. Transfusion above steady state can increase the blood viscosity and conversely worsen a vaso-occlusive crisis. Repeated blood transfusions can also lead to the development of red cell antibodies, making cross-matching blood increasingly difficult, and eventually potentially impossible. Except when clinically necessary, all blood transfusions for sickle cell patients should be discussed with the haematology team.

4. Sickle cell disease is a haemoglobinopathy resulting from a point mutation in the haemoglobin beta-chain which results in red cells that distort into the classical sickle shape under hypoxic conditions. This decreased membrane elasticity interferes with the normal red cell pliability, preventing their movement through small capillaries causing tissue hypoxia and infarction, and reducing their survival in the circulation. In sickle cell disease, the haemoglobin structure is therefore still comprised of two alpha and two beta chains, albeit with mutated beta chains. This is in contrast to thalassaemia where there is either absent or reduced production of the non-mutated alpha and beta chains resulting in the haemoglobin structure being imbalanced with an excess or lack of globin chains.

Sickle cell is phenotypically very variable, with some affected individuals never experiencing a severe sickle cell crisis, whereas others will suffer from recurrent crises and significant morbidity from sickle-related illnesses. Factors affecting the phenotype of sickle cell remain under investigation, but one well-reported association is with increased levels of HbF persisting from foetal life, which appears to be protective.

Conditions associated with sickle cell disease

- Cholecystitis
- Hyposplenism
- Avascular necrosis of the hip
- Sickle nephropathy
- Retinopathy
- Priapsim
- Stroke (including children)
- Overwhelming sepsis
- Osteomyelitis
- Chronic leg ulcers
- Pulmonary hypertension
- Chronic pain

Like other chronic conditions, sickle cell disease requires long-term management in a specialist centre, where complications can be prevented or recognized early. A care plan is usually created for patients by their tertiary centre outlining their current state of health and requirements in terms of analgesia during a crisis. The use of pethidine and intravenous opiates is no longer recommended, and well-titrated subcutaneous opiates in the safest and most effective treatment option. Figure 50.2 shows a chest x-ray from a sickle cell patient showing characteristic features of sickle cell disease. The bones are generally dense, secondary to infarction. There is sclerosis of the humeral head (arrow) consistent with avascular necrosis – this is non-weight-bearing and the bone has not fragmented as is observed in the femur. Note also the absence of spleen density in the left upper quadrant suggestive of autosplenectomy.

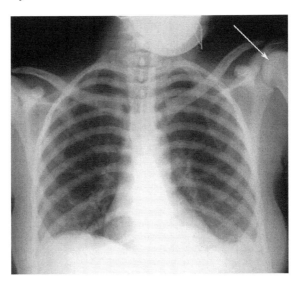

Figure 50.2

Differential diagnosis: common causes of pleuritic chest pain

- Pleural inflammation secondary to bacterial or viral chest infections
- Pulmonary embolus
- Asthma
- Rib fractures/pathology
- Subphrenic abscess/intra-abdominal sepsis
- Lung masses
- Connective tissue disorders/autoimmune disorders

Key points

- Patients with sickle cell disease require intensive treatment in a high dependency setting.
- Appropriate analgesia should be given in the acute setting, with large doses often being required in the initial phase.
- All sickle cell patients should be monitored and followed up at a tertiary centre with experience in sickle cell disease.
- Just because a sickle cell patient has presented with pain, it is not automatically a sickle cell crisis: other conditions also occur.

CASE 51: ELDERLY WOMAN WITH LIGHT-HEADEDNESS

History

A 63-year-old woman presented to the A&E with light-headedness on standing, palpitations and generalized tiredness. These symptoms came on over a period of a few hours the day prior to presentation, and were initially put down to feeling under the weather with seasonal flu. The patient also described some upper abdominal discomfort more recently, which prompted her attendance today.

Her past medical history includes type 2 diabetes mellitus on diet control only, hypertension and osteoarthritis, which has been causing increased pain in her knees recently. She has no known drug allergies, and takes bendroflumethiazide 2.5 mg/day, aspirin 75 mg/day, Gaviscon 10 mL as needed for 'indigestion', and paracetamol 1 g four times a day, as needed. On further questioning, she admits to taking her husband's diclofenac when her arthritis is severe, and has been doing so for the past week. She has no family history of note, and has smoked ten cigarettes a day for the past 40 years. She drinks one sherry at lunch-time and a gin and tonic every evening. She is independent of activities of daily living and independently mobile.

On further questioning, she denied any change in her bowel habit or stool colour, but had not opened her bowels for a couple of days. She had not been losing weight recently.

Examination

She was pale and clammy, with a supine blood pressure of 85/43 mmHg. She had a normal body mass index and was not clinically jaundiced. No lymphadenopathy was palpable. Respiratory examination revealed tachypnoea, but no wheeze or crepitations. Cardiovascular examination revealed a regular tachycardia of 115/min, with normal heart sounds and blood pressure. Her abdomen was soft, but tender in the epigastrium. Bowel sounds were normal and no ascites could be detected.

Investigations

		Reference range
Haemoglobin	7.5 g/dL	11.5–16.0 g/dL
White cell count	11.1×10^9/L	$4.0–11.0 \times 10^9$/L
Neutrophils	7.6×10^9/L	$2.0–7.5 \times 10^9$/L (40–75%)
Lymphocytes	1.9×10^9/L	$1.5–4.0 \times 10^9$/L (20–45%)
Mean corpuscular volume (MCV)	83 fL	76–96 fL
Haematocrit	0.225	0.37–0.47
Platelets	563×10^9/L	$150–400 \times 10^9$/L
Sodium	144 mmol/L	135–146 mmol/L

		Reference range
Potassium	3.7 mmol/L	3.5–5.0 mmol/L
Urea	23.1 mmol/L	2.5–6.7 mmol/L
Creatinine	101 µmol/L	79–118 µmol/L
Corrected calcium	2.53 mmol/L	2.12–2.65 mmol/L
Phosphate	0.93 mmol/L	0.42–0.8 mmol/L
Bilirubin	19 µmol/L	3–17 µmol/L
Alkaline phosphatase (ALP)	122 U/L	39–130 U/L
Alanine aminotransferase (ALT)	23 U/L	5–40 U/L
C-reactive protein (CRP)	11 mg/L	<5 mg/L
International normalized ratio (INR)	1.2	1.0–1.3
Activated partial thromboplastin time (APTT)	29 s	23–31 s

QUESTIONS

1. What is the likely cause of this woman's symptoms?
2. How should she be managed?
3. What is the cause of the elevated platelet count?

ANSWERS

1-3. This lady is shocked with hypotension and tachycardia. She is pale and clammy on examination, and light-headed on standing. These features point towards an acute pathology, as compensatory mechanisms have not yet developed. The 'indigestion' and use of aspirin and non-steroidal anti-inflammatory drugs (NSAIDs) might help point towards the aetiology here and the normocytic anaemia strongly suggests that acute blood loss from the upper gastrointestinal (GI) tract is the cause of her symptoms as chronic blood loss generally produces a microcytic anemia, although a previous blood count result would be useful in determining the duration of anaemia. Her raised platelet count is consistent with an acute bleed, although a number of other causes of thrombocytosis are possible, including infection (see below). Her biochemistry results give the strongest indication that an upper GI bleed is the cause with the elevated urea compared to the creatinine. This was traditionally thought to relate to the large protein load that blood places into the GI tract, with the resulting production of urea as a byproduct of its metabolism. Others believe that this raised urea may simply be a reflection of the prerenal impairment secondary to hypovolaemia. In reality, both mechanisms are likely to play a role in this phenomenon. Although she has not opened her bowels recently, it would be expected that fairly soon, this woman would develop melaena, but in the presence of a high bleeding rate, fresh blood may also be seen *per rectum* resulting from an upper GI bleed.

In view of the acute nature of this upper GI blood loss, this patient needs urgent medical care. Initial treatment is with the acquisition of good venous access (minimum of two large-bore cannulae), bloods to be sent for repeat full blood count, liver screening, clotting tests, along with a group and save, and a cross-match for four units of packed red cells. She should be volume replaced with colloid initially until further information and/or cross-matched blood is available. In the presence of life-threatening haemorrhage, the use of uncross-matched O RhD-negative blood can be used, but only if essential. Cross-matched blood can normally be available within 15–30 minutes, as long as no abnormal antibodies are detected.

Scoring systems for the prediction of prognosis in patients with an upper GI bleed are available (e.g. Rockall score), which take into account the patient's age, comorbidities, the presence of shock and the endoscopy findings.

After initial resuscitation, all anticoagulants, antiplatelets and other drugs potentially affecting the gastric mucosa, such as NSAIDs, should be stopped. High-dose proton-pump inhibitor therapy should be initiated and consideration of upper GI endoscopy should be made. All high-risk patients with an upper GI bleed should proceed to endoscopy within 24 hours, which may be both diagnostic and therapeutic, if the bleeding source can be located and arrested.

Differential diagnosis

- Causes of thrombocytosis:
  - Reactive causes (infection, inflammation, malignancy, blood loss, surgery, iron deficiency, post-splenectomy)
  - Myeloproliferative neoplasms (i.e. essential thrombocythaemia, polycythaemia vera, myelofibrosis)
  - Chronic myeloid leukaemia
  - Myelodysplasia
- Causes of upper gastrointestinal bleeding:
  - Peptic ulcer disease
  - Oesophagogastric varices
  - Arteriovenous malformations
  - Mallory–Weiss tears
  - Tumours and erosions
  - Dieulafoy's lesion

Key points

- Upper gastrointestinal bleeding is a medical emergency which needs early recognition and resuscitation, ideally with cross-matched blood.
- Raised urea levels in comparison with the serum creatinine can imply an upper GI bleed.
- The Rockall score can be used to predict outcome in these patients.

CASE 52: ELDERLY WOMAN WITH ANAEMIA

History

A 67-year-old woman was referred by her GP to the medical assessment unit for investigation and management of anaemia. She had been diagnosed with a borderline anaemia for some years, but over the past year she reports worsening symptoms of anaemia with constant tiredness and lethargy. She now feels lonely, being unable to leave the house, sleeping off and on for most of the day. Alongside this tiredness, she feels her arthritis has been worsening and this has also limited her mobility.

She denies any obvious blood loss either *per rectum* or vaginally, and no melaena. She says she has no dyspepsia or vomiting. She is not vegetarian, and although her appetite has worsened over the past year, she does eat meat. She denies any weight loss, night sweats or fevers. She has no pets and no recent foreign travel.

Her past medical history includes a cholecystectomy, appendicectomy, hypertension, rheumatoid arthritis and aortic stenosis. She is currently on ramipril, simvastatin, bisoprolol, and low-dose prednisolone. She has no known drug allergies, does not smoke and drinks approximately two glasses of sherry per week. There is no family history of note. She lives alone in a ground floor, warden-controlled flat, without any carers, but her family help out with shopping and cleaning. Her daughter, who is attending with her today, has expressed concerns about her mother returning home without any additional support.

Examination

She was pale but not jaundiced, with no rashes noted. Tender swelling of her metacarpophalangeal joints was present. Her pulse was of good volume and regular at 90 beats per minute. Blood pressure was 138/76 mmHg, and heart sounds revealed an ejection systolic murmur at the upper right sternal edge. Her lungs were clear, except for fine bibasal inspiratory and expiratory crepitations that did not clear with coughing. Her abdomen was soft and non-tender, with no masses or palpable organomegaly.

Investigations

		Reference range
Haemoglobin	8.5 g/dL	11.5–16.0 g/dL
White cell count	11.6×10^9/L	$4.0–11.0 \times 10^9$/L
Neutrophils	8.3×10^9/L	$2.0–7.5 \times 10^9$/L (40–75%)
Lymphocytes	1.8×10^9/L	$1.5–4.0 \times 10^9$/L (20–45%)
Mean corpuscular volume (MCV)	82 fL	76–96 fL
Mean corpuscular haemoglobin (MCH)	29 pg	27–33 pg

		Reference range
Haematocrit	0.255	0.37–0.47
Platelets	433×10^9/L	$150–400 \times 10^9$/L
Sodium	136 mmol/L	135–146 mmol/L
Potassium	4.4 mmol/L	3.5–5.0 mmol/L
Urea	4.6 mmol/L	2.5–6.7 mmol/L
Creatinine	86 µmol/L	79–118 µmol/L
Corrected calcium	2.22 mmo/L	2.12–2.65 mmol/L
Phosphate	0.63 mmol/L	0.42–0.8 mmol/L
Bilirubin	12 µmol/L	3–17 µmol/L
Alkaline phosphatase (ALP)	43 U/L	39–130 U/L
Alanine aminotransferase (ALT)	37 U/L	5–40 U/L
Total protein	72 g/L	60–80 g/L
Albumin	37 g/L	35–50 g/L
Lactate dehydrogenase (LDH)	190 IU/L	70–250 IU/L
C-reactive protein (CRP)	65 mg/L	<5 mg/L
Erythrocyte sedimentation rate (ESR)	84 mm/h	<20 mm in first hour

QUESTIONS

1. What further investigations would you initiate?
2. What is the likely cause of her anaemia?
3. How should her anaemia be managed?

ANSWERS

1-3 This woman has a history of longstanding anaemia, which is normocytic and nor-
mochromic. She appears to be symptomatic from this anaemia, although some of
her tiredness may also relate to her aortic stenosis and rheumatoid arthritis, the
latter of which is worsening. Her platelets, CRP and ESR are all elevated, consistent
with an inflammatory or infective problem, which may be a cause for her underlying anaemia.

Broadly, there are two causes of anaemia: excessive blood loss or destruction and
insufficient blood production. In the first category, she currently denies any blood
loss and her biochemistry argues against the presence of haemolysis (normal bilirubin and LDH). The likely cause of anaemia here is therefore due to insufficient
blood production. Initial investigations for this patient would be targeted at this
hypothesis, with assays for B12, folate and ferritin, to ensure no haematinic deficiencies are present, which could be easily corrected. Although traditionally iron
deficiency causes microcytic anaemia, and B12/folate deficiencies cause macrocytic
anaemia, a mixed deficiency of two or more of these can result in a normocytic
anaemia, as the MCV is a measure of the average red cell size in the blood sample,
some of which may be large and some small, giving a 'normal' MCV.

In this patient's case, no B12 or folate deficiency was present, and the ferritin level
was elevated at 432 μg/L (normal range, 6–110 μg/L), as part of the inflammatory response. It is likely, given these elevated markers of inflammation, that this
woman's increasingly active rheumatoid arthritis is the cause of her anaemia. This
is termed anaemia of chronic disease (ACD), and is often underdiagnosed, and can
sometimes be hard to distinguish from iron deficiency anaemia. In fact, serum iron
and transferrin saturation measurements are often decreased in both ACD and iron
deficiency, although for different reasons. There are four main mechanisms thought
to cause ACD, which include defective utilization of iron in the production of red
cells, a lower than normal increase in the level of the hormone erythropoietin
despite the presence of anaemia, a reduced response of the primitive red cells to
erythropoietin, and finally, reduced red cell lifespan.

In cases of ACD, treatment is best targeted at the underlying chronic condition,
if possible. In this case, it would involve treatment of the underlying rheumatoid
arthritis with disease-modifying drugs. In some instances, further treatment with
intravenous iron and/or erythropoiesis-stimulating agents can be employed to help
overcome the abnormal red cell production.

Another, less likely, cause of the anaemia is Heyde syndrome which is where chronic
blood loss occurs through angiodysplasia in the bowel, compounded by the presence of aortic stenosis – although this would likely cause a microcytic anaemia. This
blood loss is often too slow to be recognized by the patient. Treatment, if severe
enough, is with aortic valve replacement, which has been shown to be effective. It is
also important to note that some people suffering from colour-blindness will be unable to distinguish the colour of fresh red rectal bleeding from that of normal stool.

Differential diagnosis: causes of normocytic anaemia

- Anaemia of chronic disease
- Most haemolytic anaemias
- Mixed causes of anaemia

Key points

- Anaemia of chronic disease is very common and underdiagnosed.
- Differentiating between iron deficiency anaemia and ACD can sometimes be very difficult.
- Treatment involves tackling the underlying condition wherever possible.

CASE 53: MIDDLE-AGED WOMAN WITH ANAEMIA

History

A 56-year-old woman was referred by her GP to the on-call surgical team after a 1-week history of tiredness and weakness and a recent blood count showed significant anaemia. She reports having felt completely normal and well a few weeks ago at her son's wedding, but since then has not felt quite right. Although she denies any weight loss, fevers, night sweats and change in bowel habit – and has not noticed any melaena or rectal bleeding – a full blood count performed only a month earlier as part of 'routine screening' had been entirely normal. Her GP was therefore concerned about the possibility of a gastrointestinal bleed.

Other than the symptoms mentioned above, the patient denied any other complaints, nor had she been taking any anticoagulants, non-steroidal anti-inflammatory medications, or any steroids. She had experienced generally good health, and had only required medical attention during pregnancies and for support with her menopausal symptoms. She was on no regular medication, and had no drug allergies. There was a family history of asthma, but not of bowel cancer. She was independent and active, working as a lawyer in a local firm. She smoked 15 cigarettes a day, and drank two large glasses of wine every evening.

Examination

On inspection, the patient appeared pale, with slightly jaundiced sclera. There were no signs of chronic liver disease. Respiratory examination revealed a clear chest, with no crepitations or wheeze and no dullness to percussion. Cardiac auscultation revealed a regular tachycardia with an apex rate of 110 beats per minute. Abdominal examination revealed a soft, non-tender abdomen with no hepatomegaly palpable, but the suspicion of a mass just palpable in the left upper quadrant. No lymphadenopathy was palpable. Mild ankle oedema was present bilaterally.

Investigations

		Reference range
Haemoglobin	6.6 g/dL	11.5–16.0 g/dL
White cell count	8.5×10^9/L	$4.0–11.0 \times 10^9$/L
Neutrophils	6.2×10^9/L	$2.0–7.5 \times 10^9$/L (40–75%)
Lymphocytes	1.4×10^9/L	$1.5–4.0 \times 10^9$/L (20–45%)
Mean corpuscular volume (MCV)	105 fL	76–96 fL
Haematocrit	0.199	0.37–0.47
Platelets	162×10^9/L	$150–400 \times 10^9$/L

		Reference range
Sodium	142 mmol/L	135–146 mmol/L
Potassium	5.2 mmol/L	3.5–5.0 mmol/L
Urea	7.8 mmol/L	2.5–6.7 mmol/L
Creatinine	108 µmol/L	79–118 µmol/L
Corrected calcium	2.41 mmol/L	2.12–2.65 mmol/L
Phosphate	0.92 mmol/L	0.42–0.8 mmol/L
Bilirubin	112 µmol/L	3–17 µmol/L
Alkaline phosphatase (ALP)	144 U/L	39–130 U/L
Alanine aminotransferase (ALT)	55 U/L	5–40 U/L
Total protein	55 g/L	60–80 g/L
Albumin	32 g/L	35–50 g/L
C-reactive protein (CRP)	15 mg/L	<5 mg/L
Lactate dehydrogenase (LDH)	556 IU/L	70–250 IU/L
International normalized ratio (INR)	1.2	1.0–1.3

QUESTIONS

1. What is the likely diagnosis?
2. What further investigations would you like to confirm your diagnosis?
3. What is the management required for this patient?

ANSWERS

1. This patient has a significant anaemia with a haemoglobin of 6.6 g/dL which appears to have come on rapidly in view of the reportedly normal blood count performed only a month earlier. This, along with her recent symptoms of anaemia, confirms the short history. Individuals can often cope with significantly low levels of haemoglobin if they develop slowly, sometimes to levels even lower than this patient's, but rapid drops in haemoglobin always produce symptoms.

   The causes of an acute drop in haemoglobin levels include blood loss, sudden onset of ineffective blood production (e.g. aplastic crisis), or increased destruction/sequestration of red cells within the body. The blood counts provided reveal a macrocytic anaemia, which is likely to be caused by an elevation in reticulocytes: immature red cells that are larger in size than mature red cells. Reticulocyte numbers are raised in any condition where the bone marrow has to rapidly replace lost or destroyed red cells.

   The biochemistry results in this patient's case reveal a significantly raised bilirubin and LDH, which raise the possibility of haemolysis. The mass in the left upper quadrant is therefore likely to represent the spleen that has increased in size due to splenic sequestration of red cells. Causes of haemolysis are vast, but can be broadly divided into acquired and congenital. Congenital haemolytic anaemias include sickle cell disease, thalassaemia, glucose-6-phosphate dehydrogenase deficiency, hereditary spherocytosis and many others. In a woman of this age, it would be unusual for a congenital haemolytic anaemia to present *de novo*, particularly with a recent normal blood count.

   The likely diagnosis here is therefore of an acquired haemolytic anaemia. These can be caused by infections – particularly *Mycoplasma pneumoniae* or *Clostridium perfringens* – sepsis, drugs, burns, metallic heart valves and autoimmune causes. This patient has no signs of sepsis or history of burns or cardiac surgery; and is also on no regular medication. She therefore has an autoimmune haemolytic anaemia (AIHA).

2. Confirmatory testing would involve requesting a blood film, which may help determine the cause of haemolysis, reticulocyte count, a direct antiglobulin test (DAT; also known as the Coombs' test), unconjugated bilirubin and the LDH. In AIHA, red cells are coated in either antibodies (IgG) or complement (C3d) that provoke their uptake by the reticuloendothelial system and promote red cell haemolysis. AIHA can then be further divided into 'warm' – usually IgG-coated, where the antibody reacts more strongly with red cells at 37°C; and 'cold' – usually C3d-coated, where the antibody reacts more strongly at 4°C. In this woman's case, the DAT was 'IgG+++, C3d negative' confirming warm AIHA.

3. Treatment for AIHA is to remove the precipitating cause, if possible – i.e. treat any infection and remove any drugs that may be contributing to the haemolysis. Initial therapy is usually with high doses of prednisolone, such as 1 mg/kg daily, followed by a slow tapering of dose once haemolysis has decreased. In severe cases,

folic acid replacement is given to prevent depletion. Regular monitoring of the haemoglobin, LDH, bilirubin and reticulocyte count is required. In some cases with severely symptomatic anaemia, a blood transfusion may be required, but this can prove difficult to cross-match, and is usually best avoided unless necessary. Where steroids do not provide benefit, other immunosuppressive agents can be used, such as azathioprine and ciclosporin, as can immunomodulatory agents such as intra-venous immunoglobulins, and more recently rituximab – a monoclonal anti-CD20 antibody, which reduces antibody-producing B cells, thereby reducing haemolysis.

Key points

- Rapid declines in haemoglobin in the absence of obvious bleeding can be caused by autoimmune haemolytic anaemia.
- Investigations include bilirubin, LDH, reticulocytes, DAT and blood film.
- Treatment involves removing any precipitating cause, and immunosuppression with high-dose steroid therapy.

CASE 54: CONFUSED ELDERLY WOMAN

History

A 76-year-old woman was seen in A&E at her local hospital after being found that morning by her son on the floor next to her bed. She appeared confused and disoriented and accused the nursing staff of trying to poison her. Her only physical complaint was of pain in her left shoulder, which was new.

Further details from her son revealed a past history of hypertension, diet-controlled type 2 diabetes mellitus and asthma. She lived alone and was independent. Her son reported that she had been complaining of general aches and pains recently, but she had put this down to 'getting old'.

Examination

Examination of the musculoskeletal system revealed weakness of the left shoulder, with restriction of movement in all directions due to pain. She appeared dehydrated and had mild generalized abdominal tenderness, but the remainder of the musculoskeletal, cardiovascular, respiratory and abdominal examination was unremarkable.

Investigations

		Reference range
Haemoglobin	9.8 g/dL	11.5–16.0 g/dL
White cell count	6.3 × 10⁹/L	4.0–11.0 × 10⁹/L
Neutrophils	4.5 × 10⁹/L	2.0–7.5 × 10⁹/L (40–75%)
Mean corpuscular volume (MCV)	98 fL	76–96 fL
Haematocrit	0.280	0.37–0.47
Platelets	344 × 10⁹/L	150–400 × 10⁹/L
Sodium	133 mmol/L	135–146 mmol/L
Potassium	4.2 mmol/L	3.5–5.0 mmol/L
Urea	12.1 mmol/L	2.5–6.7 mmol/L
Creatinine	155 µmol/L	79–118 µmol/L
Corrected calcium	3.44 mmol/L	2.12–2.65 mmol/L
Phosphate	1.6 mmol/L	0.42–0.8 mmol/L
Bilirubin	16 µmol/L	3–17 µmol/L
Alkaline phosphatase (ALP)	225 U/L	39–130 U/L
Alanine aminotransferase (ALT)	35 U/L	5–40 U/L
Total protein	86 g/L	60–80 g/L
Albumin	29 g/L	35–50 g/L

		Reference range
Glucose	7.2 mmol/L	3.5–4.5 mmol/L (fasting)
C-reactive protein (CRP)	7 mg/L	<5 mg/L

A plain x-ray of the left shoulder was taken (Figure 54.1).

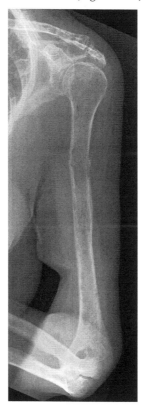

Figure 54.1

QUESTIONS

1. What does the x-ray show?
2. What is the likely diagnosis?
3. What further investigations are required?

ANSWERS

1. This patient has suffered a left humeral fracture, which can be seen on the plain x-ray in Figure 54.2. The white arrow shows the site of fracture with periosteal reaction and a large lytic lesion at its centre. Lytic lesions can also be seen throughout the humerus, with those lower down the shaft of the humerus marked with black arrows. Lytic lesions are areas of punched out lucency (appear less white) due to resorption of bone.

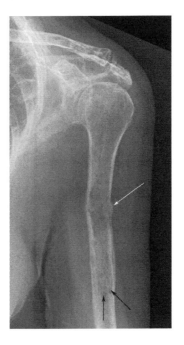

Figure 54.2

2. The diagnosis here is of a pathological humeral fracture secondary to multiple myeloma. This lady has confusion, dehydration and abdominal pain secondary to hypercalcaemia. Her laboratory results show a raised total protein with a low serum albumin, resulting in a high globulin fraction of 55 g/L (total protein–albumin). This gives a clue that there must be other proteins present, other than albumin, contributing to the high protein level.

3. Investigation of suspected myeloma includes an immunoglobulin profile, serum protein electrophoresis, urine Bence-Jones protein estimation and serum free light chains. If these indicate the possibility of myeloma, a bone marrow aspirate and trephine are required to look for plasma cell infiltration.

In this woman, an immunoglobulin profile revealed:

		Normal range
IgG	52.5 g/L	5.3–16.6 g/L
IgA	0.6 g/L	0.8–4.0 g/L
IgM	0.2 g/L	0.5–2.0 g/L

Myeloma is a malignant condition causing approximately 1 per cent of all cancers and 10–15 per cent of haematological malignancies. It is characterized by a clonal increase in plasma cells within the bone marrow. These plasma cells secrete a clonal immuno-globulin, termed a 'paraprotein' or 'M-band' when investigated with serum electropho-resis, and can be IgG, IgM or IgA. The release of various cytokines from these plasma cells causes the typical lytic lesions seen on x-rays, resulting in bone weakening and propensity to fracture, particularly with low-impact trauma.

When serum protein electrophoresis was performed on this patient, a monoclonal ('M') band of IgG protein was measured at 51 g/L. Infections and other conditions can cause an increase in immunoglobulin levels, but this increase will be polyclonal on electro-phoresis, rather than a single clone, from a clone of malignant plasma cells. When pro-ducing this IgG paraprotein, the abnormal plasma cells subsequently produce reduced levels of IgA and IgM – this is termed 'immune paresis', and is another pointer towards the diagnosis of myeloma.

The diagnostic criteria for symptomatic myeloma are:

- M-protein in serum or urine (usually at least 25 g/L in the serum or >1 g/24 h of urine light chains)
- Bone marrow infiltration with plasma cells (usually more than 10 per cent)
- Related organ or tissue impairment (CRAB: hypercalcaemia, renal insufficiency, anaemia, bone lesions).

Differential diagnosis

- Hypercalcaemia has a number of potential causes including malignancy, myeloma, hyperparathyroidism, sarcoidosis, vitamin D intoxication, milk-alkali syndrome, and familial benign hypercalciuric hypercalcaemia.

Radiological features of myeloma

Imaging in myeloma may be normal; however, there are four recognized types of skeletal involvement:
- Diffuse skeletal osteopenia – the most common radiological manifestation
- Widespread skeletal involvement with lytic lesions (seen as lucencies on plain x-ray)
- Solitary plasmacytomas
- Sclerosing myeloma – rare.

Key points

- Assessment of elderly patients post-fracture should aim to establish a cause for both the mechanism of the fall (e.g. syncope) and the fracture itself, particularly if the mechanism is low impact.
- Myeloma should be considered in any patient over the age of 50 years with an unexpected fracture, bony aches or pains, anaemia, renal impairment, hypercalcaemia or elevated serum protein.
- Initial investigations for myeloma include a serum immunoglobulin profile, serum protein electrophoresis, urinary Bence-Jones protein estimation and serum free light chain assay.

CASE 55: ELDERLY WOMAN WITH BRUISING

History

A 78-year-old woman attended her GP with spontaneous bruising over her arms. On further questioning, she admits to these bruises having occurred only over the past week, and not always in response to trauma. She does not think she has been banging into things more than usual and says she has not had any recent falls.

She admits that she has been becoming increasingly tired over the past few weeks, and does report some fresh red blood mixed with her stool on one occasion. Other than this, she is fit for her age, active and walks the dog at least 2–3 miles a day. She has a past medical history of hypertension, angina, and had two coronary stents inserted several years ago. She takes aspirin, clopidogrel, amlodipine, ramipril and simvastatin. She is allergic to septrin which causes a widespread rash. She drinks no alcohol and has never smoked. She lives alone and is independent of all activities of daily living. Her appetite is normal and she denies any problems swallowing. She does, however, report a weight loss of 6–7 kg in the past 2 months.

Examination

Several large bruises were noted over the arms and upper chest. No lymph nodes were palpable in the cervical, axillary or inguinal regions. Heart sounds were normal with no added sounds and her pulse was regular at 92 beats per minute. Her chest was clear, with no audible wheeze or crepitations. Her abdomen was soft with no palpable masses, but there was a suspicion of fullness in the left upper quadrant.

Investigations

Her GP requested clotting studies and a full blood count to investigate the bruising further, then referred the patient to the medical assessment unit (MAU) after the hospital pathology laboratory returned these results:

		Reference range
Haemoglobin	8.9 g/dL	11.5–16.0 g/dL
White cell count	1.1×10^9/L	$4.0–11.0 \times 10^9$/L
Neutrophils	0.3×10^9/L	$2.0–7.5 \times 10^9$/L (40–75%)
Lymphocytes	0.4×10^9/L	$1.5–4.0 \times 10^9$/L (20–45%)
Mean corpuscular volume (MCV)	82.5	76–96 fL
Haematocrit	0.268	0.37–0.47
Platelets	10×10^9/L	$150–400 \times 10^9$/L
Sodium	136 mmol/L	135–146 mmol/L
Potassium	3.6 mmol/L	3.5–5.0 mmol/L

		Reference range
Urea	6.9 mmol/L	2.5–6.7 mmol/L
Creatinine	92 µmol/L	79–118 µmol/L
Corrected calcium	2.59 µmol/L	2.12–2.65 µmol/L
Phosphate	0.97 mmol/L	0.42–0.8 mmol/L
Bilirubin	18 µmol/L	3–17 µmol/L
Alkaline phosphatase (ALP)	43 U/L	39–130 U/L
Alanine aminotransferase (ALT)	54 U/L	5–40 U/L
Total protein	62 g/L	60–80 g/L
Albumin	36 g/L	35–50 g/L
C-reactive protein (CRP)	25 mg/L	<5 mg/L
Lactate dehydrogenase (LDH)	353 IU/L	70–250 IU/L
International normalized ratio (INR)	1.2	1.0–1.3
Activated partial thromboplastin time (APTT)	38.3 s	23–31 s
Blood film	Confirms low blood counts, but no abnormal cells seen	

QUESTIONS

1. What investigations should be performed next?
2. What is the differential diagnosis?
3. What is the prognosis for this patient?

ANSWERS

1. This patient's blood picture is described as pancytopenia, with insufficiencies of all three major blood components (red cells, white cells and platelets). A number of different conditions can cause this picture, but the rapidity of symptoms – i.e. bruising for only 1 week – suggests a rapidly progressing condition.

   Her tiredness is likely due to her anaemia, and her bruising and fresh rectal bleeding are likely secondary to her thrombocytopenia, but not helped by her concomitant usage of aspirin and clopidogrel, which should be stopped if possible.

2. Assessment of this patient should include a full history and examination, to look for possible causes of pancytopenia (see differential diagnosis box). Examination should look for the possibility of elder abuse, including those in institutional care, and for the presence of hepatomegaly and splenomegaly. Blood tests should be repeated to ensure that the previous results are valid, and not due to sampling or laboratory error. Clotting studies should include a fibrinogen to rule out disseminated intravascular coagulation (DIC) which can occur in the presence of acute myeloid leukaemias. As the blood film here is unhelpful, the key investigation required is a bone marrow aspirate and trephine, which can be examined to look for the morphology of the cells within the bone marrow. It can also be used to send for flow cytometry, cytogenetic assessment and molecular studies which may help refine the subtype and prognosis of leukaemia, if present.

   Blast cells are immature myeloid precursor cells that should not normally be increased to any higher than 5 per cent of the total nucleated cells in a sample. In acute myeloid leukaemia (AML), the blast count is greater than 20 per cent. This woman's bone marrow blast count was 60 per cent and this was confirmed using flow cytometry on the bone marrow sample, giving a diagnosis of AML.

3. The prognosis of acute myeloid leukaemia is dependent on a number of factors, including the patient's age and performance status, cytogenetic and molecular abnormalities associated with the leukaemia, previous exposure to chemotherapy, and other underlying bone marrow disorders. However, in the elderly, AML generally has a poor prognosis with some studies showing an overall survival at three years of just 2 per cent.

   The treatment of AML depends on the patient's risk stratification and their ability to undergo intensive chemotherapy, with all its associated risks of neutropenic sepsis and organ dysfunction. Treatment options include a number of different high-dose chemotherapy regimens, including enrolment of patients into clinical trials comparing these regimens. They also include high-dose allogeneic stem cell transplant, from either a sibling or a matched unrelated donor (MUD). Finally, and most likely in this case, there is the option to use low-dose chemotherapy to prolong survival, but not cure the disease, or simple palliation with symptomatic support in the form of blood and platelet transfusion, or antibiotics where thought to be appropriate.

Differential diagnosis of pancytopenia

- Post-chemotherapy (transient)
- Haematinic deficiency (B12 or folate)
- Autoimmune conditions
- Sepsis
- Bone marrow infiltration from lymphoma or other metastatic malignancy
- Myelodysplastic syndrome
- Acute or chronic leukaemias
- Acute viral infections
- Drug induced

Key points

- Pancytopenia of short duration requires urgent and thorough investigation.
- In the absence of an obvious cause, a bone marrow aspirate and blood film are required.
- Treatment options for acute myeloid leukaemia include chemotherapy, bone marrow transplantation and supportive care.

CASE 56: ELDERLY MAN WITH HIP PAIN

History

A 69-year-old man has attended as an elective admission to the surgical ward for a total hip replacement. During his admission clerking, he reports that he has been getting increasing pain in his right hip over the past few years. After analgesia failed to help, he was referred to the orthopaedic surgeons for assessment. This led to his placement on the waiting list for a hip replacement, and he is both relieved to be having the operation and also nervous about the procedure.

His past medical history includes mild asthma, controlled with salbutamol inhalers, as needed, on-going right hip pain secondary to osteoarthritis, type 2 diabetes mellitus controlled with metformin and a previous cholecystectomy. He has no known drug allergies, and apart from the salbutamol inhalers and metformin, he takes aspirin, simvastatin and ramipril. There is no family history of note. He drinks five glasses of wine a week and has never smoked.

Other than his hip pain, he feels well and denies any night sweats, fevers or weight loss. He also denies feeling any lumps or bumps appearing.

Examination

Cardiorespiratory examination was normal, with a clear chest, equal air entry bilaterally and normal heart sounds. His abdomen was soft and non-tender, with no masses, spleen or liver palpable. Examination for lymphadenopathy revealed no enlarged lymph glands in the cervical, axillary or inguinal regions. Hip examination showed restricted movement in all planes of the right hip, secondary to pain.

Investigations

		Reference range
Haemoglobin	15.2 g/dL	13.5–18.0 g/dL
White cell count	28.2×10^9/L	$4.0–11.0 \times 10^9$/L
Neutrophils	5.1×10^9/L	$2.0–7.5 \times 10^9$/L (40–75%)
Lymphocytes	21.7×10^9/L	$1.5–4.0 \times 10^9$/L (20–45%)
Mean corpuscular volume (MCV)	92 fL	76–96 fL
Haematocrit	0.48	0.40–0.54
Platelets	251×10^9/L	$150–400 \times 10^9$/L
Sodium	139 mmol/L	135–146 mmol/L
Potassium	3.6 mmol/L	3.5–5.0 mmol/L
Urea	8.1 mmol/L	2.5–6.7 mmol/L
Creatinine	99 µmol/L	79–118 µmol/L
Corrected calcium	2.41 mmol/L	2.12–2.65 mmol/L

		Reference range
Phosphate	0.79 mmol/L	0.42–0.8 mmol/L
Bilirubin	18 µmol/L	3–17 µmol/L
Alkaline phosphatase (ALP)	88 U/L	39–130 U/L
Alanine aminotransferase (ALT)	15 U/L	5–40 U/L
Total protein	77 g/L	60–80 g/L
Albumin	44 g/L	35–50 g/L
C-reactive protein (CRP)	11 mg/L	<5 mg/L

Peripheral blood smear was taken (Figure 56.1).

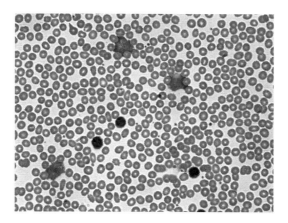

Figure 56.1

QUESTIONS

1. What is the key abnormality in the blood count?
2. What is the likely diagnosis in this patient?
3. Should this condition prevent his operation from going ahead?

ANSWERS

1. The key abnormality in this case is the presence of leukocytosis in the full blood count. When looking at the white cell differential, it is shown that there is a rise in the lymphocyte count which comprises most of this leukocytosis.

2. The most common causes of a peripheral blood lymphocytosis are acute viral infections, particularly Epstein–Barr virus infection (glandular fever) and rarer bacterial infections. However, in these cases you would expect the patient to symptomatic. Other causes include both acute and chronic lymphocytic leukaemia (CLL). In acute lymphocytic leukaemia (ALL), you would also expect the patient to be very symptomatic and unwell and other blood indices would be affected, for example, with anaemia, neutropenia or thrombocytopenia. The likely diagnosis here is therefore CLL.

    The diagnosis of CLL is supported by the blood film (Figure 56.2) showing small, round (mature) lymphocytes with a nucleus that is approximately the same size as a normal red cell (arrowhead). There are also smear cells present, which are lymphocytes that have been destroyed during the production of the blood film, which commonly occurs in patients with CLL (arrows). The definitive diagnosis rests with peripheral blood or bone marrow immunophenotyping, which gives a characteristic profile of monoclonal B lymphocytes. Once diagnosed, other genetic mutations are usually requested to aid diagnosis and staging of the condition.

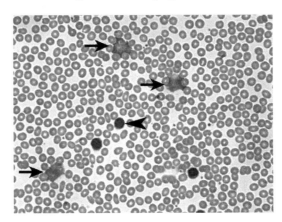

Figure 56.2

CLL is a condition of the elderly, with the median age at diagnosis of 72 years. Men are affected twice as often as women and it is also more common in the Caucasian population. The condition causes a peripheral blood lymphocytosis that can range anywhere between 5 and 300 × 10^9/L and in a proportion of patients will result in lymphadenopathy and splenomegaly. Many patients will have little or no progression of their lymphocytosis and require no treatment for this condition. However, in some the condition progresses, with increasing lymphadenopathy, reduction in platelet, haemoglobin and other white cell counts due to marrow infiltration, splenomegaly, and increased susceptibility to infection. CLL remains incurable, but many treatment options are available, depending on the patient's performance status.

3. This patient is asymptomatic and has no lymphadenopathy or splenomegaly. It would be useful to obtain previous full blood counts from his record to see if this lymphocytosis has been noted before, is stable, and may already have been diagnosed as CLL. There are two staging systems for CLL – Rai and Binet – and in both systems the patient has early stage disease. The involvement of the local haematology team would be useful, but in the absence of any bone marrow suppression, recurrent infections, or progressive lymphadenopathy, no treatment would be indicated and there is no reason why his operation should not progress as normal.

Differential diagnosis

- Acute viral infection (e.g. glandular fever)
- Chronic lymphocytic leukaemia
- Atypical bacterial or fungal infection
- Acute lymphoblastic leukaemia

Key points

- Chronic lymphocytic leukaemia is a common but incurable malignancy of mature B cells.
- CLL does not always require treatment and in some may follow an indolent course, but always requires monitoring.
- Despite being called 'leukaemia', it does not always imply a significantly reduced life expectancy and should therefore not automatically interfere with normal medical or surgical procedures.

CASE 57: TEENAGER WITH UNEXPLAINED BRUISES

History

A 16-year-old male was encouraged by his boyfriend to see his GP after developing a number of unexplained bruises. These bruised areas were not painful, and the patient could not remember having experienced any trauma that might have produced them. He denied any nose bleeds or rectal bleeding. On further questioning, it became clear that for the past few weeks he had been feeling generally lethargic and felt as though he had flu. He complained of a sore throat and for the past few days a worsening headache accompanied by nausea.

His past medical history was remarkable only for a tonsillectomy that had been performed a few years earlier. He otherwise denied any long-term medical conditions. He reported that at a visit to the genitourinary medicine (GUM) clinic last year, he was given a 'clean bill of health'. He had no known drug allergies and took no regular medication, except for the occasional paracetamol, and no illicit drug use. He drank 35 units of alcohol a week and smoked ten cigarettes a day. He was a pupil at college studying accountancy. No family history was known.

Examination

On inspection, he was underweight, pale and had a number of bruises over his limbs. No rash was present. His temperature was elevated at 38.5°C and examination of the oropharynx revealed erythema throughout. Some lymph nodes were palpable in the cervical and axillary regions, measuring up to 2 cm in diameter, but were not tender. His chest was clear to auscultation, and his heart sounds were normal. His abdomen was soft and non-tender, with mild hepatosplenomegaly palpable. No neck stiffness was present nor was photophobia, and Kernig's sign was negative.

Investigations

		Reference range
Haemoglobin	6.8 g/dL	13.5–18.0 g/dL
White cell count	16.0 × 10⁹/L	4.0–11.0 × 10⁹/L
Neutrophils	0.2 × 10⁹/L	2.0–7.5 × 10⁹/L (40–75%)
Lymphocytes	15.1 × 10⁹/L	1.5–4.0 × 10⁹/L (20–45%)
Mean corpuscular volume (MCV)	80 fL	76–96 fL
Haematocrit	0.200	0.40–0.54
Platelets	7 × 10⁹/L	150–400 × 10⁹/L
Sodium	133 mmol/L	135–146 mmol/L
Potassium	4.2 mmol/L	3.5–5.0 mmol/L

		Reference range
Urea	15.2 mmol/L	2.5–6.7 mmol/L
Creatinine	94 µmol/L	79–118 µmol/L
Corrected calcium	2.71 mmol/L	2.12–2.65 mmol/L
Phosphate	0.75 mmol/L	0.42–0.8 mmol/L
Bilirubin	13 µmol/L	3–17 µmol/L
Alkaline phosphatase (ALP)	121 U/L	39–130 U/L
Alanine aminotransferase (ALT)	12 U/L	5–40 U/L
Total protein	65 g/L	60–80 g/L
Albumin	34 g/L	35–50 g/L
C-reactive protein (CRP)	265 mg/L	<5 mg/L
Lactate dehydrogenase (LDH)	690 IU/L	70–250 IU/L
International normalized ratio (INR)	1.2	1.0–1.3
Activated partial thromboplastin time (APTT)	27 s	23–31 s

QUESTIONS

1. What further investigations would you initiate?
2. What is the likely diagnosis?
3. What is the cause of this patient's headaches?

ANSWERS

1. This man is clearly unwell from the history, and the main differential here is between an acute viral illness, which would include a human immunodeficiency virus (HIV) seroconversion illness and a primary bone marrow problem with immune suppression leading to infections.

2. The available blood counts clearly show a significant anaemia with an elevated lymphocyte count, which would not fit with an HIV seroconversion, where such an anaemia would be very unusual. Further investigation with a blood film would reveal the presence of primitive lymphoid cells (blasts) within the peripheral blood, making the diagnosis of an acute leukaemia more likely. Final confirmation of the diagnosis would require a bone marrow aspirate and biopsy, where samples of bone marrow liquid and cores of the bone – usually taken from the posterior superior iliac crest – are analysed to determine what the predominant cells are within the bone marrow. Flow cytometry and cytogenetic testing can be performed on these samples to further delineate the diagnosis of acute lymphoblastic leukaemia (ALL) and further subclassifications.

    ALL is a disorder affecting either the T-lymphocytes, or more commonly the B-lymphocytes, resulting in uncontrolled production of primitive lymphoid blast cells. This accelerated production of blasts impairs the bone marrow's ability to produce normal cells – erythrocytes, leukocytes and platelets – hence the presentation with infection (due to neutropenia), tiredness (due to anaemia) and bruising (due to thrombocytopenia).

3. Most cases of ALL occur in childhood, with a median age at diagnosis of 13 years, where the 5-year survival with intensive chemotherapy is 70–80 per cent, whereas in adults the disease is much harder to treat and there is a 5-year survival of just 30–40 per cent. Presentation is with fevers, weakness, malaise, lymphadenopathy, bruising, bleeding, bone pain and headaches. Two to three per cent of patients present with symptoms of disease affecting the central nervous system, resulting in headaches and other neurological symptoms, which can be diagnosed through examination of cerebrospinal fluid during the diagnostic work up. A further 30 per cent will have evidence of central nervous system (CNS) involvement on cerebrospinal fluid (CSF) examination, but will be asymptomatic.

    Treatment of ALL depends on the subclassification, but generally involves three phases of treatment: induction of remission, consolidation and continuation treatment. These phases can take up to two years to complete. CNS-directed therapy is also required, in the form of either cranial irradiation, and/or intrathecal chemotherapy, where chemotherapy is injected into the CSF space through a lumbar puncture needle at regular intervals.

Differential diagnosis

- Primary HIV infection
- Acute viral infections (infectious mononucleosis, pertussis)
- Acute myeloid leukaemia
- Non-Hodgkin/Hodgkin lymphoma

Key points

- New spontaneous bruising with anaemia is nearly always pathological.
- Blood film examination can often be helpful, if not diagnostic.
- Treatment of ALL in the young has a good prognosis.

CASE 58: TEENAGER WITH PANIC ATTACKS

History

A 17-year-old male has been attending his GP over the past couple of months complaining of malaise, weight loss and panic attacks. His initial presentation takes place during the weeks leading up to his A-level examinations, and he admits to his GP that he is anxious about taking them and has a lot of pressure placed on him at home. They agree to monitor the situation and general advice is given about coping with stress.

Two weeks later, the day before his first exam, he again attends his GP with on-going malaise, sweats and weight loss. He reports feeling some lumps around his neck, but examination is reported as unremarkable. Further questioning about his weight loss reveals a poor diet and anorexia, which he puts down to exam nerves. The patient and GP again agree to monitor the situation and reassess after his exams have finished.

Four weeks later he reattends. Now his sweats have become drenching and mostly at night. He has lost enough weight to notice the difference in his belt size at school. He continues to report malaise and tiredness and now reports shortness of breath on exertion. Blood tests are requested (see below) and the patient is referred to the medical team for further investigation.

When seen in the medical assessment unit, his history is as above. He has never had any major illnesses, and takes no regular medication. He has no known drug allergies. He does not smoke, but admits to a few beers at the weekends, although he is drinking less than he used to as it now makes his neck ache. There is no family history of note and he denies any recent unprotected sexual contacts.

Examination

The patient appeared pale and thin, with no obvious rashes. Examining for lymphadenopathy revealed bulky lymph nodes in the cervical and axillary regions. His chest was clear with no audible wheeze or crepitations. Heart sounds were normal, and his pulse was regular at 100 bpm. His abdomen was soft and non-tender with a spleen tip palpable 4 cm below the costal margin. Inguinal lymph nodes were also palpable bilaterally. A chest x-ray confirmed bilateral hilar and paratracheal lymphadenopathy.

Investigations

		Reference range
Haemoglobin	10.2 g/dL	13.5–18.0 g/dL
White cell count	5.2×10^9/L	$4.0–11.0 \times 10^9$/L
Neutrophils	2.4×10^9/L	$2.0–7.5 \times 10^9$/L (40–75%)
Lymphocytes	1.1×10^9/L	$1.5–4.0 \times 10^9$/L (20–45%)

		Reference range
Mean corpuscular volume (MCV)	78 fL	76–96 fL
Haematocrit	0.332	0.40–0.54
Platelets	152×10^9/L	$150–400 \times 10^9$/L
Sodium	133 mmol/L	135–146 mmol/L
Potassium	4.9 mmol/L	3.5–5.0 mmol/L
Urea	4.2 mmol/L	2.5–6.7 mmol/L
Creatinine	69 µmol/L	79–118 µmol/L
Corrected calcium	2.67 mmol/L	2.12–2.65 mmol/L
Phosphate	0.75 mmol/L	0.42–0.8 mmol/L
Bilirubin	11 µmol/L	3–17 µmol/L
Alkaline phosphatase (ALP)	153 U/L	39–130 U/L
Alanine aminotransferase (ALT)	43 U/L	5–40 U/L
Total protein	63 g/L	60–80 g/L
Albumin	34 g/L	35–50 g/L
C-reactive protein (CRP)	12 mg/L	<5 mg/L
Lactate dehydrogenase (LDH)	523 IU/L	70–250 IU/L
International normalized ratio (INR)	1.3	1.0–1.3
Activated partial thromboplastin time (APTT)	27 s	23–31 s
Glandular fever test	Negative	

QUESTIONS

1. What are the three most likely diagnoses in this young man?
2. How should his case be managed?

ANSWERS

1. This patient's history and examination have so far revealed him to be suffering from tiredness, night sweats and lymphadenopathy. Investigations reveal anaemia, a borderline hypercalcaemia and an elevated LDH. His chest x-ray shows bilateral mediastinal adenopathy. The three most common causes for bilateral hilar lymphadenopathy are sarcoidosis, lymphoma and tuberculosis (tends to be asymmetric with the latter).

    The most common cause of malaise and lymphadenopathy in teenagers is glandular fever, but other infections can cause a similar picture, including sexually transmitted infections such as HIV, so an accurate history relating to these risk factors is important. Other causes of lymphadenopathy broadly include autoimmune disorders and malignancies.

2. With infection being the usual culprit for malaise and lymphadenopathy in young people, they can normally be followed up to monitor symptoms over 1–2 weeks. Infectious symptoms should normally settle within this time-frame, and some regression of the lymphadenopathy would be expected as the infection resolves. However, prolonged or progressive symptoms require prompt investigation. In this case, the GP elected to perform some blood tests, the results of which have already been outlined above. Simple infections alone should not normally cause anaemia and a raised LDH is suggestive of an underlying malignancy. The chest radiograph is suspicious of lymphadenopathy within the mediastinum to an extent that is not consistent with infection.

    Investigations at this point would include a computed tomography (CT) scan of the chest, abdomen and pelvis, to investigate and 'stage' the lymphadenopathy, along with virology studies to rule out infectious mononucleosis and HIV. The definitive test here is a lymph node biopsy which in this case would confirm the clinical suspicion of Hodgkin lymphoma.

    The classification of lymphoma was updated by the World Health Organization in 2008 and is split into three broad categories: (1) mature B-cell neoplasms (such as chronic lymphocytic leukaemia and non-Hodgkin lymphoma of various types), (2) mature NK-cell/T-cell neoplasms (more rare variants), and (3) Hodgkin lymphoma. The primary difference between these lymphomas diagnostically is based on their histological appearances on biopsy, along with confirmatory immunological staining. Hodgkin lymphomas (also known as Hodgkin's disease) generally arise in lymph nodes, affect young adults and tissue usually contains Reed–Sternberg cells (bilobed or multinucleate cells).

    Treatment of Hodgkin lymphoma is with intravenous chemotherapy administered in cycles over a period of several months. The outlook is generally good, particularly for young adults, with a 4-year overall survival of greater than 90 per cent.

Causes of raised LDH

- Myocardial injury
- Malignancy (especially lymphoma)
- Liver disease
- Lung disease
- Haemolysis

Differential diagnosis

- Infections, including infectious mononucleosis and HIV
- Autoimmune conditions
- Malignancies, especially Hodgkin lymphoma

Key points

- The most common cause of malaise and lymphadenopathy in young people is infection.
- Even if Hodgkin lymphoma is diagnosed, assessment of HIV status is essential due to the possibility of HIV-related lymphomas, which are managed differently.
- The incidence of Hodgkin lymphoma is greatest in the 15–29-year age group.

CASE 59: ELDERLY MAN WITH NOSE BLEEDS

History

An 82-year-old man presents to his GP with epistaxis that has been occurring on and off for the past couple of days. At worst it has been torrential, lasting a few hours before settling and then only with packing. He has not suffered particularly with nose-bleeds in the past, however he has been unwell recently with a lower respiratory tract infection – for which he also consulted his GP – and wonders if his persistent coughing has resulted in this nose bleeding.

The patient has been referred into the medical assessment unit for on-going care and appears a little muddled. He is unable to tell you much about his past medical history, and unfortunately the referral letter from the GP has gone missing. Nevertheless, his neighbour, Betty, has come in to visit and knows some of his history. He apparently lives alone without any carers. He has a history of 'heart problems' having once been admitted for an irregular heartbeat and is diabetic on tablet medication only. He takes a lot of medications throughout the day and Betty is sure that he once had to stop a cholesterol tablet because of leg pains. She also thinks he has an allergy to penicillin. He has no family history of note and smokes ten roll-ups a day. When you ask Betty about the patient, she reports that he is not normally this muddled, but he has been a bit under the weather with this chest infection.

Examination

A number of bruises are present over his arms and forehead. His nose is packed with blood-stained tissues. Examination of his chest reveals bronchial breathing at the left base, with associated dullness to percussion. His heart sounds are normal, but his pulse is irregular at approximately 100 bpm and blood pressure 155/80 mmHg. His abdomen is soft and non-tender with no masses and no hepatosplenomegaly. No lymph nodes are palpable. His calves are soft and non-tender with mild pitting oedema of both ankles.

Investigations

		Reference range
Haemoglobin	11.1 g/dL	13.5–18.0 g/dL
White cell count	15.6×10^9/L	$4.0–11.0 \times 10^9$/L
Neutrophils	12.5×10^9/L	$2.0–7.5 \times 10^9$/L (40–75%)
Lymphocytes	1.5×10^9/L	$1.5–4.0 \times 10^9$/L (20–45%)
Mean corpuscular volume (MCV)	88 fL	76–96 fL
Haematocrit	0.333	0.40–0.54
Platelets	466×10^9/L	$150–400 \times 10^9$/L

		Reference range
Sodium	128 mmol/L	135–146 mmol/L
Potassium	3.9 mmol/L	3.5–5.0 mmol/L
Urea	8.5 mmol/L	2.5–6.7 mmol/L
Creatinine	123 μmol/L	79–118 μmol/L
Corrected calcium	2.22 mmol/L	2.12–2.65 mmol/L
Phosphate	0.67 mmol/L	0.42–0.8 mmol/L
Bilirubin	5 μmol/L	3–17 μmol/L
Alkaline phosphatase (ALP)	121 U/L	39–130 U/L
Alanine aminotransferase (ALT)	32 U/L	5–40 U/L
Total protein	74 g/L	60–80 g/L
Albumin	38 g/L	35–50 g/L
C-reactive protein (CRP)	73 mg/L	<5 mg/L

QUESTIONS

1. What further information do you require?
2. What is the likely problem, and how has it occurred?
3. What other issues concern you?

ANSWERS

1. This patient is experiencing significant bleeding problems and the clinical information is currently lacking, requiring some detective work to be carried out. From the information provided by Betty and from your clinical examination it is apparent that this patient suffers from atrial fibrillation (AF). Using the CHADS-VASc calculator for risk of stroke in atrial fibrillation, he scores 3 on the information provided alone and is therefore already into the moderate/high-risk category where warfarin is likely to be recommended for prevention of stroke due to his AF.

2. It would therefore be useful to determine this man's international normalized ratio (INR) result to assess his level of anticoagulation. Further detective work would lead you to suspect that he had been prescribed antibiotics for his current chest infection and with his penicillin allergy, it is likely that he will have been prescribed a macrolide, such as erythromycin or clarithromycin. These both interact with warfarin and reduce its metabolism and can sometimes result in elevated INRs, which is most likely the cause of his nose bleeds. All this information could be gained by telephoning the GP or his/her receptionist and asking for a patient record sheet to be faxed through.

3. In this case, the INR was 11.5. Betty also admitted that the patient was not usually as confused as this and the clinical findings included bruising over his forehead. There is therefore a significant concern that any trauma to the head while over-anticoagulated could result in an intracranial bleed, such as a subdural haematoma. A computed tomography (CT) scan of the head would be essential.

   Warfarin is a vitamin K antagonist and works by inhibiting the production of clotting factors II, VII, IX and X. Dosing of warfarin varies between patients and is affected by a number of other drugs due to its metabolism by the cytochrome P450 system. Careful monitoring of patients taking warfarin is the main drawback of what is otherwise a very effective anticoagulant. The target INR for most indications is 2–3, although exceptions occur. Further information about target ranges is available on the British Committee for Standards in Haematology website (www.bcshguidelines.com).

   This patient requires reversal of his raised INR and further examination and investigation to rule out an intracranial bleed. For those with non-life-threatening bleeding, this can be reversed using 1–3 mg of intravenous vitamin K, which will result in a reduction in INR within 6–8 hours. For life- or limb-threatening bleeding, immediate reversal of warfarin anticoagulation can be achieved with the use of prothrombin complex concentrates (PCC), of which only octaplex and beriplex are currently licensed within the UK for this indication. A dose of 25–50 units/kg is generally used and achieves reversal of anticoagulation within 10 minutes. PCCs contain the missing factors II, VII, IX and X, but these clotting factors have a set half-life, so vitamin K should also be given to reverse the effects of warfarin 6–8 hours later, once the PCC has started to decrease in efficacy.

Fresh-frozen plasma is no longer recommended in the reversal of warfarin as it contains only dilute concentrations of the missing clotting factors, and large volumes need to be given to produce an effect, with the resulting risk of volume overload. It is also a donated product, which has a small but finite risk of viral transmission and infection with new-variant Creutzfeldt–Jakob disease (CJD).

Key points

- Warfarin has a number of potential interactions with food and drugs, so care must always be taken when prescribing for patients taking it.
- Reversal of the effects of warfarin involves the use of vitamin K and PCC depending on the circumstances.
- Fresh-frozen plasma is not recommended in the reversal of warfarin-induced anticoagulation.

CASE 60: TEENAGER WITH A SWOLLEN KNEE

History

A 15-year-old boy presents to the A&E after falling over and injuring his knee on a school trip. His teacher had become concerned as the knee had swollen dramatically in size since the injury a few hours earlier. This swelling was accompanied by significant joint pain and tenderness, which the patient remembers having experienced a few times several years ago, but cannot remember what exactly happened around that time.

His medical information was not known by the school, but the boy reported no significant past medical history. He denied any drug allergies and admitted to receiving injections from his parents twice a week into a subcutaneous port, which he thinks may relate to his previous joint pains and swellings, but he is not entirely sure about this. His mother has been unwell recently and had to go into hospital herself, so he thinks he may have missed one of his injections.

He does not smoke, drink or take illicit drugs. He is in year 10 at school and progressing normally. He is not aware of any family history, but he was adopted as a young child. He lives with his adoptive parents and has been engaging with the doctors and nurses appropriately.

Examination

On examination, his left knee is significantly swollen and tender to touch, with over-lying erythema. He is unable to bend his knee without pain, or weight-bear. There is no obvious restriction of movement in the hip or ankle joints on the left side. Other large joints in his upper and lower limbs appear normal.

Examination of the cardiovascular and respiratory systems is normal. His abdomen is soft and non-tender, with no masses and no hepatosplenomegaly. Examination of the chest wall reveals a likely Portacath present under the left clavicle.

Investigations

		Reference range
Haemoglobin	12.4 g/dL	13.5–18.0 g/dL
White cell count	7.5×10^9/L	$4.0–11.0 \times 10^9$/L
Neutrophils	5.9×10^9/L	$2.0–7.5 \times 10^9$/L (40–75%)
Lymphocytes	0.9×10^9/L	$1.5–4.0 \times 10^9$/L (20–45%)
Mean corpuscular volume (MCV)	83 fL	76–96 fL
Haematocrit	0.373	0.40–0.54
Platelets	263×10^9/L	$150–400 \times 10^9$/L

		Reference range
Sodium	141 mmol/L	135–146 mmol/L
Potassium	4.2 mmol/L	3.5–5.0 mmol/L
Urea	4.4 mmol/L	2.5–6.7 mmol/L
Creatinine	66 µmol/L	79–118 µmol/L
Bilirubin	15 µmol/L	3–17 µmol/L
Alkaline phosphatase (ALP)	156 U/L	39–130 U/L
Alanine aminotransferase (ALT)	39 U/L	5–40 U/L
Total protein	79 g/L	60–80 g/L
Albumin	45 g/L	35–50 g/L
C-reactive protein (CRP)	16 mg/L	<5 mg/L
International normalized ratio (INR)	1.2	1.0–1.3
Activated partial thromboplastin time (APTT)	54 s	23–31 s

QUESTIONS

1. What is the likely diagnosis?
2. How should this case be managed?

ANSWERS

1. This young man has experienced a traumatic haemarthrosis secondary to a fall. He thinks this has happened before, although he is not clear about when or how often. Bleeding into joints is not common in young people and, in the absence of a bleeding disorder, should only normally occur with significant trauma rather than a simple fall.

    The vague information with regards to injections every couple of days likely relates to prophylactic intravenous injection of clotting factors through a Portacath, such as in haemophilia A. This is supported by the prolonged APTT in the presence of a normal INR (which implies a normal prothrombin time (PT)).

    A prolonged APTT in the presence of a normal PT can indicate either a deficiency in one of the clotting factors measured by the APTT, such as VIII, IX, XI and XII; the presence of something inhibiting the action of these clotting factors – which occurs in acquired haemophilia; or the presence of something interfering with the APTT test *in vitro*, such as heparin contamination of a sample, or the presence of antiphospholipid antibodies (lupus anticoagulants), which prolong the APTT but clinically are associated with thrombosis *in vivo*. Mixing of the plasma from a patient with prolonged APTT, with that of a normal subject should increase levels of any clotting factors if absent and result in a 'correction' of the APTT towards the normal range. In those patients where an inhibitor is present, or a lupus anticoagulant, this mixing will not normally correct the APTT. Although this technique is useful, the improved availability of specific clotting factor assays has largely superseded its use.

    Haemophilias A and B are the deficiencies of clotting factors VIII and IX respectively, and are both congenital X-linked recessive disorders. Haemophilia A, confirmed in this case by a specific assay for factor VIII, therefore predominantly affects males, although rarely women can be affected where lionization occurs. Haemophilia A classically causes joint haemarthroses (see Figure 60.1) that can be spontaneous, along with intramuscular bleeding. The severity of phenotype is related with the factor VIII levels, with increasingly severe bleeding symptoms as the baseline factor VIII level falls towards undetectable.

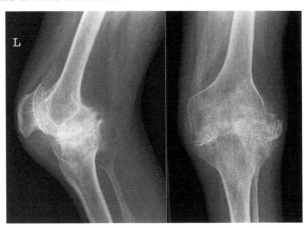

Figure 60.1

2. Treatment for haemophilia A can be either prophylactic or demand-based. Prophylactic therapy is where injections of recombinant factor VIII are given intravenously once to four times a week, usually instigated at an age before significant joint problems have begun. This is a long-term commitment with significant costs associated in terms of time for patients and expense for the health system. Demand therapy requires the infusions to be delivered as soon as any bleed is suspected, often before any investigations can take place to confirm the bleed. Concern does exist with regard to the development of inhibitors against clotting factors, and for that reason it is best for each individual patient to only be treated with the brand of factor replacement upon which they are started. In the emergency situation, however, the pragmatic approach should be employed. It is also important to note that the production of factor VIII concentrates between approximately 1978 and 1985 was sadly virally contaminated and many severe haemophiliacs treated within that time-frame are infected with HIV and/or hepatitis C as a result.

Some patient with mild forms of haemophilia A can be treated with desmopressin (DDAVP) which temporarily increases levels of factor VIII and von Willebrand factor (VWF) by provoking their release from endothelial cells.

Figure 60.1 is a left knee x-ray in an adult showing classical features of haemophilic arthropathy – there is joint effusion with osteopenic bones and there are florid knee joint degenerative changes with squaring of the condyles. The appearances are due to recurrent haemorrhage with abnormal bone development and modelling with secondary arthritis.

Key points

- Haemophilia A is a congenital X-linked recessive disorder.
- Treatment can be either prophylactic in nature, or on demand.
- Awareness of previous HIV/hepatitis C contamination of clotting factor products is important.

CASE 61: WOMAN WITH A HEAVY PERIOD

History

A 35-year-old Caucasian woman presented to her GP with symptoms of an unusually heavy period, but without any significant change in her usual abdominal pain. She had not been planning any pregnancies and she and her partner were always very careful to use barrier contraceptives.

The patient had only been seen a few times in the surgery, mostly for coughs and colds, over the past ten years as a registered patient. She was planning on visiting prior to this vaginal bleeding as she had started to experience bilateral symmetrical joint pains in her hands and was concerned that she might be developing arthritis. Apart from these symptoms, she is currently clinically well.

Otherwise, there was no past medical history of note and no surgical or gynaecological history either. She was on no regular medication, and had no known drug allergies. There was a family history of thyroid gland problems, but she did not know their exact nature.

Examination

Examination of the abdomen was normal, with no tenderness, guarding or rebound. Bowel sounds were present and normal. However, on further examination small petechial bruises were present on the arms and legs, particularly over exposed areas.

Cardiorespiratory examination and gross neurological examination were both unremarkable. A full blood count and clotting studies were requested by the GP and can be reviewed below.

Investigations

		Reference range
Haemoglobin	12.4 g/dL	11.5–16.0 g/dL
White cell count	6.3×10^9/L	$4.0–11.0 \times 10^9$/L
Neutrophils	4.4×10^9/L	$2.0–7.5 \times 10^9$/L (40–75%)
Lymphocytes	1.1×10^9/L	$1.5–4.0 \times 10^9$/L (20–45%)
Mean corpuscular volume (MCV)	82 fL	76–96 fL
Haematocrit	0.38	0.37–0.47
Platelets	4×10^9/L	$150–400 \times 10^9$/L
Sodium	143 mmol/L	135–146 mmol/L
Potassium	3.8 mmol/L	3.5–5.0 mmol/L
Urea	4.4 mmol/L	2.5–6.7 mmol/L

		Reference range
Creatinine	66 µmol/L	79–118 µmol/L
Corrected calcium	2.38 mmol/L	2.12–2.65 mmol/L
Phosphate	0.65 mmol/L	0.42–0.8 mmol/L
Bilirubin	12 µmol/L	3–17 µmol/L
Alkaline phosphatase (ALP)	42 U/L	39–130 U/L
Alanine aminotransferase (ALT)	11 U/L	5–40 U/L
Total protein	72 g/L	60–80 g/L
Albumin	39 g/L	35–50 g/L
C-reactive protein (CRP)	6 mg/L	<5 mg/L

QUESTIONS

1. What is the main abnormality in the full blood count?
2. What is the initial treatment of choice in this woman?
3. What is the significance of her joint pains?

ANSWERS

1. This patient has presented with bleeding and bruising problems, and has a platelet count of 4×10^9/L, which is significantly thrombocytopenic. Investigation of profound thrombocytopenia should include a thorough history and examination, a repeat full blood count to rule out sampling error and a blood film to look for any signs of a haematological malignancy that might be present.

2 and 3. In this case, as the remainder of the full blood count is normal, it is unlikely that this thrombocytopenia is secondary to an underlying haematological malignancy, such as acute leukaemia or myelodysplastic syndrome. The presence of long-standing joint pains raises the possibility of another underlying autoimmune condition, such as rheumatoid arthritis or systemic lupus erythromatosus (SLE). As she denies any regular drug use, drug-induced thrombocytopenia is unlikely, but it is always worthwhile questioning her further about any over-the-counter, illicit or herbal medicines used. We do not know her full sexual history, but it would appear unlikely that she has acquired HIV or hepatitis, however, testing for these viruses in at-risk groups should be considered routinely. Finally, she reports feeling generally well, so glandular fever or other acute viral infections would be unlikely. The most likely diagnosis here is immune thrombocytopenic purpura (ITP).

The treatment of ITP generally requires the involvement of the on-call haematology team and depends on the severity of bleeding or bruising, especially if mucosal bleeding has occurred. Initial therapy is aimed at suppressing the immune response that is causing immune destruction of the patient's own platelets. The immunosuppressant of choice is usually high-dose prednisolone (1 mg/kg daily), but may also include immune modulatory doses of intravenous immunoglobulins. Response to this treatment is usually rapid and platelet counts can improve significantly after only 24 hours, but failure of treatment is not usually determined until no response has been achieved after 2–3 weeks' treatment. A number of other immunosuppressant drugs, monoclonal antibodies, other treatment modalities and even splenectomy are options for those patients failing or relapsing after first-line therapy.

Platelet transfusion is rarely used, as antibodies for autologous platelets will destroy any transfused platelets just as rapidly as they destroy the patient's own platelets. Their use is restricted to significant haemorrhage and should be discussed with the haematology team.

Differential diagnosis
• Immune thrombocytopenic purpura
• Drug-induced thrombocytopenia
• Acute viral infection (e.g. HIV, hepatitis C)
• Sepsis
• Underlying haematological malignancy/myelodysplastic syndrome

Key points

- In ITP, the rest of the full blood count is normal, unless significant blood loss has resulted in anaemia.
- Treatment of ITP involves immune suppression or modulation, rather than platelet transfusion unless severe haemorrhage is present.
- A large number of patients with a successfully treated episode of ITP will have recurrent thrombocytopenia when the initial therapy is tapered.

CASE 62: YOUNG WOMAN WITH LEG PAIN AND SWELLING

History

A 22-year-old female presents to the medical assessment unit with a 2-day history of increasing right leg pain and swelling. It was present upon waking one morning, and despite walking around and taking simple analgesia, the pain and swelling has not settled. She has never had anything like this happen before and denies any trauma to the limb. She is 32 weeks' pregnant in her first pregnancy, with no current concerns from her midwife according to her maternity notes.

Her past medical history includes an admission at the age of 16 for a paracetamol overdose and a couple of other A&E attendances for minor injuries. She has no known drug allergies and has been taking paracetamol for her leg pain and Gaviscon for indigestion as needed. She has no family history of note, although she does not know her parents well, having been adopted at an early age. She smokes 20 cigarettes a day and has managed to cut down her alcohol intake to about 8 units a week while pregnant. She lives with her boyfriend in a council flat with two flights of stairs.

On direct questioning, she denies any increased shortness of breath, palpitations, dizziness or chest pain.

Examination

On examination, she has an elevated body mass index, and an obviously gravid uterus. Her right leg is swollen, with an increased mid-calf circumference by 3 cm compared with the left. It is tender to touch, but not erythematous.

The remainder of her systemic examination is unremarkable with a clear chest, normal heart sounds, but for a mammary soufflé. Her abdomen was soft and non-tender, but palpation of organs was difficult in view of the uterus. No inguinal lymphadenopathy was palpable.

Investigations

		Reference range
Haemoglobin	11.2 g/dL	11.5–16.0 g/dL
White cell count	5.5×10^9/L	$4.0–11.0 \times 10^9$/L
Neutrophils	3.1×10^9/L	$2.0–7.5 \times 10^9$/L (40–75%)
Lymphocytes	1.3×10^9/L	$1.5–4.0 \times 10^9$/L (20–45%)
Mean corpuscular volume (MCV)	79 fL	76–96 fL
Haematocrit	0.34	0.37–0.47
Platelets	165×10^9/L	$150–400 \times 10^9$/L

		Reference range
Sodium	139 mmol/L	135–146 mmol/L
Potassium	4.2 mmol/L	3.5–5.0 mmol/L
Urea	2.8 mmol/L	2.5–6.7 mmol/L
Creatinine	69 µmol/L	79–118 µmol/L
Glucose	5.2 mmol/L (random)	3.5–4.5 mmol/L (fasting)
C-reactive protein (CRP)	11 mg/L	<5 mg/L
International normalized ratio (INR)	1.2	1.0–1.3
Activated partial thromboplastin time (APTT)	25 s	23–31 s

QUESTIONS

1. What is the likely diagnosis?
2. What investigations would help reach this diagnosis?
3. Is a thrombophilia screen indicated in the acute situation?

ANSWERS

1. The likely diagnosis here is of a deep vein thrombosis (DVT) affecting the right lower limb. Venous thromboembolism (VTE) manifesting either as a DVT or pulmonary embolus (PE) is increasingly prevalent in pregnancy due in part to the hormonal changes during pregnancy, but also to immobility and compression of pelvic blood vessels by the gravid uterus. Virchow's triad describes the commonly quoted conditions associated with an increased risk of VTE: venous stasis, hypercoagulable state and endothelial damage. These risks are all increased in pregnancy, but also in situations such as prolonged immobility and surgery.

2. A number of protocols exist for the investigation and management of VTE that take into account factors such as medical and surgical history, clinical features with regard to the affected leg, among others. One such assessment tool is the Wells' score (see below), which provides a pre-test probability of VTE in patients under investigation and can be combined with a D-dimer blood test to help decide which patients are likely to be suffering from a VTE. Unfortunately, most of these assessment tools have not been validated in pregnancy and D-dimer results are often increased in pregnancy in the absence of VTE, so imaging is necessary in those suspected of having a DVT. D-dimers are the products of fibrin when degraded by plasmin which occurs during the clot formation in venous thrombosis. They are mainly used for their negative predictive value, and help exclude DVT in a patient with low probability of VTE, but they may be positive in acute illness, trauma, post-surgery, the elderly and in pregnancy.

   In this case, a compressive ultrasound Doppler of the affected limb is required to rule out the presence of VTE. The presence of a non-compressible vein is more than 95 per cent sensitive and specific for a DVT. It is a safe, non-invasive test, involves no ionizing radiation and is therefore the best investigation both in pregnancy and in the general population. Other investigations available include venography, magnetic resonance venography and impedance plethysmography, although these are not used frequently in the diagnosis of DVT.

   The treatment of a DVT generally involves systemic anticoagulation, although more recently there has been renewed interest in intravascular localized thrombolysis. Initial treatment often takes the form of low-molecular-weight heparins (LMWH), as they have a rapid onset of action, when compared to vitamin K antagonists, such as warfarin, but they are contraindicated in patients with renal impairment. Once DVT has been confirmed, warfarin can be started with the LMWH continued until the INR has reached the therapeutic range (usually 2–3) for 2 consecutive days. Warfarin is contraindicated in the first trimester of pregnancy and is used with caution in the second and third trimesters. LMWH is therefore usually continued throughout pregnancy when a VTE occurs pre-partum. Pregnant patients need monitoring of their LMWH use during pregnancy due to the variations in volume of distribution and renal clearance of the drug throughout pregnancy. This monitoring takes the form of anti-Xa levels measured 4 hours post-dose. This monitoring should normally be performed by your hospital's anticoagulation service or directly through the haematology clinic. The duration of anticoagulant therapy for a first provoked DVT is generally 3 months.

3. The risk of VTE is five times greater during pregnancy than in age-matched non-pregnant controls. This risk increases to as high as 60 times greater during the 3 months post-partum. There is clearly an increased risk, therefore, for VTE during pregnancy. Testing for a heritable thrombophilia would not change your management of this patient either acutely, or in the long term, and is therefore not currently recommended. Further information about testing for heritable thrombophilias is available from the British Committee for Standards in Haematology website (www.bcshguidelines.com).

Wells' score

- Active cancer (treatment on-going, administered within previous 6 months or palliative) (1 point)
- Paralysis, paresis or recent plaster immobilization of the lower extremities (1 point)
- Recently bedridden >3 days or major surgery within previous 12 weeks requiring general or regional anaesthesia (1 point)
- Localized tenderness along the distribution of the deep venous system (1 point)
- Swelling of entire leg (1 point)
- Calf swelling >3 cm larger than asymptomatic side (measured 10 cm below tibial tuberosity) (1 point)
- Pitting oedema confined to the symptomatic leg (1 point)
- Collateral superficial veins (non-varicose) (1 point)
- Previously documented DVT (1 point)
- Alternative diagnosis at least as likely as DVT (–2 points)

A score of 2 or higher indicates that the probability of DVT is 'likely'; a score of <2 indicates that the probability is 'unlikely'.

Differential diagnosis

- Deep vein thrombosis
- Deep vein compression of other causes (e.g. lymphadenopathy, tumour, ruptured Baker's cyst)
- Muscular tear/strain
- Cellulitis

Key points

- The risk of VTE is greatly increased in pregnancy.
- Prognostic scores for DVT assessment have not been validated in pregnancy.
- Treatment is with low-molecular-weight heparins.
- Thrombophilia testing is not generally recommended.

CASE 63: ELDERLY WOMAN WITH FEVER AND LETHARGY

History

A 62-year-old woman presents to A&E on a Saturday morning, having experienced a 12-hour history of fevers, lethargy and general deterioration. As a result, she is no longer able to give you a coherent history and the remainder of the information is obtained from her husband.

He tells you that up to yesterday she had been feeling well, except for some long-standing tiredness. However, since yesterday evening she has become increasingly tired and weak and went to bed early last night. Overnight she awoke twice with fevers and sweats and they measured her temperature at 39.6°C on one occasion. She has not been drinking or eating well during this time, as everything tasted 'like cardboard'.

The husband informs you that his wife has been undergoing chemotherapy for non-Hodgkin lymphoma and had her second cycle just over a week ago. She did not have any problems like this with her last course. Her husband tells you that she has not complained of a cough, diarrhoea or dysuria. She has a past medical history of type 2 diabetes, hypertension and hypothyroidism. She has an allergy to non-steroidal anti-inflammatory drugs and takes allopurinol, lansoprazole, metoclopramide, metformin, gliclazide, losartan and levothyroxine. She has a family history of heart disease and is a non-smoker and non-drinker. Prior to her chemotherapy, she was active and independent, running 5 miles on a daily basis.

Examination

On examination she is lethargic, drowsy, responding to voice on the AVPU (alert, voice, pain, unresponsive) scale. Her temperature is 38.8°C, blood pressure is 96/54 mmHg and her pulse is weak but regular at 122/min. Auscultation of the chest reveals no wheeze or crepitations and pulse oximetry is 96 per cent on high flow oxygen. Heart sounds are rapid, but no discernible murmur is heard. Her abdomen is soft, non-tender, and bowel sounds are present. Her fingers and toes are cool to the touch, but no calf tenderness or ankle swelling is evident.

INVESTIGATIONS

		Reference range
Haemoglobin	8.6 g/dL	11.5–16.0 g/dL
White cell count	0.6×10^9/L	$4.0–11.0 \times 10^9$/L
Neutrophils	0.1×10^9/L	$2.0–7.5 \times 10^9$/L (40–75%)
Lymphocytes	0.3×10^9/L	$1.5–4.0 \times 10^9$/L (20–45%)

		Reference range
Mean corpuscular volume (MCV)	81 fL	76–96 fL
Haematocrit	0.27	0.37–0.47
Platelets	42×10^9/L	$150–400 \times 10^9$/L
Sodium	148 mmol/L	135–146 mmol/L
Potassium	4.4 mmol/L	3.5–5.0 mmol/L
Urea	11.1 mmol/L	2.5–6.7 mmol/L
Creatinine	120 µmol/L	79–118 µmol/L
Corrected calcium	2.70 mmol/L	2.12–2.65 mmol/L
Phosphate	0.81 mmol/L	0.42–0.8 mmol/L
Bilirubin	8 µmol/L	3–17 µmol/L
Alkaline phosphatase (ALP)	93 U/L	39–130 U/L
Alanine aminotransferase (ALT)	42 U/L	5–40 U/L
Total protein	62 g/L	60–80 g/L
Albumin	33 g/L	35–50 g/L
C-reactive protein (CRP)	195 mg/L	<5 mg/L
Urate	220 µmol/L	150–390 µmol/L

QUESTIONS

1. What is the diagnosis here?
2. How should her case be managed?
3. Why is this patient taking allopurinol?

ANSWERS

1. This woman is suffering from neutropenic sepsis as defined by signs of sepsis (hypotension, tachycardia, fever, peripheral shut-down) and neutropenia (neutrophils $<1.0 \times 10^9/L$). Neutropenic sepsis is a medical emergency, requiring urgent assessment and management. It is the most treatable cause of mortality related to chemotherapy. The major morbidity and mortality of neutropenic sepsis results from the patient's inability to mount an immune response to a bacterial pathogen.

   The usual time-frame for neutropenia is between 7 and 10 days post-chemotherapy. This is often termed the 'nadir' and is when patients are most at risk from neutropenic sepsis. People most at risk of profound neutropenia are those with lower bone marrow reserve, such as the elderly and those who have had many previous courses of chemotherapy. Haematology patients are also at greater risk than those treated with chemotherapy for solid tumours.

   Early signs of neutropenic sepsis include a fever of greater than 38°C, tachycardia, hypotension, shivers/rigors and diarrhoea. These may progress to include restlessness, clamminess, confusion, hypothermia, severe hypotension and tachypnoea.

2. The management of neutropenic sepsis involves the early administration of high doses of broad-spectrum antibiotics to those thought to be at risk from neutropenia, often even before a full blood count has been performed to confirm the neutropenia. Broad-spectrum antibiotic usage will depend on local protocols, and depends on patient allergies, but often includes piperacillin/tazobactam (tazocin) with or without gentamicin/ciprofloxacin. If you are involved in the initial management of patients with neutropenic sepsis, it would be beneficial to familiarize yourself with local policies.

   After gaining venous access and taking blood cultures – including cultures from any indwelling central line – administration of antibiotics is the first priority. Further investigations, including urine and sputum culture, should be performed when possible and a chest radiograph should be taken. Other investigations are guided by any signs or symptoms present. Neutropenic patients often display no localizing signs because, for example, the production of sputum/chest crepitations requires the presence of neutrophils to migrate to the site of infection and these are absent in neutropenic patients. It is often only when a patient's neutrophil count is recovering that it becomes clear exactly from where the offending infection has arisen.

   As with other acutely ill patients, neutropenic sepsis patients require supportive treatment varying from fluid resuscitation to inotrope administration, depending on the clinical scenario, and should always be nursed in areas with expertise in neutropenic sepsis, and areas where higher nurse:patient ratios are available. It is recommended that intensive care or high dependency units, where available, are made aware of these patients early as deterioration can be rapid and unpredictable.

3. Allopurinol, a xanthine oxidase inhibitor, is commonly used in the UK to treat chronic gout, but in patients undergoing chemotherapy it is used to prevent tumour lysis syndrome from occurring. This is a condition where chemotherapy agents cause rapid destruction of large numbers of tumour cells resulting in intracellular proteins and metabolites entering the circulation in concentrations that overcome normal physiological clearance mechanisms. Allopurinol is therefore used prophylactically to help prevent uric acid build up in patients either undergoing or about to undergo chemotherapy, such as in this case.

Key points

- Neutropenic sepsis is an acute medical emergency.
- Treatment with broad-spectrum antibiotics should be initiated early.
- Early involvement of intensive care teams is recommended.

CASE 64: WOMAN WITH AN EMERGENCY HIP REPAIR

History

A 67-year-old woman is currently an inpatient under the orthopaedic team after falling at home and sustaining a fractured neck of femur on the right side. She was admitted for an emergency repair with a dynamic hip screw. As part of the medical team on call, the orthopaedics team have contacted you because her platelet count has been consistently dropping, and they are now concerned that it is too low for her to continue with the heparin infusion that she is currently receiving for her metallic heart valve, which was started 6 days ago. During her admission she has been generally well, but had experienced a urinary tract infection, treated with gentamicin. The operation had gone smoothly without any significant bleeding and there was no haematoma at the wound site.

Her past medical history included type 2 diabetes mellitus, on metformin and a metallic aortic valve for which she was normally on warfarin. She had been placed on a heparin infusion pump on admission as her usual anticoagulation with warfarin had to be reversed prior to surgery. She was on candesartan, metformin, aspirin and warfarin, the aspirin also having been stopped on admission. She did not smoke or drink and denied any relevant family history. She was previously living alone and entirely independent.

Examination

On examination, she was drowsy due to analgesia which was partly for her post-operative pain, but also for some new left foot/calf pain. She had no unusual bruises or a petechial rash. Her chest was clear and heart sounds confirmed the presence of a prosthetic valve. Her abdomen was soft and non-tender with no spleen or liver palpable. Her left foot was cold, pale and pulseless.

Investigations

Recent blood count results are shown below. On admission, her platelet count was normal at 225×10^9/L.

		Reference range
Haemoglobin	9.6 g/dL	11.5–16.0 g/dL
White cell count	10.6×10^9/L	$4.0–11.0 \times 10^9$/L
Neutrophils	8.9×10^9/L	$2.0–7.5 \times 10^9$/L (40–75%)
Lymphocytes	0.9×10^9/L	$1.5–4.0 \times 10^9$/L (20–45%)
Mean corpuscular volume (MCV)	88 fL	76–96 fL
Haematocrit	0.285	0.37–0.47

		Reference range
Platelets	34×10^9/L	$150–400 \times 10^9$/L
Sodium	129 mmol/L	135–146 mmol/L
Potassium	4.4 mmol/L	3.5–5.0 mmol/L
Urea	10.1 mmol/L	2.5–6.7 mmol/L
Creatinine	94 µmol/L	79–118 µmol/L
Bilirubin	19 µmol/L	3–17 µmol/L
Alkaline phosphatase (ALP)	122 U/L	39–130 U/L
Alanine aminotransferase (ALT)	12 U/L	5–40 U/L
Total protein	64 g/L	60–80 g/L
Albumin	32 g/L	35–50 g/L
C-reactive protein (CRP)	45 mg/L	<5 mg/L
International normalized ratio (INR)	1.2	1.0–1.3
Activated partial thromboplastin time (APTT)	49 s	23–31 s

QUESTIONS

1. What is the cause of her thrombocytopenia?
2. Why does she have new symptoms in her left foot/calf?
3. What treatment is required?

ANSWERS

1. This patient has sustained a fractured neck of femur and during her admission to have this surgically corrected, has developed a significant thrombocytopenia. The normal blood count on admission with platelet count of 225×10^9/L is useful as it rules out pre-existing thrombocytopenia, and confirms this as a new development. The most common cause of thrombocytopenia in hospital patients is infection/sepsis, which can result in quite a profound drop in platelet count. This woman has been treated for a urinary tract infection, but this appears to no longer be an issue. Another common cause of thrombocytopenia is drug therapy and it would therefore be useful to review the drug chart to rule out drugs that could cause this. Another concern is the heparin infusion – for two opposing reasons. First, it is generally accepted that when platelet counts drop below 50×10^9/L, the risk of therapeutic anticoagulation increases significantly, often outweighing the benefits gained. In this patient, the presence of a metallic heart valve and the significant consequences of it thrombosing – which could prove fatal – mean that the balance between risks and benefits is more difficult to achieve, but needs to be considered carefully. The second concern regarding heparin is its role as a possible cause of the thrombocytopenia, a condition known as heparin-induced thrombocytopenia (HIT).

2. HIT is caused by the body's production of antibodies to heparin/platelet complexes that results in further platelet activation and consumption within the circulation. It usually occurs 5–14 days after initiating heparin, which relates to the time taken for the immune response to develop. However, in those with previous exposure to heparin, the development of thrombocytopenia can occur 24 hours after exposure due to preformed antibodies. Any amount of heparin can induce HIT, but newer low-molecular-weight heparins (LMWHs), such as enoxaparin and tinzaparin, are much less likely to result in HIT. Signs and symptoms that suggest the presence of HIT include skin necrosis, particularly at the site of subcutaneous heparin injections, venous or arterial thromboses (which may be the cause of this patient's cold pulseless left leg) and anaphylactic reactions. It is unusual for HIT to cause a platelet count of less than 20×10^9/L, but this is not an absolute rule.

The diagnosis of HIT can be aided with the '4Ts' scoring system:

Thrombocytopenia:

   2 points for platelet count fall of >50 per cent from baseline and nadir $\geq 20 \times 10^9$/L
   1 point for platelet count fall of 30–50 per cent or platelet nadir $10–19 \times 10^9$/L
   0 points for platelet count fall of <30 per cent or platelet nadir $<10 \times 10^9$/L

Timing of platelet count fall:

   2 points for a clear onset between day 5 and 14 after heparin onset (or ≤ 1 day for exposure within the last 30 days)
   1 point for a fall consistent with 5–14 days, but incomplete data available, or onset after 14 days, or fall within ≤ 1 day with exposure 30–100 days previously
   0 points for platelet count fall ≤ 4 days without recent exposure

Thrombosis:

2 points for new confirmed thromboses; skin necrosis at injection sites; anaphylactic reaction after i.v. heparin bolus
1 point for progressive or recurrent thrombosis; non-necrotizing skin lesions; suspected, but unconfirmed thrombosis

Other causes of thrombocytopenia:

2 points if no other causes are apparent
1 point if possible causes present
0 points for definite alternative causes

A score of 6–8 points indicates a high probability of HIT, with 4–5 indicating intermediate probability and 3 or fewer indicating low probability.

Further investigation involves immunoassays for the heparin/platelet factor 4 antibodies, but these tests are not always readily available and management of suspected HIT should not wait for these results.

3. Initial treatment of HIT involves immediate cessation of the heparin infusion/injections. No further heparin should be administered to the patient and this includes the use of small volumes of heparin to flush indwelling catheters. Warfarin must not be initiated until the platelet count has returned to normal as it is procoagulant when first started, due to its effect on the production of naturally occurring anticoagulants, such as protein C. Treatment with alternative anticoagulants without cross-reaction with the heparin/PF4 antibody is essential and these include lepirudin, danaparoid, fondaparinux, argatroban and bivalirudin, although not all of these drugs are licensed in HIT in the UK. Warfarin can be restarted cautiously once the platelet count has returned to normal. Platelet transfusions should not be given routinely to patients with HIT as they are considered to increase the risk of thrombosis, but they may be necessary in significant bleeding episodes, but should always be discussed with a haematologist.

Differential diagnosis

- Infection/sepsis
- Immune thrombocytopenic purpura (ITP)
- Drug-induced ITP

Key points

- Heparin-induced thrombocytopenia usually occurs 5–14 days after exposure to heparin.
- HIT induces a procoagulant state even when platelet counts are low.
- All heparin products must be discontinued as soon as HIT is suspected.

CASE 65: MIDDLE-AGED WOMAN WITH RIGHT-SIDED WEAKNESS

History

A 55-year-old woman presented with sudden-onset right-sided weakness on the acute medical take. Her history is difficult to obtain, but you can ascertain that she has never had a stroke before and denies any risk factors for stroke, such as hypertension, hyper-cholesterolaemia, or previous vascular disease, but she does smoke 30 cigarettes a day and has done so for the past 30 years. She does not drink alcohol.

Her past medical history includes systemic lupus erythematosus (SLE), for which she has been having various courses of immunosuppressants, most recently mycophenolate mofetil, under the care of the rheumatologists. She has no other past medical history and lives with her husband. She was previously independent of activities of daily living. There was no family history of note. Medication included mycophenolate mofetil, aspirin and warfarin, although this had recently been temporarily stopped in preparation for an upcoming colonoscopy.

On admission, her computed tomography (CT) scan of the head was reported as normal, so aspirin had been started as per the stroke protocol for presumed ischaemic stroke. Due to on-going neurological symptoms, a magnetic resonance imaging (MRI) scan of the brain was performed the next day which confirmed a left parietal infarct. Further information was sought from relatives, and the blood results below were obtained.

Examination

Examination of the cardiovascular system was normal with no audible murmurs and a regular pulse with a rate of 76 bpm. The chest was clear to auscultation and the abdomen was soft and non-tender with no spleen or liver palpable. Neurological examination revealed increased tone, decreased power and hyper-reflexia in the right arm and leg. No carotid bruits were audible.

Investigations

		Reference range
Haemoglobin	12.1 g/dL	11.5–16.0 g/dL
White cell count	9.2×10^9/L	$4.0–11.0 \times 10^9$/L
Neutrophils	6.6×10^9/L	$2.0–7.5 \times 10^9$/L (40–75%)
Lymphocytes	2.1×10^9/L	$1.5–4.0 \times 10^9$/L (20–45%)
Mean corpuscular volume (MCV)	77 fL	76–96 fL
Haematocrit	0.363	0.37–0.47
Platelets	151×10^9/L	$150–400 \times 10^9$/L
Sodium	136 mmol/L	135–146 mmol/L

		Reference range
Potassium	4.7 mmol/L	3.5–5.0 mmol/L
Urea	10.1 mmol/L	2.5–6.7 mmol/L
Creatinine	87 µmol/L	79–118 µmol/L
Corrected calcium	2.55 mmol/L	2.12–2.65 mmol/L
Phosphate	0.63 mmol/L	0.42–0.8 mmol/L
Bilirubin	5 µmol/L	3–17 µmol/L
Alkaline phosphatase (ALP)	44 U/L	39–130 U/L
Alanine aminotransferase (ALT)	22 U/L	5–40 U/L
Total protein	77 g/L	60–80 g/L
Albumin	39 g/L	35–50 g/L
Glucose	3.8 mmol/L	3.5–4.5 mmol/L (fasting)
C-reactive protein (CRP)	31 mg/L	<5 mg/L
International normalized ratio (INR)	1.2	1.0–1.3
Activated partial thromboplastin time (APTT)	51 s	23–31 s

QUESTIONS

1. What is the main abnormality on the blood results?
2. What is the likely diagnosis here?
3. What precipitated this patient's stroke?

ANSWERS

1. This presentation is of a young woman experiencing an ischaemic stroke, as confirmed by MRI brain imaging. The only obvious precipitating factor is her significant smoking history. The blood results are mostly normal, including her INR, indicating complete reversal of her warfarin therapy prior to her planned procedure. The main abnormality on the results is the APTT which is significantly prolonged at 51 seconds, which seems counterintuitive in the presence of ischaemic stroke symptoms. Nevertheless, in a patient with an autoimmune condition, such as SLE, the diagnosis of antiphospholipid syndrome should be entertained. Here, the presence of a lupus anticoagulant in the blood can cause an *in vitro* abnormality where the antiphospholipid antibody slows clot formation, causing artificial prolongation of the APTT. The presence of a lupus anticoagulant is not always pathological, but in some cases it can produce a procoagulant state resulting in arterial or venous thrombosis, such as this case.

2. Antiphospholipid syndrome is an acquired autoimmune condition causing arterial or venous thromboses, or pregnancy complications and failure. It is characterized by the presence of auto-antibodies directed at negatively charged phospholipids, such as anticardiolipin antibodies, lupus anticoagulant, or anti-β2-glycoprotein I antibodies. The diagnostic criteria for the syndrome can be seen below and require the presence of at least one clinical and one laboratory feature to be present:

   - Clinical criteria
     - Vascular thrombosis – one or more episodes of arterial, venous or small vessel thrombosis
     - Pregnancy morbidity:
       o One or more unexplained deaths of a morphologically normal foetus at or beyond the 10th week of gestation
       o One or more preterm births of a morphologically normal neonate before the 34th week of gestation because of (1) eclampsia or severe pre-eclampsia or (2) recognized features of placental insufficiency
       o Three or more unexplained consecutive spontaneous miscarriages before the 10th week of gestation, with maternal anatomic or hormonal abnormalities and paternal and maternal chromosomal abnormalities excluded.

   - Laboratory criteria
     - Lupus anticoagulant present in plasma on two or more occasions at least 12 weeks apart
     - Anticardiolipin antibodies (IgM or IgG medium/high titre) on two or more occasions at least 12 weeks apart
     - Anti-β2-glycoprotein I antibodies (IgM or IgG) present on two or more occasions at least 12 weeks apart

3. It is likely that this woman was already known to have antiphospholipid syndrome due to previous vascular thromboses which instigated her treatment with warfarin, as no other obvious indication for warfarin has been revealed. The current stroke

may therefore have resulted from under-anticoagulation, while the warfarin was stopped pre-colonoscopy.

Treatment of this patient's acute stroke will require input from experts in stroke medicine and haematology, as therapeutic anticoagulation will be required at an earlier time point than that which is usually recommended in stroke. This increases the risk of haemorrhagic transformation, but there are some cases where the risk of further thrombosis is greater. The decisions regarding long-term anticoagulation are multidisciplinary and include considerations about the intensity of anticoagulation (INR range 2–3 versus 3–4).

Key points

- Prolonged APTT can indicate either a propensity to bleed due to clotting factor deficiency, or an *in vitro* abnormality affecting the assay.
- Antiphospholipid syndrome is a clinicopathologic entity comprising vascular thromboses and pregnancy complications along with laboratory evidence of antiphospholipid antibodies.
- Initial treatment of acute thrombosis is with systemic anticoagulation, where possible, and early involvement of specialists in the condition.
- Antiphospholipid syndrome may occur in other autoimmune conditions, but it may present *de novo*.

CASE 66: MIDDLE-AGED MAN WITH INCREASING TIREDNESS

History

A 56-year-old teacher presented to his GP with increasing tiredness and lethargy, which had come on progressively over the preceding 4–6 months. He had been experiencing early satiety recently and feels that this may explain his recent weight loss. He denies any change in bowel habit or obvious blood loss, but does report easy bruising on minimal trauma. Apart from this, he has recently experienced recurrent chest infections that took three courses of antibiotics to clear. On systems review, he reports hearing a whooshing noise in his ears most evenings.

Before the last 6 months, he has experienced good health with no significant past medical history. There is no family history of note. He has no known drug allergies and takes only occasional paracetamol for abdominal discomfort.

Examination

On examination, he was pale. His pulse was regular at 92 bpm, normotensive. An occasional right basal crepitation was audible on his chest and cardiovascular examination was normal. His abdomen was soft and non-tender with a large mass palpable in the left upper quadrant extending down to the umbilicus, the top edge of which was not palpable.

Investigations

His GP sent him for some blood tests to look for the cause of his symptoms (see below), then referred him to the medical assessment unit for further management.

		Reference range
Haemoglobin	5.8 g/dL	13.5–18.0 g/dL
White cell count	3.2×10^9/L	$4.0–11.0 \times 10^9$/L
Neutrophils	1.8×10^9/L	$2.0–7.5 \times 10^9$/L (40–75%)
Lymphocytes	1.1×10^9/L	$1.5–4.0 \times 10^9$/L (20–45%)
Mean corpuscular volume (MCV)	101 fL	76–96 fL
Haematocrit	0.168	0.40–0.54
Platelets	522×10^9/L	$150–400 \times 10^9$/L
Sodium	138 mmol/L	135–146 mmol/L
Potassium	4.8 mml/L	3.5–5.0 mmol/L
Urea	6.6 mmol/L	2.5–6.7 mmol/L
Creatinine	83 µmol/L	79–118 µmol/L
Corrected calcium	2.22 mmol/L	2.12–2.65 mmol/L
Phosphate	0.86 mmol/L	0.42–0.8 mmol/L

		Reference range
Bilirubin	22 µmol/L	3–17 µmol/L
Alkaline phosphatase (ALP)	210 U/L	39–130 U/L
Alanine aminotransferase (ALT)	32 U/L	5–40 U/L
Total protein	69 g/L	60–80 g/L
Albumin	38 g/L	35–50 g/L
C-reactive protein (CRP)	9 mg/L	<5 mg/L
Lactate dehydrogenase (LDH)	622 IU/L	70–250 IU/L
International normalized ratio (INR)	1.1	1.0–1.3
Activated partial thromboplastin time (APTT)	26 s	23–31 s

QUESTIONS

1. What is the cause of this patient's anaemia?
2. How should his case be managed?
3. What is the long-term outcome in this condition?

ANSWERS

1. This patient has leukopenia with macrocytic anaemia, a raised LDH, and spleno-megaly with a gradual onset of symptoms, such that the presentation only occurred once the haemoglobin had decreased to 5.8 g/dL. Very few conditions, other than chronic bone marrow pathologies, can present in this chronic manner, although haematinic deficiencies, such as B12 and folate, should be excluded initially. Chronic haemolytic anaemias may present in this manner, but would be unusual in the presence of leukopenia and thrombocytosis. Examination of the blood film might help with the diagnosis which in this case showed tear drop poikilocytes (red cells in the shape of tear drops), and immature red and white cells – the so-called 'leukoerythroblastic blood picture'. Bone marrow investigations are the next step in diagnosis and would reveal the presence of fibrosis within the marrow, among other typical features. The cause of this patient's anaemia is likely to be myelofibrosis.

    Myelofibrosis is a clonal myeloproliferative neoplasm which commonly develops in the sixth and seventh decades. It has occasionally been linked to ionizing radiation and benzene exposure, but is generally idiopathic. Proliferation of granulocyte and platelet precursors occurs within the bone marrow and results eventually in bone marrow fibrosis, which interferes with normal blood cell production. Due to reduced capacity for blood production within the marrow, other tissues within the body are taken over to produce it, including the spleen and liver. This is termed 'extramedul-lary haematopoiesis'.

    The presentation is either asymptomatic, or with anaemia, leukocytosis or throm-bocytosis. Symptoms are those of fatigue, weight loss, tiredness, sweats, fevers and bleeding problems. Splenomegaly is usually present and hepatomegaly is commonly found. The spleen can increase in size significantly and lead to abdominal discom-fort and early satiety.

    Approximately half of all patients with myelofibrosis test positive for the JAK2 V617F mutation. Janus kinase 2 (JAK2) is a tyrosine kinase and mutated forms have been associated with myeloproliferative neoplasms and are used in the diag-nostic criteria for myelofibrosis.

2 and 3. Treatment is generally with supportive measures that reduce symptoms, such as blood transfusion and analgesia. The only curative option is an allogeneic stem cell transplant, but the majority of people diagnosed with myelofibrosis are unsuitable for such intensive treatment. Newer JAK2 inhibitors are currently in development and may prove useful in the management of this condition. Life expectancy is very variable and depends on a number of factors, but can range from just 13 months median survival up to 93 months.

Differential diagnosis

- Chronic myeloid leukaemia and other haematological malignancies such as lymphoma
- Myelofibrosis
- Infections
- Inflammatory/autoimmune conditions
- Metastatic malignancies

Key points

- Gradual onset of symptoms suggests a gradually progressive condition.
- Anaemia with splenomegaly, thrombocytosis and a raised LDH are suggestive of myelofibrosis.
- Treatment is generally supportive, but newer agents are in development.

CASE 67: ELDERLY MAN WITH ABNORMAL BLOOD TEST RESULTS

History

A 62-year-old man was referred to the general outpatient clinic for further investigation and management of abnormal blood test results. He had been for a preoperative assessment for a hernia repair and, as part of the assessment, a full blood count had been performed which produced the results below.

In himself he feels fine and has only been to his GP with regard to a urinary tract infection a few years ago. He is frustrated that his hernia operation has been postponed due to these results and is keen to find out what is wrong.

Examination

On examination, he appeared well with no lymphadenopathy and no rashes present. He was afebrile with stable observations. Cardiovascular, respiratory and abdominal examinations were entirely normal, except for a reducible direct right inguinal hernia.

Investigations

		Reference range
Haemoglobin	19.2 g/dL	13.5–18.0 g/dL
White cell count	14.1×10^9/L	$4.0–11.0 \times 10^9$/L
Neutrophils	9.8×10^9/L	$2.0–7.5 \times 10^9$/L (40–75%)
Lymphocytes	1.3×10^9/L	$1.5–4.0 \times 10^9$/L (20–45%)
Mean corpuscular volume (MCV)	90.2 fL	76–96 fL
Haematocrit	0.577	0.40–0.54
Platelets	1077×10^9/L	$150–400 \times 10^9$/L
Sodium	141 mmol/L	135–146 mmol/L
Potassium	6.6 mmol/L	3.5–5.0 mmol/L
Urea	8.2 mmol/L	2.5–6.7 mmol/L
Creatinine	97 µmol/L	79–118 µmol/L
Corrected calcium	2.22 mmol/L	2.12–2.65 mmol/L
Phosphate	0.74 mmol/L	0.42–0.8 mmol/L
Bilirubin	20 µmol/L	3–17 µmol/L
Alkaline phosphatase (ALP)	72 U/L	39–130 U/L
Alanine aminotransferase (ALT)	26 U/L	5–40 U/L
Total protein	71 g/L	60–80 g/L
Albumin	38 g/L	35–50 g/L
C-reactive protein (CRP)	6 mg/L	<5 mg/L

QUESTIONS

1. What is the diagnosis here?
2. What further investigations are required?
3. How is this condition managed?

ANSWERS

1. This patient has polycythaemia – an increase in red cell mass – as indicated by the elevated haemoglobin and haematocrit. Polycythaemia may be 'apparent' due to a decreased plasma volume, giving the appearance of polycythaemia but with a normal red cell mass; or it may be 'true' polycythaemia.

   True polycythaemia is further divided into primary (polycythaemia vera) or secondary. Secondary polycythaemias may be due to increased erythropoietin production with or without hypoxia as a driving force. Primary polycythaemia (polycythaemia vera (PV)) is a myeloproliferative neoplasm, and almost always occurs in conjunction with the mutated form of the tyrosine kinase, JAK2, which forms a major part of the diagnostic criteria for PV. True PV is often associated with a neutrophilia and thrombocytosis, as in this case, whereas other causes of polycythaemia often lack these features.

   Presentation of PV is often asymptomatic, as in this case, but other features include venous and arterial thromboses, headaches, dizziness, visual disturbances, and itchiness – particularly after hot showers/baths. Splenomegaly is present in less than half of patients and gout is a common complaint.

2. Diagnosis in JAK2-positive patients requires the presence of a raised haematocrit of >0.52 in men and >0.48 in women, or a raised red cell mass (>25% above predicted). In JAK2-negative patients, the diagnosis is more complicated and is outlined in the British Committee for Standards in Haematology guideline (www.bcshguidelines.com).

3. Treatment is directed at mitigating the risks associated with PV, in particular the thrombotic risk. In patients with elevated platelet counts, such as here, drug treatments including hydroxycarbamide, interferon and anegralide can be used to reduce the platelet count. The polycythaemia itself is treated with regular venesection, initially every few weeks, aiming to reduce the haematocrit to 0.45 or less. Treated PV has a life expectancy of over ten years.

   For this patient, as the operation is elective, it may prove beneficial for his platelet count and haemoglobin to be better controlled preoperatively, rather than risk the increased thrombotic risk associated with untreated PV. His elevated potassium is likely to be a pseudohyperkalaemia which is associated with polycythaemia. This is defined as a difference between serum and plasma potassium levels of >0.4 mmol/L. Pseudohyperkalaemia is thought to be due to the loss of potassium from cells as blood clots due to high numbers of blood components in PV and relatively smaller volume of distribution due to the raised haematocrit.

Differential diagnosis

Causes of secondary polycythaemia:

- Chronic hypoxia (lung disease, heart disease, high altitude)
- Long-term smoking
- Abnormal haemoglobins
- Increased erythropoietin production (renal tumours, other malignancies)

Key points

- Polycythaemia may be 'true' or 'apparent'.
- Primary polycythaemia is associated with an increased risk of venous and arterial thrombosis.
- Nearly all patients with primary polycythaemia are JAK2-positive.
- Treatment includes venesection and drugs aimed at platelet count reduction.

CASE 68: MIDDLE-AGED MAN WITH CELLULITIS

History

A 46-year-old man presented to his GP after feeling generally under the weather, while suffering from cellulitis over the left thigh. The cellulitis had developed over the past few days and by now was bright red, painful and hot to touch. He denied any other symptoms of infection, or any bleeding or bruising problems. He had not had any recent insect bites or skin breaks, and was not diabetic. He had been given a course of flucloxacillin from his GP for a week without any improvement in the erythema, so blood tests were arranged.

His past medical history included hypertension and recently diagnosed rheumatoid arthritis. He had no known drug allergies and was on ramipril, diclofenac and sulphasalazine, which had been started 10 weeks previously for his rheumatoid arthritis. He drank 3–4 pints of beer a week and did not smoke. He lived with his wife and worked in sales for a local double glazing firm.

Examination

On examination, he was febrile at 39.2°C and sweaty. He had obvious erythema over his left upper anterior thigh, along with a couple of small sub-centimetre tender lymph nodes in the left groin. His chest was clear to auscultation. His pulse was 110 bpm regular and heart sounds and blood pressure were normal. His abdomen was soft and non-tender, with no liver or spleen palpable. Calves were soft and non-tender with no ankle oedema present.

Investigations

		Reference range
Haemoglobin	12.2 g/dL	13.5–18.0 g/dL
White cell count	0.2×10^9/L	$4.0–11.0 \times 10^9$/L
Neutrophils	0.0×10^9/L	$2.0–7.5 \times 10^9$/L (40–75%)
Lymphocytes	0.2×10^9/L	$1.5–4.0 \times 10^9$/L (20–45%)
Mean corpuscular volume (MCV)	81 fL	76–96 fL
Haematocrit	0.38	0.40–0.54
Platelets	225×10^9/L	$150–400 \times 10^9$/L
Sodium	143 mmol/L	135–146 mmol/L
Potassium	4.0 mmol/L	3.5–5.0 mmol/L
Urea	8.2 mmol/L	2.5–6.7 mmol/L
Creatinine	92 µmol/L	79–118 µmol/L

		Reference range
Bilirubin	16 µmol/L	3–17 µmol/L
Alkaline phosphatase (ALP)	41 U/L	39–130 U/L
Alanine aminotransferase (ALT)	7 U/L	5–40 U/L
Total protein	72 g/L	60–80 g/L
Albumin	45 g/L	35–50 g/L
Glucose	5.1 mmol/L	3.5–4.5 mmol/L (fasting)
C-reactive protein (CRP)	263 mg/L	<5 mg/L

QUESTIONS

1. What is the primary abnormality on the blood count?
2. What is the likely cause of this abnormality?
3. What treatment is required?

ANSWERS

1 and 2. This man has developed cellulitis compounded by profound neutropenia, making it difficult to treat, and producing constitutional symptoms. His profound neutropenia is occurring in the face of a normal platelet count, and near normal haemoglobin. A recent full blood count would be useful to determine the rapidity of neutrophil decline and to ensure it is a new phenomenon. There are many possible causes of neutropenia (see list below), but not many cause such an isolated low neutrophil count. The likely diagnosis here is therefore a drug-induced neutropenia/marrow failure secondary to sulphasalazine, which had only recently been started.

3. Treatment in suspected drug-induced bone marrow failure/neutropenia is to immediately withdraw the suspected drug wherever possible. Antibiotic therapy will be required for the cellulitis and, in view of the neutropenia, an admission to a side room for intravenous antibiotics with broad-spectrum cover is imperative, in case other underlying infections are present. There may be a role for granulocyte colony-stimulating factor (G-CSF) injections in an attempt to raise the neutrophil count faster, although this is not supported by high quality data. The neutropenia usually recovers within a few days to a few weeks, with the median time to neutrophil recovery being 10 days. In cases where the diagnosis is unclear, or where neutrophil recovery is slow, a bone marrow examination may be required to rule out other underlying pathologies, such as aplastic anaemia, acute leukaemia or myelodysplastic syndromes.

In younger patients, the possibility of inherited bone marrow failure syndromes (inherited aplastic anaemia) should be considered, although a pancytopenia would be more usual as an outcome, rather than just neutropenia. These conditions include Fanconi anaemia, dyskeratosis congenita, and Schwachman–Diamond syndrome, among others. Referral to a specialist paediatric haematology centre would be required if considering these diagnoses.

Differential diagnosis

- Drugs
- Haematinic deficiencies
- Viral infections
- Primary bone marrow pathologies (myelodysplastic syndrome, acute leukaemia, aplastic anaemia)
- Autoimmune conditions

Key points

- Isolated neutropenia is usually caused by acute viral infections, autoimmune conditions or drugs, whereas bone marrow disorders tend to cause reductions in two or more cell lines.
- Prolonged neutropenia not responding to therapy should be investigated by bone marrow examination.
- Broad-spectrum antibiotics should be used in the management of neutropenic sepsis patients, in line with local protocols.

SECTION 4: CARDIOLOGY

Case 69: Elderly man with palpitations

Case 70: Elderly man with chest pain

Case 71: Middle-aged man with syncope

Case 72: Middle-aged woman with chest pain

Case 73: Middle-aged man with light headedness

Case 74: Young woman with palpitations

Case 75: Elderly woman with chest pain

Case 76: Elderly man with syncope

Case 77: Middle-aged woman with chest pain

Case 78: Young woman with syncope

Case 79: Middle-aged man with abdominal pain

Case 80: Elderly man with palpitations

Case 81: Elderly woman with fever and weight loss

Case 82: Young man with shortness of breath

Case 83: Young man undergoing army medical

Case 84: Woman with increasing shortness of breath

Case 85: Elderly man with atrial fibrillation

Case 86: Elderly man with kidney disease

Case 87: Young man with central chest pain

Case 88: Young man with palpitations

CASE 69: ELDERLY MAN WITH PALPITATIONS

History

A 75-year-old retired mechanic presents with shortness of breath on exertion and palpitations present for 1 week. He has had minimal ankle swelling, but no paroxysmal nocturnal dyspnoea, orthopnoea or chest pain. He has a past medical history of hypertension for which he takes bendrofluazide 2.5 mg/daily. He is an ex-smoker (gave up 12 years ago smoking 30/day from the age of 15). He drinks four cups of tea a day and drinks three pints of strong lager per night.

Examination

He is comfortable at rest with warm well-perfused peripheries. His pulse is 120 irregularly irregular, blood pressure (BP) 160/90 mmHg, jugular venous pressure (JVP) +3 cm, apex beat is not displaced, the first heart sound is variable and no murmurs are heard. The chest is clear and there is minimal ankle oedema. The rest of his examination is normal. His electrocardiogram (ECG) is shown in Figure 69.1.

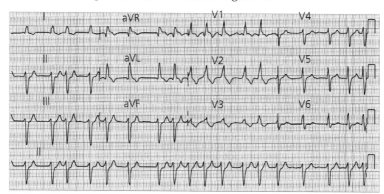

Figure 69.1

Blood results

Full blood count is normal.

		Reference range
Sodium	143 mmol/L	135–146 mmol/L
Potassium	3.2 mmol/L	3.2–5.1 mmol/L
Urea	4.1 mmol/L	1.7–8.3 mmol/L
Creatinine	97 µmol/L	62–106 µmol/L
Troponin T	80 ng/L	<14 ng/L

QUESTIONS

1. What is the ECG diagnosis?
2. Give three factors that would contribute to the causation of this condition?
3. What treatment options are available acutely for this condition?
4. What measures should be taken in the long term?
5. What is his pack-year total?
6. Give three causes for the positive tropinin T result?

ANSWERS

1. The ECG shows:

   a. Fast atrial fibrillation. There are irregularly timed QRS complexes with the absence of p-waves. Any rate over 100 bpm is deemed tachycardic.
   b. Left axis deviation: negative QRS complex in lead aVF and lead II with a positive QRS complex in lead I.
   c. Right bundle branch block: broad QRS (over three small squares) and rSR pattern in V1 (see Figure 69.2).

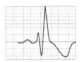

Figure 69.2

- **Bundle branch block.** Left and right ventricular co-ordinated contraction is mediated by the specialized electrical conduction tissue. This originates in the AV node and then is transmitted along the His tissue which broadly separates into a left and right bundle. This organized ventricular depolarization occurs in no longer than 120 ms, hence the QRS complex should be no broader than three small squares (3×40 ms = 120 ms). In cases of bundle branch block, there is a delay in the conduction along one of the branches (the left or right bundle) compared with the other. This results in a lengthening of the time taken for complete ventricular depolarization and hence widening of the QRS complex to 120 ms or greater.
- **Left bundle branch block (LBBB).** LBBB is always pathological. Causes include hypertension, aortic stenosis, acute myocardial infarction, coronary artery disease and primary conducting system disease. Along with the widening of the QRS V1 should have a QS or rS pattern and RsR' in V6.
- **Right bundle branch block (RBBB).** RBBB can be a normal finding in young slim men. The QRS is broad. In contrast to LBBB, there is a rSR' pattern seen in V1 and a qRs pattern seen in V6.

A mnemonic to remember the difference in ECG findings between LBBB and RBBB is:

	V1		V6
LBBB, WiLLiaM	(QS or rS) W	iLLia	M (RsR')
RBBB, MaRRoW	(rSR') M	aRRo	W (qRs)

2. Contributing factors to the atrial fibrillation in this case include age, alcohol, hypertension, caffeine and hypokalaemia. Other common causes include acute insult (medical, surgical or traumatic), valvular heart disease, ischaemic heart disease and thyroid disease.

3. Acute treatment. The patient is haemodynamically stable as evidenced by his warm peripheries and blood pressure. He has had symptoms of atrial fibrillation for over a week and therefore acute cardioversion is not appropriate due to the embolic stroke risk. The goal of treatment should therefore be rate control in the first instance.

   a. Drug therapy. The main drugs used are β-blockers and calcium-channel antagonists. Digoxin can be used, but is less effective. Digoxin should not be used alone (except in immobile patients) for rate control in atrial fibrillation as it loses all effectiveness on exercise. Amiodarone and flecainide should be reserved for attempting chemical cardioversion. Dronedarone should not be used for cardioversion (dronedarone is a new anti-arrhythmic agent used for paroxysmal atrial fibrillation which has similar properties to amiodarone but with a reduced side-effect profile). This patient would need to be anticoagulated (warfarin would be most appropriate) for at least 4 weeks before considering cardioversion.

   b. Electrical therapy. As with chemical cardioversion, DC (direct current) electrical cardioversion should only be attempted in the context of a clear history of atrial fibrillation lasting no more than 24 hours, if the patient has been adequately warfarinized for at least 4 weeks or if they have had a transoesophageal echocardiogram (TOE) demonstrating absence of left atrial thrombus. The exception to this is if the patient is haemodynamically unstable in which case electrical cardioversion should be performed as a matter of urgency. This is true of any tachyarrhythmia.

   c. Other factors. The hypokalaemia which is likely to be secondary to his thaizide diuretic should be treated. Acute medical insults, such as pneumonia and pulmonary embolism, should be looked for and treated, most physicians would use low-molecular-weight heparin in these patients to try to reduce the stroke risk.

4. Long term management. This would include tight blood pressure control, reduce/cease alcohol intake and stop caffeine intake. The patient must be adequately rate controlled. The patient should be anticoagulated with warfarin. Rhythm control could be considered – this can be drug therapy – amiodarone, flecainide, dronedarone and/or DC cardioversion and/or ablation therapy. If rhythm control is not attempted or fails, then rate control would be essential. This is usually achieved with medication, but may require a pacemaker and AV node ablation. Other investigations would include blood tests especially thyroid function and a chest x-ray, an echocardiogram, assessment for cardiac ischaemia, (stress test, cardiac magnetic resonance imaging or nuclear medicine scan). Coronary computed tomography (CT) scan is used to evaluate coronary artery patency.

5. Pack-years. This is worked out according to number of years smoked and number of cigarettes smoked per day. Smoking 20/day for one year is one pack-year. Here, number of years smoking is 75 minus years not smoking (i.e. 15, started at this age and 12, gave up 12 years ago), he smoked 30 a day for these 48 years. 72 pack-years ($75 - 12 - 15 = 48$ years, 48 years $\times$ 30/20 = 72).

6. Positive troponin T: In this case, the following causes should be considered:

   a. Cardiac ischaemia
   b. Cardiac arrhythmia
   c. Pneumonia
   d. Pulmonary embolism.

   The degree of troponin elevation does correlate with overall mortality, whatever the cause. In this case troponin is only mildly raised (<100 ng/L), so the elevation is unlikely to relate to true cardiac ischaemia.

CASE 70: ELDERLY MAN WITH CHEST PAIN

History

A 73-year-old man presents to his GP with exertional chest discomfort. The pain is sharp and central. The pain does not radiate and there are no associated autonomic symptoms. He has a history of hypertension and hypercholesterolaemia. He is taking ramipril and simvastatin. He has no family history of note.

Examination

Examination is normal. He proceeds with an exercise treadmill test (Figure 70.1).

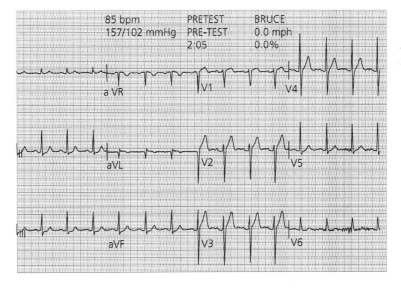

Figure 70.1 (a) At rest.

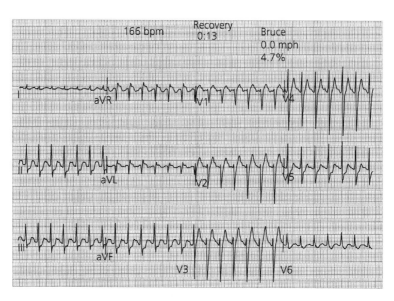

Figure 70.1 (b) At 7 minutes.

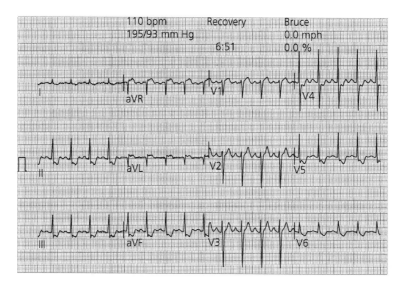

Figure 70.1 (c) At recovery.

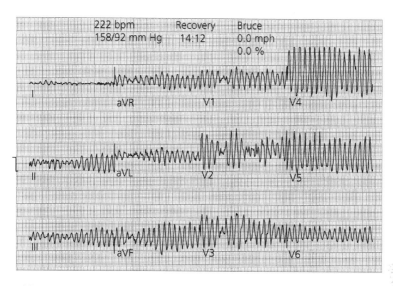

Figure 70.1 (d) At 14 minutes.

QUESTIONS

1. What does the resting electrocardiogram (ECG) show?
2. What does it show in recovery?
3. What does it show at 14 minutes?
4. What is the immediate management?
5. What is the likely underlying diagnosis?

ANSWERS

1. The resting ECG shows:

    a. Normal sinus rhythm
    b. Normal axis
    c. Rate 86 bpm
    d. Left ventricular hypertrophy – S wave in V2 + R wave in V5 >35 mm.

2. The recovery ECG shows deep ST depression inferiorly – arrowed (II, III and aVF) and depression in V5 and V6 with ST elevation in aVL (the lateral territory) (Figure 70.2).

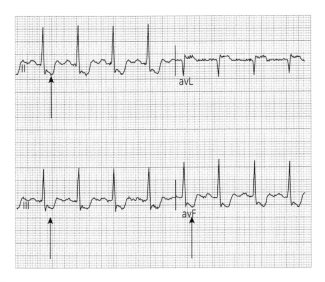

Figure 70.2

3. Ventricular fibrillation.

4. DC (direct current) cardioversion.

5. Severe ischaemic heart disease.

Figure 70.3 shows the normal ECG complex and how the varying key measurements are obtained.

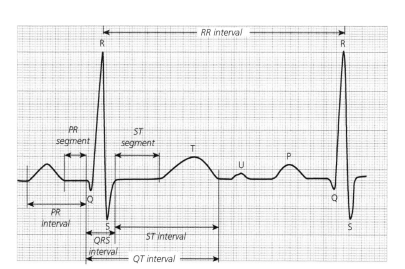

Figure 70.3

CASE 71: MIDDLE-AGED MAN WITH SYNCOPE

History and Investigations

You are called to see a 54-year-old man on the ward who has become acutely dizzy. He was admitted with syncope 4 hours ago. He has a history of intermittent dizziness for the last 3 weeks. He has a history of hypertension and was started on a medication by his GP recently for this, but cannot remember its name. His admission examination was recorded as normal. His admission blood tests were normal as was his chest x-ray. Figure 71.1 shows his admission electrocardiogram (ECG) and Figure 71.2 is his current ECG tracing.

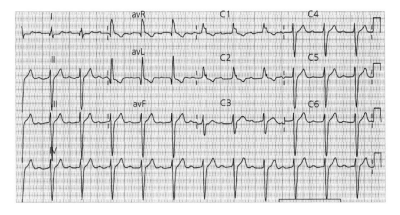

Figure 71.1

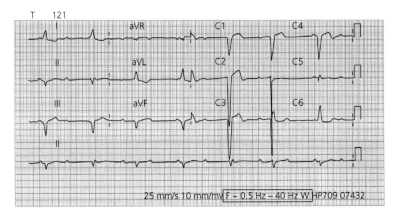

Figure 71.2

While you are looking at the ECG, the patient loses consciousness. The senior sister has bleeped your senior doctor, but she is at an arrest call and will be delayed for 5 minutes.

QUESTIONS

1. What does the admission ECG show?
2. What does the ECG show now?
3. Given the patient's condition, what medication might the GP have started?
4. What are the immediate treatment options (list three) while awaiting senior support?

ANSWERS

1. The admission ECG shows:
   a. Sinus rhythm
   b. Rate 67 bpm
   c. Left axis deviation
   d. First-degree heart block (PR interval = 360 ms)
   e. Right bundle branch block (QRS width = 160 ms, RSR pattern in V1)

ECG features of first-degree heart block
• PR interval >5 small squares/200 ms   • No dropped beats (all p-waves conducted)   • Stable PR interval

   The ECG pattern in this case indicates trifascicular block (proximal conductive tissue disease) and is associated with a 2 per cent per year risk of complete heart block.

2. The ECG now shows complete heart block (third-degree heart block). The P-waves are dissociated from the QRS complexes indicating complete AV block. Other clues are the broad QRS complexes (over three small squares) and the heart rate (between 30 and 40 beats per minute). Beware that if the escape rhythm originates from high up in the bundle of His, then the QRS may be narrow and the rate will be nearer 50 bpm, therefore the AV dissociation will be the only clue. Note that the computer interpretation on the ECG is incorrect. Dissociated p-waves are shown in Figure 71.3. In the first ECG, the origin of the ventricular beat is through the AV node via the bundle of His causing a RBBB (right bundle branch block) pattern. In the second ECG, the QRS morphology has changed, due to a different origin of the ventricular beat (due to the complete heart block).

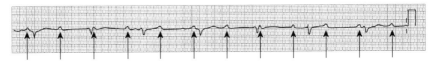

Figure 71.3

3. Drugs that are used for hypertension and cause AV block include beta-blockers and the non-dihydropyridine calcium-channel antagonists, such as verapamil.

4. Immediate treatment options are atropine (parasympathetic inhibitor), chronotropic drugs, e.g. isoprenaline (sympathetic agonist), percussion pacing (as described in Advanced Life Support) and transcutaneous pacing via a defibrillator.

   This patient is in extreme peril and immediate action is required. A temporary pacing wire would take too long to insert. The above methods allow rapid return to a more acceptable heart rate and buy time for more complex treatments. You should familiarize yourself with the hospital defibrillators as they may vary between trusts. Transcutaneous pacing via a defibrillator can be life-saving.

CASE 72: MIDDLE-AGED WOMAN WITH CHEST PAIN

History

You are asked to see a 57-year-old woman who has presented to A&E with central chest pain, sweats and pallor. The nurse acquired an electrocardiogram (ECG) just as you arrive and the patient passes out (Figure 72.1).

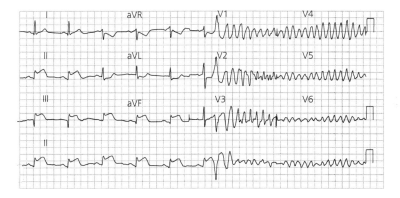

Figure 72.1

QUESTIONS

1. Can you describe the ECG findings from the limb leads?
2. What is the diagnosis from the limb leads?
3. What arrhythmia is present in the chest leads?
4. What event provoked this arrhythmia?
5. What is the immediate treatment?

ANSWERS

1. The ECG shows:

    a. Normal sinus rhythm
    b. Rate 60 bpm
    c. Normal axis
    d. ST elevation in leads II, III and aVF.

2. Acute inferior myocardial infarction.

3. Ventricular fibrillation (VF).

4. R on T phenomenon: during the repolarization period, an ectopic beat occurs triggered by the unstable infarcting myocardium. This is turn initiates VF (Figure 72.2).

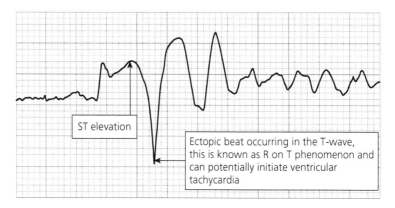

Figure 72.2

5. Direct current (DC) cardioversion.

CASE 73: MIDDLE-AGED MAN WITH LIGHT HEADEDNESS

History

A 45-year-old man presents to A&E with light headedness. He has otherwise been fit and well. He has no past medical history and is on no medications. He has not lost consciousness.

Examination

On examination, his pulse is 40 bpm and regular. All other examination findings are normal.

His electrocardiogram (ECG) is shown in Figure 73.1.

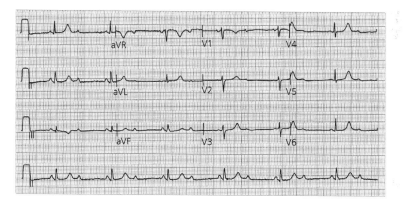

Figure 73.1

QUESTIONS

1. What does his ECG show?
2. What are the possible causes of this condition?
3. What treatment is indicated in this man?

ANSWERS

1. The ECG shows:

   a. Sinus rhythm
   b. Rate 40 bpm
   c. Normal axis
   d. 2:1 heart block (second-degree heart block).

ECG features of second-degree heart block
Unlike complete heart block where there is complete dissociation between P-wave and the QRS, in second-degree block P-wave conduction is intermittent (AV node refractory), usually a 2:1 ratio (can be 3:1, 4:1, variable or lengthening, the Wenckebach phenomenon).

2. The possible causes of this condition are ischaemic heart disease, sarcoidosis, Lyme disease, thyroid disease, strong parasympathetic response, drugs such as digoxin and verapamil.

3. Initial management: admission, investigation and observation are required in the first instance. Symptomatic 2:1 block with no reversible cause will require a dual-chamber permanent pacemaker. There has been no syncope, so a temporary pacing wire is not required at this stage.

CASE 74: YOUNG WOMAN WITH PALPITATIONS

History

A 24-year-old woman presents with rapid palpitations and shortness of breath. These came on very suddenly. She has suffered short episodes in the past, but these have always self-terminated. She has no other past medical history, is on no medications and does not use recreational drugs.

Examination

She is warm and well perfused. Her pulse is 180 bpm regular, blood pressure (BP) 100/60 mmHg, jugular venous pressure (JVP) +2 cm, apex beat is normal, no heaves or thrills, heart sounds are normal. The rest of the examination is entirely normal.

Figure 74.1 shows her admission electrocardiogram (ECG) and Figure 74.2 her ECG after treatment.

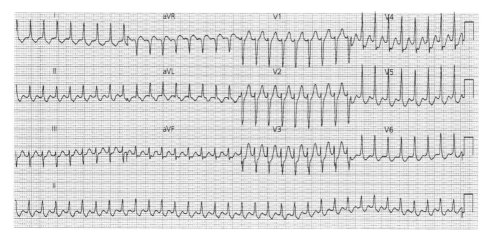

Figure 74.1

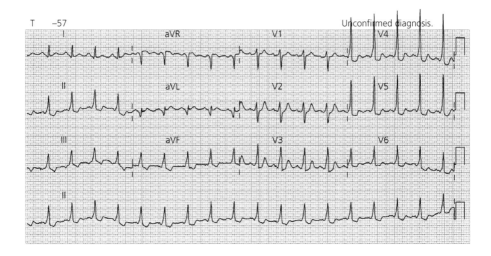

Figure 74.2

QUESTIONS

1. What does the admission ECG show (Figure 74.1)?
2. What treatment could she have received (list three different modes of treatment)?
3. What does the post-treatment ECG show (Figure 74.2)?
4. What is the underlying diagnosis?
5. Which drug therapy is contraindicated for treatment of her arrhythmia?
6. What is the definitive treatment for her condition?

ANSWERS

1. The admission ECG shows:

   a. Narrow complex tachycardia – probable SVT (supraventricular tachycardia). The differential diagnosis includes sinus tachycardia, atrial fibrillation with a fast ventricular rate (although the rhythm is regular, so this is unlikely) and atrial flutter (which often has a ventricular rate of 150 bpm)
   b. Rate 180–200 bpm
   c. Normal axis.

2. Treatment options. Vagal manoeuvres (blowing hard against closed lips, cold water splashed into face, carotid massage), adenosine, beta-blockers/calcium-channel antagonists/flecanide/amiodarone (not digoxin) and direct current (DC) cardioversion.

3. Post-treatment ECG shows:

   a. Sinus tachycardia
   b. Rate 105 bpm
   c. Normal axis
   d. Short PR interval – 80 ms (normal 3–5 small squares = 120–200 ms)
   e. Delta wave most prominent V3–V4. The delta wave is a slurred upstroke of the QRS complex, causing apparent QRS widening (see Figure 74.3). Note the slurred QRS upstroke (arrowed – the delta wave). The short PR interval and delta waves are signs of pre-excitation.

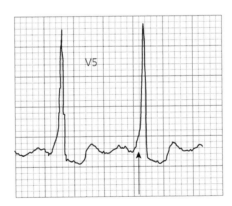

Figure 74.3 Arrow shows delta wave

4. Underlying diagnosis. Wolff–Parkinson–White (WPW) syndrome – congenital accessory pathway conduction between the atria and ventricles.

5. Contraindicated medication. Digoxin – this drug will slow AV (atrioventricular) node conduction exclusively and therefore encourage conduction along the accessory pathway. The accessory pathway in this example conducts at a very high

rate – far faster than the AV node, encouraging conduction along the accessory pathway. If atrial fibrillation develops, uncontrolled conduction along the accessory pathway can lead to ventricular fibrillation and death.

6. Definitive treatment. Electrophysiological studies with accessory pathway ablation would be appropriate.

CASE 75: ELDERLY WOMAN WITH CHEST PAIN

History

A 62-year-old woman presents with 1 hour of central crushing chest pain radiating into her neck. She is sweaty and pale. She has a past medical history of diet-controlled diabetes and hyperlipidaemia.

Examination

She is pale and diaphoretic, pulse 50 regular, blood pressure (BP) 110/70 mmHg, jugular venous pressure (JVP) has cannon waves, normal apex beat, normal heart sounds. The chest is clear and the abdomen is soft and non-tender. Figure 75.1 shows her electrocardiogram (ECG).

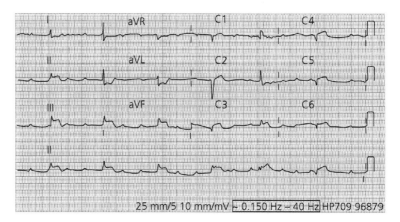

Figure 75.1

QUESTIONS

1. Describe the ECG.
2. What is the diagnosis?
3. Can you describe why the complication has occurred and what other potential complications are there of this acute condition (give four complications)?
4. What is the definitive treatment plan?
5. Explain the JVP appearance and what is the normal upper value?

ANSWERS

1. The ECG shows:

   a. Narrow complex regular rhythm
   b. Rate 38 bpm
   c. Normal axis
   d. Dissociated P-waves and QRS complexes (complete heart block)
   e. ST elevation II, III, aVF.

   Once you find the obvious P-waves be sure to recheck for 'hidden' P-waves often buried in QRS complexes and T-waves. The P-wave rate is often regular and therefore gaps in the easily identified P-waves will reveal their 'hiding spots' (see Figure 75.2 arrowed).

   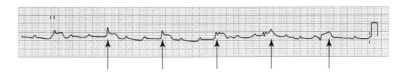

Figure 75.1 Arrows on p waves

2. Inferior STEMI with complete heart block (STEMI: ST elevation myocardial infarction).

3. The right coronary artery has a branch to the AV node. The inferior wall of the heart is often supplied by the right coronary artery which is likely blocked in this case. The presence of complete heart block suggests the branch to the AV node is also blocked.

   Other complications include ventricular arrhythmia, reduced left ventricular function leading to acute left ventricular failure, right ventricular failure, ischaemic ventricular septal defect and acute mitral regurgitation due to papillary muscle rupture.

4. Right coronary artery occlusion is the most likely underlying cause for this presentation and therefore opening of this vessel should be the priority. Primary percutaneous intervention is now the gold standard treatment. If the complete heart block does not resolve, a temporary pacing wire might be required.

5. The presence of AV dissociation causes the right atrium to contract against a closed tricuspid valve resulting in a column of blood shooting up the jugular vein – a cannon wave.

CASE 76: ELDERLY MAN WITH SYNCOPE

History

An 81-year-old man presents with a single syncopal attack. There was no warning, it lasted about 30 seconds and he felt well on regaining consciousness. He states that he has been struggling with stairs due to his breathing over the last two months.

Examination

He has a slow rising pulse with a blood pressure of 110/85 mmHg. On auscultation, he has an ejection systolic murmur radiating to the carotids. Figure 76.1 shows his electrocardiogram (ECG) results.

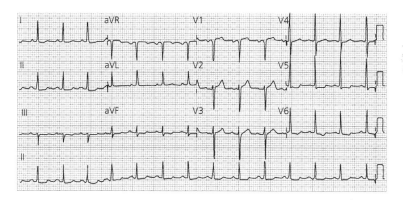

Figure 76.1

QUESTIONS

1. What does the ECG show?
2. What is the diagnosis?
3. What are the long-term treatment options?

ANSWERS

1. The ECG shows:

   a. Sinus rhythm
   b. Rate 90 bpm
   c. Normal axis
   d. P-mitrale (bifid P-wave, best seen in lead II, may signify enlarged left atrium)
   e. Left ventricular hypertrophy (LVH–S-wave in V2 + R-wave in V5 = 37 mm, over 35 mm = LVH) (see Figure 76.2, showing (a) V2 S-wave = 16 mm and (b) V5 R-wave = 21 mm, ST depression is present).
   f. ST depression and T-wave inversion V5 and V6.

   The ST changes and T-wave inversion do not represent ischemia. In the context of LVH these usually represent changes in repolarization due to the hypertrophy. This is described as LVH with strain.

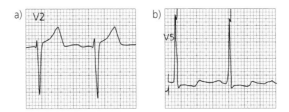

Figure 76.2

2. This patient has the correct history, examination and ECG consistent with severe aortic stenosis, namely syncope, shortness of breath, slow rising pulse, narrow pulse pressure and an ejection systolic murmur radiating to the carotids.

3. The reference standard therapy is open heart surgical replacement of the valve. Alternatively, a transcatheter valve implant (TAVI) can be performed percutaneously. Aortic balloon valvuloplasty is a palliative option.

CASE 77: MIDDLE-AGED WOMAN WITH CHEST PAIN

History

A 48-year-old woman presents with central crushing chest pain that radiates to her back. She has a history of poorly controlled hypertension. She is pale and sweaty. Blood pressure (BP) is 210/120 mmHg in both arms, pulse is 110 bpm regular, chest is clear, jugular venous pressure (JVP) and heart sounds are normal. She has been given 10 mg of i.v. morphine by the A&E staff with little improvement in her pain.

Examination

Figure 77.1 shows the results of her electrocardiogram (ECG). An AP (anteroposterior) chest x-ray was also undertaken (Figure 77.2).

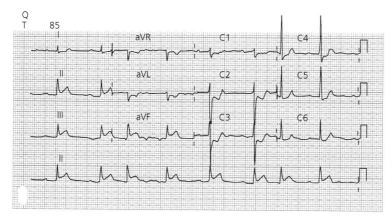

Figure 77.1

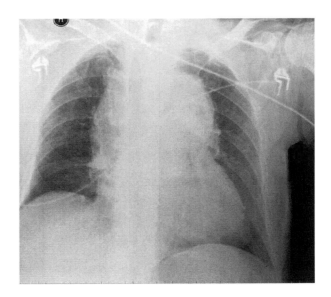

Figure 77.2

QUESTIONS

1. What are the ECG findings?
2. What does the chest x-ray show?
3. How can you explain the ECG findings?
4. What is the most likely diagnosis?
5. What investigation is needed urgently?
6. What is the immediate treatment?
7. What is the mortality of this condition if untreated?

ANSWERS

1. This ECG shows:

   a. Sinus bradycardia
   b. Rate 47 bpm
   c. Normal axis
   d. First-degree heart block (PR interval = 360 ms)
   e. Left ventricular hypertrophy (LVH) (S-wave in V2 + R-wave in V5 = 47 mm)
   f. ST elevation leads II, III and aVF.
   g. ST depression with biphasic T-waves in leads V1, V2, V3 and aVL.

   The ECG shows an acute inferior STEMI (STEMI: ST elevation myocardial infarction). The changes in the other leads may be reciprocal or may represent posterior
   wall involvement. When considering posterior wall involvement turn the ECG paper
   upside down and look through from the back of the paper at lead V1 or V2 –
   consider posterior involvement if ST elevation is seen (see Figure 77.3).

   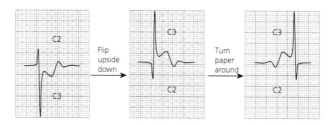

   Figure 77.3

2. This is an AP chest radiograph. This projection does cause some magnification of
   the heart size and mediastinal contour. Allowing for this, there is a widening of the
   mediastinum suggestive of mediastinal haematoma.

3. (Answers 3 and 4). The primary diagnosis is likely type A aortic dissection that is
   involving the right coronary artery (RCA) causing the secondary problems of acute
   inferior infarction with posterior wall involvement and first-degree heart block
   (arterial branch to the AV node from the RCA). Besides the dissection, LVH confirms
   end organ damage from hypertension. Aortic dissection can be divided into type A
   (involves ascending aorta/arch proximal to the origin of the left subclavian artery)
   or type B (where the dissection involves the aorta distal to the left subclavian artery
   origin). The division is important as type A lesions require surgical repair, type B
   can be managed conservatively (medical treatment of hypertension). Aortic stents
   can be used in some cases.

5. Computed tomography (CT) scan of the aorta (emergency transoesophageal echocardiography can also be of use if available faster than CT scanning and also can
   visualize the ascending aorta if CT is of poor quality). Figure 77.4 is an axial post-
   contrast CT in a patient with a type A dissection. Note intimal dissection flap in the
   ascending (paired arrows) and descending (single arrow) aorta.

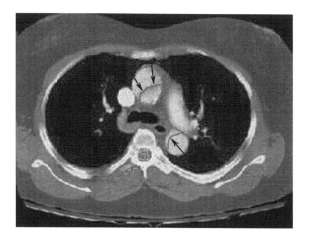

Figure 77.4

6. Urgent surgery is required to repair the dissection; in the interim the hypertension should be treated aggressively.

7. Mortality is approximately 1 per cent for each hour untreated.

CASE 78: YOUNG WOMAN WITH SYNCOPE

History

A 22-year-old woman has had several episodes of unexplained syncope. She undergoes a tilt table test (Figures 78.1 and 78.2).

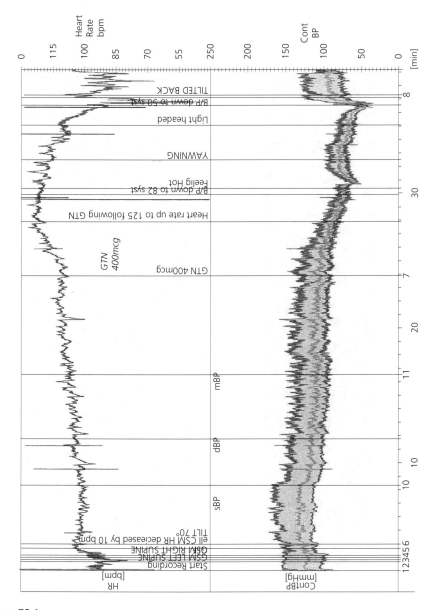

Figure 78.1

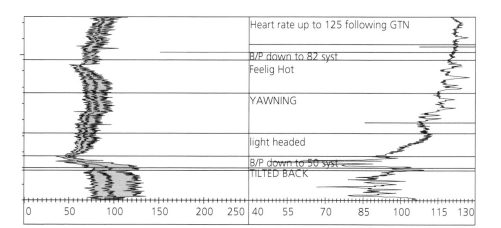

Figure 78.2

QUESTIONS

1. What physiological effect does glyceryl trinitrate (GTN) have?
2. Can you describe the vital signs during the test?
3. What is the diagnosis?
4. What is the management of this condition?

ANSWERS

Tilt table testing is used to measure and test an individual's autonomic response (in particular blood pressure and pulse) to certain stimuli, namely supine to upright manoeuvre and a vasodilatory medication. It is most commonly performed on patients with suspected vasovagal syncope. Typically, the patient's measurements are recorded while lying supine and the patient is then tilted upright to 70° on a special 'tilt table'. The patient is then monitored for 20 minutes before administering a vasodilating agent, such as GTN, and then monitored for a further 20 minutes. The test is stopped after 40 minutes or when the patient develops syncope or a near syncopal attack. A drop in pulse and blood pressure associated with syncope/near syncope is highly suggestive of vasovagal syncope.

1. (Answers 1 and 2). The blood pressure and pulse are fairly stable until the GTN is given. At this point, there is a modest increase in pulse rate. This is a normal physiological response to maintain blood pressure (BP). To understand these two formulae are important:

   BP = systemic resistance × cardiac output

   Cardiac output = stroke volume × pulse rate.

   GTN vasodilates therefore reducing the systemic resistance. Therefore, to maintain BP, the cardiac output must increase. This is achieved by an increase in pulse rate.

   Following this, the blood pressure drops very low at which point the patient would faint. The BP drop is followed by a drop in the pulse rate.

3. This case is classical for a vasovagal response.

4. About 50 per cent of the population will suffer from a vasovagal attack during their lifetime. They are benign and therefore reassurance is important. Some patients unfortunately suffer from frequent attacks. Adequate hydration and salt intake is important. Advice on isometric exercises before standing, standing slowly and preparing to sit or lie down, if symptoms develop, is important. Stopping medications, such as beta-blockers, opiates, antidepressants, angiotensin-converting enzyme (ACE) inhibitors, that slow the normal physiological responses should be considered. The evidence for medication to prevent attacks or tilt training is weak.

CASE 79: MIDDLE-AGED MAN WITH ABDOMINAL PAIN

History

A 56-year-old man is admitted under the surgeons with upper abdominal pain, nausea and lethargy. He has a past medical history of hypertension, but is on no medications.

Examination

He is found to have a pulse of 110 bpm regular, blood pressure (BP) 100/50 mmHg, jugular venous pressure (JVP) at 6 cm above the sternoclavicular joint, a strong apical thrill with a loud pan-systolic murmur throughout the precordium. The respiratory rate is 20 per minute and the chest is clear. The upper abdomen is tender, but there is no guarding and bowel sounds are normal. He is referred for a medical review after the blood results are obtained. The medical registrar has reviewed the history and elicited a history of some vague chest discomfort about a week prior to admission.

Investigations

		Reference range
Sodium	138 mmol/L	135–146 mmol/L
Potassium	3.8 mmol/L	3.2–5.1 mmol/L
Urea	14 mmol/L	1.7–8.3 mmol/L
Creatinine	160 µmol/L	62–106 µmol/L
Haemoglobin (Hb)	15.1 g/dL	13.5–18.0 g/dL
White blood cells (WBC)	14.2×10^9/L	$4.0–11.0 \times 10^9$/L
Neutrophils	12.3×10^9/L	$2.0–7.5 \times 10^9$/L
Troponin T	2 ng/L	<14 ng/L
Alkaline phosphatase (ALP)	300 IU/L	40–129 IU/L
Alanine aminotransferase (ALT)	230 IU/L	<41 IU/L

Figure 79.1 shows his electrocardiogram (ECG) and Figure 79.2 shows his echocardiogram.

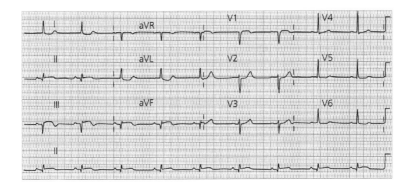

Figure 79.1

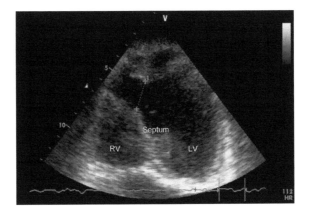

Figure 79.2

QUESTIONS

1. What does the ECG show?
2. What does the echocardiogram show (see calipers)? (RV, right ventricle; LV, left ventricle). The ventricular septum is labelled.
3. What complication has occurred?
4. How would you describe this patient's condition?
5. Describe and give an explanation for the patient's blood results.
6. What is the prognosis and definitive treatment for this patient?

ANSWERS

1. The ECG shows:

   a. Sinus bradycardia
   b. Rate 57 bpm
   c. Borderline left axis deviation
   d. Q-waves II, III and aVF
   e. 1–2 mm ST elevation II, III and aVF
   f. Biphasic T-waves II, III and aVF.

   These findings are consistent with an evolving inferior myocardial infarction (Figure 79.3), note ST elevation leads II, III, aVF.

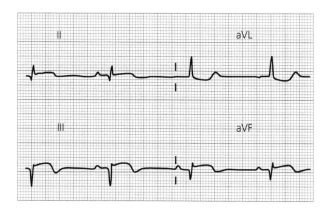

Figure 79.3

2. On this view, there is a defect in the ventricular septum, see the calipers.

3. The clinical findings and the echocardiogram are consistent with a ventricular septal defect (VSD).

4. The patient is tachycardic (not at the time of the ECG), tachypnoeic with cool peripheries. The blood pressure is low (especially considering he is normally hypertensive) and there are signs of organ failure from the blood results. This patient is therefore in shock and, given the likely mechanism is from the VSD, this should be classified as cardiogenic shock.

5. The liver function tests and urea and electrolyte abnormalities are likely to represent hypoperfusion of the organs as a result of cardiogenic shock. The raised neutrophil count is common post-myocardial infarction as the body mounts an immune response to aid repair.

6. The patient's prognosis is poor with 90 per cent of patients succumbing to cardiogenic shock. The only option for this patient is urgent referral to a cardiothoracic surgical team for consideration of VSD repair.

CASE 80: ELDERLY MAN WITH PALPITATIONS

History

A 72-year-old man presents to A&E with palpitations and dizziness on standing.

Examination

On examination, his pulse is 150 bpm and blood pressure (BP) 120/60 mmHg. His jugular venous pressure (JVP) shows cannon waves. Heart sounds are difficult to auscultate clearly or interpret. Figure 80.1 shows his electrocardiogram (ECG).

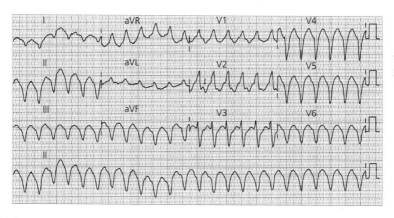

Figure 80.1

QUESTIONS

1. List the ECG findings.
2. Explain what features can be used to indicate the rhythm.
3. What are the treatment options?

ANSWERS

1. The ECG shows:

   a. Broad complex tachycardia (QRS width 190 ms)
   b. Rate 150 bpm
   c. North-west axis
   d. The differential diagnosis for a broad complex tachycardia is ventricular tachycardia or a supraventricular tachycardia with bundle branch block
   e. Positive R-wave in aVR.

2. This rhythm is ventricular tachycardia. Any broad complex tachycardia should be assumed to be ventricular tachycardia until proven otherwise. The features that indicate this rhythm is ventricular tachycardia are:

   AV dissociation (P-waves can be seen in the QRS complexes, arrowed, indicating that the rhythm is independent of the atrial activity, see Figure 80.2). Note that cannon waves on examination also indicate atrioventricular (AV) dissociation as the atrium contracts against a closed tricuspid valve.

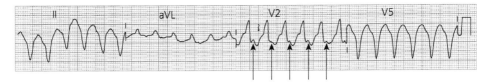

Figure 80.2 Arrows on p waves

3. The patient is currently stable and therefore therapeutic options include:

   a. Medical therapy: correct electrolytes, amiodarone, beta-blockers
   b. Direct current (DC) cardioversion.

   If the patient were to become more unwell (systolic BP below 90 mmHg or signs of cardiogenic shock or heart failure) then electrical cardioversion should be performed immediately.

CASE 81: ELDERLY WOMAN WITH FEVER AND WEIGHT LOSS

History

A 76-year-old woman is referred to the medical team with a history of fever and weight loss over 3 weeks.

Examination

Electrocardiogram (ECG) on admission is shown in Figure 81.1, while Figure 81.2 shows the ECG 2 days after admission. Her echocardiogram is shown in Figure 81.3 (RA, right atrium; LA, left atrium; Ao, aortic root).

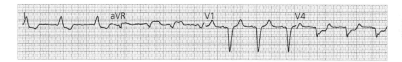

Figure 81.1

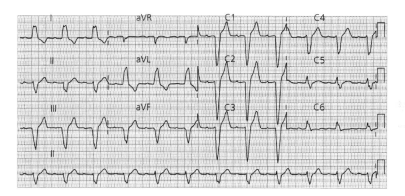

Figure 81.2

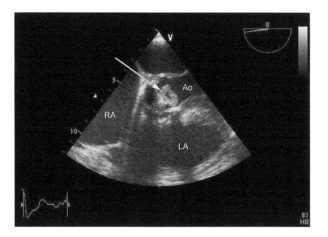

Figure 81.3

QUESTIONS

1. What does the arrow indicate in the echocardiogram and what is the diagnosis?
2. Name three likely causative organisms?
3. Describe the changes on the second ECG?
4. Why is this of concern in this case?
5. What investigation is required?
6. What treatment is required if the suspected complication is confirmed?

ANSWERS

1. Subacute infective endocarditis (see box 'Duke Criteria'). The arrow on the echocardiogram shows a large vegetation on the aortic valve.

2. Three most likely organisms:

    a. *Staphylococcus aureus*
    b. *Streptococcus viridans*
    c. *Enterococcus* spp.

3. The ECG shows:

    a. Sinus rhythm
    b. Rate 73 bpm
    c. Left axis deviation
    d. Left bundle branch block (QRS width 190 ms, RSR in V6)
    e. First-degree heart block (PR interval 260 ms; normal is 120–200 ms).

4. In the first ECG (Figure 81.4a), the PR interval equals 3.5 small squares, which equals 140 ms (40 ms × 3.5). In the second ECG (Figure 81.4b), the PR interval equals 6.5 small squares, which equals 260 ms (40 ms × 6.5). The PR interval has increased (from 140 to 260 ms) since admission which in the context of aortic valve infective endocarditis may indicate an aortic root abscess, see Figure 81.4.

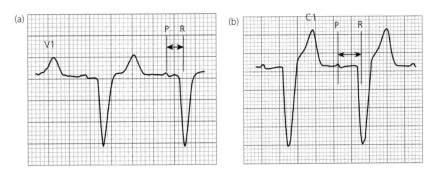

Figure 81.4

5. This patient requires a thorough examination of the heart valves and in particular the aortic root. Initially, a transthoracic echocardiogram may shed some light, but it is likely a transoesophageal echocardiogram will be necessary to fully evaluate the aortic valve and root.

6. The patient should be referred for urgent surgical intervention.

Duke criteria

Established in 1994 by the Duke Endocarditis Society and revised in 2000, the Duke criteria are a collection of major and minor criteria used to establish a diagnosis of endocarditis. A diagnosis can be reached in any of three ways: two major criteria, one major and three minor criteria, or five minor criteria.

A simplified version is listed below:

- Major criteria include:
  - Positive blood culture with typical infective endocarditis microorganism
  - Evidence of endocardial involvement with positive echocardiogram.
- Minor criteria include:
  - Predisposing factor: known cardiac lesion, recreational drug injection
  - Fever >38°C
  - Evidence of embolism: arterial emboli, pulmonary infarcts, Janeway lesions, conjunctival haemorrhage
  - Immunological problems: glomerulonephritis, Osler's nodes
  - Positive blood culture (that does not meet a major criterion) or serologic evidence of infection with organism consistent with infective endocarditis, but not satisfying major criterion.

CASE 82: YOUNG MAN WITH SHORTNESS OF BREATH

History and examination

A 26-year-old man presents to A&E with chest pain and shortness of breath on exertion. He has previously been well and there is nothing to find on examination other than a resting tachycardia. Routine bloods are normal. Figure 82.1 shows results of his electrocardiogram (ECG) and his chest radiograph is shown in Figure 82.2.

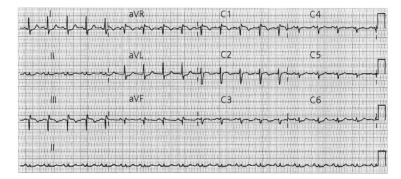

Figure 82.1

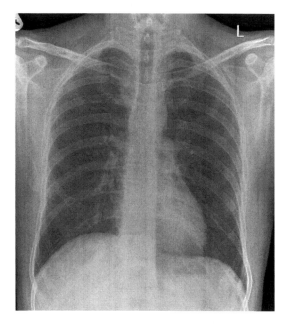

Figure 82.2

QUESTIONS

1. Can you describe the ECG?
2. What is the likely diagnosis?
3. How would you report his chest x-ray?
4. List five potential risk factors?
5. What further investigations may be warranted?

ANSWERS

1. The ECG shows:

    a. Sinus tachycardia
    b. Rate 104 bpm
    c. Normal axis, −26° (normal axis from −30 to +90°)
    d. S-wave lead I, Q-wave lead III, T-wave inversion III (see Figure 82.3).

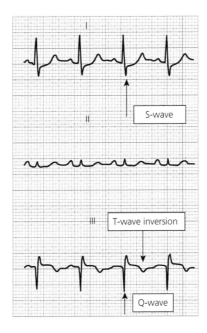

Figure 82.3

2. Pulmonary embolism.

3. His chest x-ray is normal. This is common in patients with pulmonary embolism. Other abnormalities may include:

    a. Areas of linear atelectasis or focal consolidation
    b. A mass which can cavitate
    c. In a large embolus enlargement of the involved pulmonary artery may occur with relative pulmonary oligaemia
    d. Unilateral pleural effusion.

4. Long periods of immobility, long haul flights, recent injury to leg, dehydration, thrombophilic disorders, recent surgical operations, particularly involving lower limb or pelvis.

5. A negative D-dimer in a patient with a low index of clinical suspicion can be useful in exclusion of thromboembolic disease. In patients where there is clinical concern

(Wells score), further investigation is required. The Wells score is an algorithm based on clinical history and examination findings to assess the relative risk of thromboembolic disease in a patient. Computed tomography pulmonary angiography (CTPA) has largely replaced ventilation/perfusion (V/Q) scanning in diagnosis. CTPA is widely available in and out of hours and can directly visualize thrombus. V/Q scans are reserved for patients where contrast-enhanced computed tomography (CT) scan is inappropriate or contraindicated, e.g allergy to iodinated contrast or renal impairment. Some departments use perfusion (Q) scanning alone in pregnant patients (check local protocols).

Figure 82.4 demonstrates a positive CTPA study; note low-density thrombus in the pulmonary arteries. This is a saddle embolus – thrombus is seen in the left pulmonary artery (white arrow) and bifurcation/right pulmonary artery (black arrows).

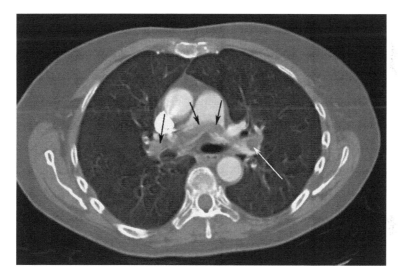

Figure 82.4

Treatment involves anticoagulation and warfarinization. Patients who are haemodynamically compromised with large emboli may need thrombolysis (either peripherally i.v. or directly into thrombus under radiological guidance using femoral vein catheterization) or surgical thrombectomy (depending on local availability of these resources).

CASE 83: YOUNG MAN UNDERGOING ARMY MEDICAL

History and examination

This is a routine electrocardiogram (ECG) on a 19-year-old fit man who has applied to join the army. He is completely well. His physical examination is normal, except his heart sounds are quiet and his apex is not palpable (Figure 83.1).

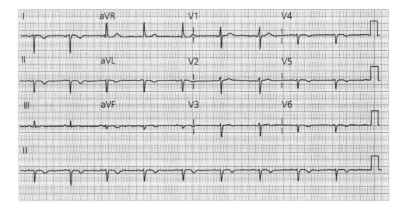

Figure 83.1

QUESTIONS

1. Describe the ECG.
2. Can you explain the physical examination findings?
3. How could you confirm your diagnosis?
4. What is the differential diagnosis for the findings in V1?

ANSWERS

1. The ECG shows:

   a. Sinus bradycardia
   b. Rate 57 bpm
   c. North-west axis
   d. Positive R-wave in V1
   e. Diminishing R-wave across the chest leads
   f. Positive aVR.

2. This ECG suggests dextrocardia. This would explain why the heart sounds are quiet and the apex is impalpable.

3. A chest x-ray and/or placing the ECG leads on the right side of the chest will help confirm your suspicions. The right chest ECG below shows normal R-wave progression across the chest leads (Figure 83.2).

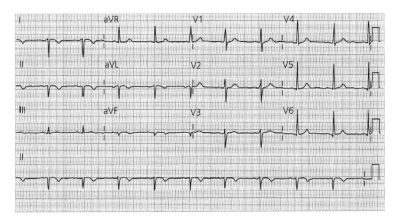

Figure 83.2

4. A positive R-wave in V1 suggests one of the following diagnoses:

   a. Incorrect lead placement
   b. Dextrocardia
   c. Right bundle block
   d. Right ventricular hypertrophy
   e. Posterior myocardial infarction (MI)
   f. WPW (Wolff–Parkinson–White) syndrome.

CASE 84: WOMAN WITH INCREASING SHORTNESS OF BREATH

History

A 36-year-old woman presents with increasing shortness of breath and fatigue. Her symptoms have come on over the last 3 months. She has no medical history of note, except previous treatment for pulmonary tuberculosis 9 months ago.

Examination

She is pale and clammy, pulse is 110 bpm regular, blood pressure (BP) 80/40 mm/Hg, jugular venous pressure (JVP) is raised to the ear lobes and increases on inspiration, the heart sounds are quiet but normal and the cardiac apex not palpable. The lungs sound clear and there is mild ankle oedema.

An electrocardiogram (ECG) (Figure 84.1) and chest x-ray (Figure 84.2) are performed and displayed below. Figure 84.1 includes the V5 rhythm strip.

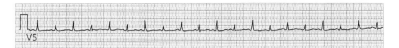

Figure 84.1

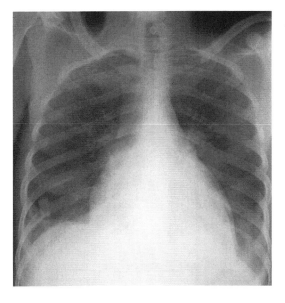

Figure 84.2

QUESTIONS

1. How would you describe her JVP?
2. What would you call the collection of clinical signs?
3. What does the ECG show and how would you account for these changes?
4. What does the chest x-ray show?
5. Which further investigation would be useful?
6. What is the immediate treatment?

ANSWERS

This woman has a pericardial effusion almost certainly secondary to incomplete treatment of her tuberculosis. Her clinical presentation indicates cardiac tamponade – a life-threatening complication.

1. The JVP would normally drop on inspiration as thoracic pressure drops with chest expansion. In this case, the JVP rising is known as Kussmaul's sign and is suggestive of a pericardial effusion. There is a paradoxical rise in the JVP with inspiration suggesting impaired filling of the right ventricle. Restrictive cardiomyopathy and constructive pericarditis are other causes.

2. Muffled heart sounds with hypotension and dilated neck veins/engorged JVP is known as Beck's triad and indicates likely pericardial effusion.

3. The ECG shows:

   a. Rate 120 bpm
   b. Rhythm: sinus rhythm
   c. Axis: normal
   d. Small QRS complexes
   e. Alternating QRS complex size best seen in V5 – electrical alternans (Figure 84.1).

   If the QRS complexes differ from beat to beat this is usually because the origin of the ventricular beat is different. In this case, however, the heart is able to move in the pericardial fluid and hence the QRS size changes beat to beat depending on the location within the chest cavity.

4. The chest x-ray shows globular enlargement of the cardiac shadow. These findings would be consistent with a pericardial effusion.

5. An echocardiogram would be useful in confirming the diagnosis of effusion (Figure 84.4, effusion shown with arrows).

6. Given the patient's immediate life-threatening state, emergency pericardial drainage is warranted, fluid also being sent for culture (including acid-fast bacilli) and cytology. Tuberculosis was confirmed in this case.

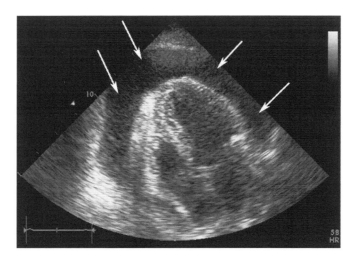

Figure 84.4

CASE 85: ELDERLY MAN WITH ATRIAL FIBRILLATION

History and examination

A 72-year-old man with a history of paroxysmal atrial fibrillation was started on flecainide 4 weeks ago. He has presented to A&E with palpitations and shortness of breath on exertion. He is currently on warfarin, flecainide and ramipril. He has a previous medical history of hypertension. On examination, he looks sweaty with an initial pulse of 150 bpm regular, blood pressure (BP) 140/90mmHg, jugular venous pressure (JVP) is rapidly pulsating and difficult to interpret, his chest is clear and there is no ankle oedema.

Figure 85.1 shows the results of his electrocardiogram (ECG).

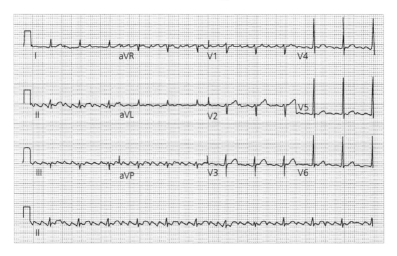

Figure 85.1

QUESTIONS

1. What does the ECG show?
2. What are the immediate treatment options?
3. Name one life-threatening risk from medical treatment of this condition?
4. What treatment option could be considered once he has been discharged?
5. Describe two ways in which this condition may be related to his paroxysmal atrial fibrillation?
6. Is the stroke risk for this condition lower, the same or higher than that of atrial fibrillation?

ANSWERS

1. The ECG shows:

   a. Rate: 100 bpm
   b. Rhythm: regular, saw tooth P-waves with 3:1 heart block (i.e. atrial rate, 300; ventricular rate, 100)
   c. Axis: normal
   d. The ECG shows classical atrial flutter (Figure 85.2).

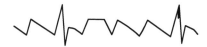

Figure 85.2

2. If the patient is adequately warfarinized, direct current (DC) cardioversion may be appropriate. The patient is already on flecainide so care must be taken on further anti-arrhythmic therapy. The conventional choices would be amiodarone or sotalol, but given the previous flecainide use, a β-blocker or calcium-channel blocker would be a good choice to help control the rate, as they help control rate without significant anti-arrhythmic effects. Digoxin is not a good drug alone, should not be combined with flecanide and should not be used in paroxysmal arrhythmias (it does not cardiovert and can be pro-arrhythmic).

3. The primary risk of medical therapy of atrial flutter is that, as the atrial rate slows from 300, the AV node may allow 1:1 conduction. It is therefore essential that if this arrhythmia is medically treated then the patient is monitored. The table below explains why this might occur if the AV node can conduct at 240 bpm.

Atrial rate	AV block (assuming it can conduct at 240 bpm)	Ventricular rate
300	2:1	150
280	2:1	140
260	2:1	130
240	1:1	240

The top row shows the classical presentation with a rate of 150 beats per minute. This most commonly occurs when the patient is on no rate control medication. If the rate control therapy does not block the AV node as efficiently as it slows the atrial rate, there can be a paradoxical rise in pulse to potentially life-threatening ventricular rates.

4. A very effective long-term therapy for atrial flutter is radiofrequency ablation. The success rates are approximately 90 per cent and the risks are relatively low.

5. Patients with atrial flutter have at least a 40 per cent chance of developing atrial fibrillation. The mechanism is unclear, but atrial abnormalities due to the fast atrial rates may be responsible. It is also well known that anti-arrhythmic drugs, such as flecanide, can change the electrical properties of the atria to promote atrial flutter – i.e. anti-arrhythmic drugs for atrial fibrillation may also be pro-arrhythmic. In this case, the initiation of flecanide may have provoked the atrial flutter.

6. The stroke risk is the same for atrial flutter and fibrillation and patients should be anticoagulated accordingly.

CASE 86: ELDERLY MAN WITH KIDNEY DISEASE

History

A 76-year-old man with a history of hypertensive kidney disease was recently started on a new medication for his blood pressure. He has felt nausea and palpitations over the last 24 hours.

Examination

The only finding on clinical examination is regular ectopic beats and hypertensive retinal changes (grade 2). An electrocardiogram (ECG) is performed while you are awaiting his blood tests (Figure 86.1).

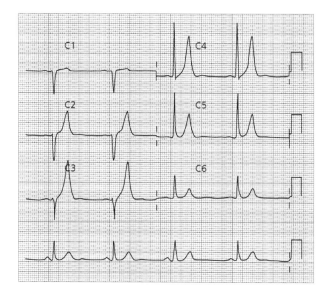

Figure 86.1

QUESTIONS

1. What do the chest leads of this ECG show?
2. What is the differential diagnosis for this appearance (give at least two)?
3. Which blood test is going to be most useful?
4. Name four classes of medication the patient may have been started on and how they may have provoked this ECG appearance?
5. If your suspicions are confirmed, what are the treatment options?

ANSWERS

1. The ECG shows:

    a. Rate: 50 bpm
    b. Rhythm: sinus rhythm
    c. Hyper-acute/peaked T-waves (Figure 86.2).

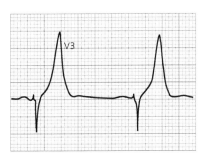

Figure 86.2

2. Tall T-waves can represent a normal variant (especially in young thin males), acute ischemia (this can be a precursor to ST elevation) and hyperkalaemia.

3. Serum potassium levels. Given that this patient has had nausea with risk factors for ischaemic heart disease, the cardiac markers should also be examined. Hyperkalaemia was the cause in this case.

4. Angiotensin-converting enzyme inhibitors, angiotensin receptor blockers and spironolactone will all increase serum potassium by reducing excretion in the distal tubule. These drugs and other drugs, such as furosemide or bendrofluazide, may also provoke renal impairment and increase serum potassium indirectly through reduced glomerular filtration rather than directly affecting the tubule itself.

5. Stop the offending drugs. Use i.v. fluid to help 'wash out' the potassium, especially if the patient is dehydrated. Administer calcium gluconate to protect the cardiac muscle. Intravenous dextrose and insulin will promote potassium intake into the cells. Salbutamol nebulizers will also encourage cellular uptake of potassium. Furosemide will increase renal excretion and calcium resonium orally is useful in the longer term to increase excretion through the bowel.

CASE 87: YOUNG MAN WITH CENTRAL CHEST PAIN

A 22-year-old man presents to A&E with severe central chest pain. He has had a recent cold, but no other medical history. He describes the pain as heavy and stabbing. It is worse when lying down at night and is relieved by sitting forward.

Examination

On examination, pulse is 60 bpm and regular, blood pressure (BP) 120/60 mmHg, jugular venous pressure (JVP) is raised at 2 cm, heart sounds are normal with a clear chest, a soft non-tender abdomen and no ankle swelling. He undergoes an electrocardiogram (ECG) (Figure 87.1).

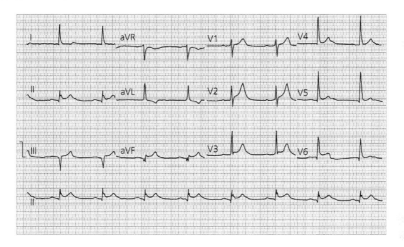

Figure 87.1

QUESTIONS

1. What does the ECG show?
2. What is the most likely diagnosis?
3. What are the causes of this condition?
4. What is the differential diagnosis?
5. What is the first-line treatment?
6. What possible complications are there of this condition?

ANSWERS

1. The ECG shows:

    a. Rate: 50 bpm and regular
    b. Rhythm: sinus rhythm
    c. Axis: normal axis
    d. Global saddle-shaped ST elevation (Figure 87.2).

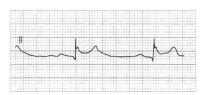

Figure 87.2

2. Given the history and the ECG appearance, this is almost certainly a case of acute pericarditis. PQ depression is another ECG sign of pericarditis – this is not present in this case.

3. Most cases are idiopathic or thought to be from undetected viral infections.

    a. Viral – in particular coxsackie, cytomegalovirus, herpes virus and HIV
    b. Immune conditions, such as systemic lupus erythematosus
    c. Myocardial infarction (MI) (Dressler's syndrome – usually occurring 2 weeks post-MI)
    d. Trauma to the heart
    e. Uraemia
    f. Malignancy (as a paraneoplastic phenomenon)
    g. Side effect of some medications
    h. Post-pericardiotomy syndrome.

4. Myocardial ischemia or myocardial infarction can both mimic pericarditis. Other conditions, such as pulmonary embolism, can cause a similar pain with non-specific ST changes. The worsening of pain when lying down, alleviated on sitting forward is characteristic of perdicardial inflammation.

5. Non-steroidal anti-inflammatory medication and rest are advised. Colchicine can be helpful. In autoimmune cases, steroids may have a role though their use is controversial. Where pericardial bleeding may be an issue, opiate or other methods of pain relief should be administered, rather than non-steroidals which can increase the risk of bleeding.

6. The most important acute complication is pericardial effusion with associated tamponade. In the long term, the condition occasionally becomes chronic or recurrent. Multiple or prolonged episodes can increase the risk of the pericardium becoming 'tight' resulting in a constrictive pericarditis. This condition may require surgery to allow the underlying cardiac muscle to function correctly.

CASE 88: YOUNG MAN WITH PALPITATIONS

History

A 23-year-old male has been referred to A&E with palpitations and dizzy spells suggestive of pre-syncopal attacks. Four months ago he had an episode of syncope when watching a horror movie. There is no past medical history of note, except mild hay fever. There is a family history of sudden unexpected death (his father died at aged 29).

Examination

On examination, the pulse is 60 bpm and regular, blood pressure (BP) 110/70 mmHg, jugular venous pressure (JVP) is not raised, normal heart sounds with a clear chest and soft non-tender abdomen. He undergoes an electrocardiogram (ECG) (Figure 88.1).

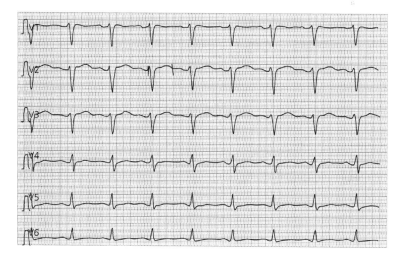

Figure 88.1

QUESTIONS

1. What does the ECG show?
2. What is the probable diagnosis?
3. What may have provoked the symptoms?
4. What would be the next step?

ANSWERS

1. The ECG shows:

   a. Rate: 50 bpm
   b. Rhythm: regular sinus rhythm
   c. QT: 680 ms (17 small squares × 40 ms). The RR interval is 1200 ms (30 small squares × 40 ms)
   d. QTc: 621 ms (QTc = QT/√RR interval (sec) 680/√1.2) (Figure 88.2).

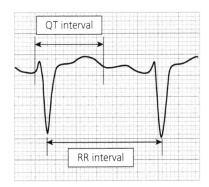

Figure 88.2

QT interval

QT interval is defined as the time from the start of the QRS complex to the end of the T-wave. It is affected by heart rate (the faster the heart, the shorter the interval) and therefore the absolute value is corrected for the heart rate – this is known as the QTc. The correction is derived by dividing the absolute QT interval by the square root of the R–R interval in seconds, e.g at a heart rate of 60 bpm, the R–R interval is 1 s and therefore the QT is divided by the square root of one, i.e QT = QTc at a heart rate of 60 bpm.

The normal values are hard to define because 2.5 per cent of people will have a long QT interval without ill effect and the QT interval can change between ECGs without an obvious cause. The following values are generally accepted as normal:

   Male QTc, 430 ms
   Female QTc, 450 ms

---

2. Long QT syndrome (congenital).

3. There is a history of hay fever and antihistamines can provoke QT prolongation. There are a large number drugs associated with prolonged QT, including certain antimicrobials, antifungal and psychiatric medications, which should be avoided in known cases of prolonged QT interval.

4. The patient will need a specialized review. This will allow confirmation of the diagnosis, screening of other family members and patient risk assessment. This man has several high-risk features and should be considered for an implantable cardiac defibrillator. Beta-blockade is usually the first line of therapy. These help by reducing the chance of arrhythmia directly, as well as reducing sympathetic output from unexpected events (such as may occur while watching a horror movie) that can provoke arrhythmia.

SECTION 5:
MISCELLANEOUS

Case 89: Elderly woman with COPD

Case 90: Elderly man with increasing confusion

Case 91: Elderly man with respiratory distress

Case 92: Young woman with cough

Case 93: Elderly man with progressive leg swelling

Case 94: Woman suspected of attempted suicide

Case 95: Man with chest pain and weight loss

Case 96: Young woman with pain in her legs and back

Case 97: Middle-aged man with severe headache

Case 98: Middle-aged man with epigastric pain

Case 99: Elderly woman with fever and mild confusion

Case 100: Elderly woman admitted following a fall

CASE 89: ELDERLY WOMAN WITH COPD

History

A 78-year-old woman was sent via ambulance to her local A&E by her residential home. She had been seen the preceding week by her GP and treated for an infective exacerbation of chronic obstructive pulmonary disease (COPD). She had not improved with the prescribed course of treatment and had become increasingly drowsy and withdrawn. She continued to cough green sputum.

Further details on telephoning the residential home revealed a past history of hypertension, diet-controlled type 2 diabetes and mild COPD (chronic obstructive pulmonary disease). She was mobile with a stick and required assistance with washing and dressing.

Examination

Examination revealed an elderly dehydrated woman with confusion and stupor. Her pulse was 120/minute, blood pressure (BP) 100/68 mmHg, oxygen saturations 98 per cent on air, respiratory rate 23 per minute and temperature 37.8°C. Respiratory examination revealed coarse crackles at the left base and mild scattered wheeze.

Investigations

		Reference range
Haemoglobin	13.2	13.5–18 g/dL
White cell count	15.4×10^9/L	$4.0–11.0 \times 10^9$/L
Neutrophils	10.4×10^9/L	$2.0–7.5 \times 10^9$/L
Platelets	440×10^9/L	$150–450 \times 10^9$/L
Sodium	155 mmol/L	135–146 mmol/L
Potassium	4.5 mmol/L	3.2–5.1 mmol/L
Urea	21 mmol/L	1.7–8.3 mmol/L
Creatinine	110 mmol/L	62–106 mmol/L
Glucose	45 mmol/L	3.2–6.0 mmol/L (fasting)
C-reactive protein (CRP)	120 mg/L	<5 mg/L
pH	7.36	7.35–7.45
pO_2	11.4 kPa	11.1–14.4 kPa
pCO_2	4.8 kPa	4.7–6.4 kPa
HCO_3	27 mmol/L	22–29 mmol/L

Urinalysis, ketones ±
Chest x-ray, patchy consolidation at the left base
Electrocardiogram (ECG), sinus tachycardia.

QUESTIONS

1. What is the diagnosis?
2. What calculation can be used to help confirm the diagnosis?
3. What is the treatment?

ANSWERS

1. The diagnosis here is of hyperosmolar hyperglycaemic state (HHS) precipitated by a left lower lobe pneumonia.

   Hyperosmolar hyperglycaemic state is characterized by hyperglycaemia, hyperosmolality and dehydration without evidence of acidosis. HHS usually presents in older patients with type 2 diabetes, however up to 20 per cent have no diagnosis of diabetes at presentation. It carries a mortality of 10–20 per cent which is significantly higher than that associated with diabetic ketoacidosis (DKA) <5 per cent.

   The cause of the biochemical abnormalities is thought to be due to a net deficiency of insulin and an elevation of counter-regulatory hormones (e.g. cortisol, catecholamines and glucagon). In HHS, there is sufficient endogenous insulin to prevent lipolysis and therefore ketoacidosis, unlike in DKA.

   The biochemical features of both DKA and HHS are summarized in the table below.

	DKA	HHS
Sodium (mmol/L)	140	155
Potassium (mmol/L)	5	5
Urea (mmol/L)	8	15
Glucose (mmol/L)	30	50
Arterial pH	<7.0–7.30	7.35
Serum HCO_3 (mmol/L)	<10–18	>15
Anion gap	>10	<12
Osmolality (mOsm/kg)	Variable	>320
Urine ketones	Positive	Small

   HHS is usually precipitated by concurrent medical illness including chest infection, urinary tract infection (UTI), myocardial infarction, pancreatitis and stroke. It can also be associated with medication including steroids, thiazide diuretics and second-generation atypical antipsychotics. Elderly patients are particularly vulnerable as they experience thirst less acutely and are likely to have a restricted fluid intake due to being incapacitated by the concurrent illness.

   HHS usually develops over several days to weeks, unlike DKA which develops more rapidly. In this case, the contributing factors are the partially treated pneumonia; it is also likely that the GP prescribed a course of steroids for the presumed COPD exacerbation. Patients may complain of polyuria, thirst, fatigue and weight loss. The most common clinical presentation of HHS is of altered cerebral function. This can include a variety of both focal and global neurological features:

   a. Drowsiness and lethargy
   b. Hemiparesis
   c. Hemianopia

    d. Delirium

    e. Seizures (usually partial, rather than general)

    f. Coma.

HHS was previously termed hyperosmolar non-ketotic coma (HONK); however, terminology has changed based on the observation that coma is evident in fewer than 20 per cent of cases. Clinical examination reveals signs of dehydration including dry mucous membranes, decreased skin turgor, tachycardia and hypotension.

2. Typically significant hypernatraemia is present in HHS; however, due to severe hyperglycaemia, pseudohyponatraemia may be present as glucose draws water into the vascular space. If this is suspected, a corrected Na^+ can be calculated:

Corrected $Na^+ = Na^+ + 1.6 \times ([\text{plasma glucose} - 5.5] \div 5.5)$

Hypo- or hyper-kalaemia may be present. Relative insulin deficiency causes extracellular flux of potassium into the vascular space leading to an elevated serum potassium despite low total body potassium. If serum potassium is measured as low, this suggests dangerously low levels of total body potassium requiring close monitoring and vigorous replacement to prevent life-threatening arrhythmia.

In this case, it is important to calculate the serum osmolality to help confirm the diagnosis.

$$\text{Osmolality} = 2(Na^+ + K^+) + \text{glucose} + \text{urea}$$

$$= 2(155 + 4.5) + 45 + 21$$

$$= 385 \ (275 - 299 \ \text{mmol/L})$$

Studies have demonstrated a linear relationship between serum osmolality and degree of cerebral dysfunction.

3. Treatment is not dissimilar to that of DKA. Patients may be up to 9 litres deficient in total body water. Treatment should be aimed at correcting dehydration, electrolyte imbalance, hyperglycaemia and any other co-morbid factors, e.g. pneumonia. Initial fluid resuscitation should be with 0.9 per cent saline 1 L over 1 hour. Continuous reassessment of fluid status is imperative to avoid iatrogenic fluid overload particularly in the elderly. The aim should be to replace estimated fluid losses within 24–48 hours and should be guided by BP, pulse and urine output. Potassium should be replaced with 20–40 mmol/L of KCl in each litre of i.v. fluid aiming to keep serum potassium between 4 and 5 mmol/L.

Prior to initiating insulin sliding scale, it is imperative to ensure serum potassium >3.2 mmol/L to reduce the risk of arrhythmia. Insulin therapy should be delayed until this has been achieved. Patients with HHS tend to be extremely sensitive to insulin, and glucose levels can plummet precipitously. Rapid changes in both serum osmolality and serum glucose can cause significant cerebral damage; therefore it is important to measure glucose and electrolytes closely, i.e. every 2–4 hours until stable. Once glucose levels have fallen to 10–12 mmol/L fluid should be changed from saline to dextrose.

The risk of venous thromboembolism is exaggerated in cases of HHS due to the hyperosmolar state, and therefore prophylactic low-molecular-weight heparin should be used to reduce the risk of deep venous thrombosis (DVT) or pulmonary embolism (PE). In this case, treatment should also include the precipitating cause, i.e. antibiotics to cover pneumonia.

Unlike DKA, HHS is not an absolute indication for insulin therapy and many patients are well managed on diet and oral medications. Education is key to prevent recurrence and particular attention should be paid to blood sugars during the time of illness.

CASE 90: ELDERLY MAN WITH INCREASING CONFUSION

History

A 75-year-old Nigerian man is admitted to hospital with a history of increasing confusion. This has been progressively worsening over the last few months. His daughter has become increasingly concerned that he is not able to cope at home. He has a past medical history of hypertension, cataract surgery and has been told he has a leaky heart valve. His current medication includes amlodipine 5 mg/day and atorvastatin 10 mg/day. He has no allergies. He lives alone in a first floor flat and is normally independent in all activities of daily living. He grew up in Nigeria and moved to the UK ten years ago when his wife died. He is a non-smoker and drinks a measure of whisky every night.

Examination

On examination he looks well. His observations are within normal limits. His abbreviated mental test score is 6/10. Cardiovascular examination reveals a quiet early diastolic murmur heard best at the left sternal edge in end expiration. Respiratory and abdominal examinations are unremarkable.

Investigations

		Reference range
Haemoglobin	13.5 g/dL	13.5–18 g/dL
White cell count	6.0×10^9/L	$4.0–11.0 \times 10^9$/L
Neutrophil count	5.0×10^9/L	$2.0–7.5 \times 10^9$/L
Platelets	400×10^9/L	$150–450 \times 10^9$/L
Sodium	136 mmol/L	135–146 mmol/L
Potassium	4.5 mmol/L	3.2–5.1 mmol/L
Urea	7.0 mmol/L	1.7–8.3 mmol/L
Creatinine	83 mmol/L	62–106 mmol/L
C-reactive protein (CRP)	33 mg/L	<5 mg/L
Calcium	2.35 mmol/L	2.15–2.55 mmol/L
Thyroid-stimulating hormone (TSH)	3.5 mU/L	0.3–4.2 mU/L
B12	300 pg/mL	197–866 pg/mL
Folate	7.6 ng/mL	4.6–18.7 ng/mL

Treponema pallidum enzyme immunoassay (EIA): reactive.

QUESTIONS

1. What is the differential diagnosis?
2. What further investigations would be useful?
3. What are the clinical features and classification of acquired syphilis?
4. What tests are used in the diagnosis of syphilis?
5. What is the treatment of syphilis?

ANSWERS

1. The differential diagnosis here remains wide. The common causes of a confusional
    state are shown in the table below. There is insufficient information to reach a con-
    clusive diagnosis from the information given. The aetiology may be infective, such
    as urinary tract infection (UTI), related to alcohol excess (one measure of whisky
    per day is likely to be an underestimate), the subacute history could be suggestive
    of dementia. The reactive EIA test raises the possibility of tertiary syphilis, although
    we are not given details of the neurological examination findings.

Common causes of confusional state

Infection	Any infection, including UTI, particularly in the elderly
Metabolic disturbance	Electrolyte imbalance Liver failure Renal failure Hypoxia
Endocrine disturbance	Hypothyroidism Cushing syndrome
Vitamin deficiency	B12 deficiency Thiamine deficiency (Wernicke – Korsakoff syndrome)
Drugs	Alcohol withdrawal Recreational drugs Digoxin Tricyclic antidepressants Anticonvulsants
Intracranial causes	Dementia Tumour Abscess Epilepsy Subdural haematoma Subarachnoid haemorrhage

2. In order to help narrow the wide differential, further tests are necessary. A full neu-
    rological examination is imperative and may elucidate a neurological cause for his
    confusion. Liver function tests (including clotting) would be useful given the history
    of regular alcohol use. Urinalysis would establish whether urinary tract infection is
    contributing. A computed tomography (CT) scan of his brain would help elucidate
    an intracranial cause of his confusion. In the absence of any diagnosis following
    the above steps, a lumbar puncture ought to be considered.

3. Syphilis is an uncommon chronic infection that can be congenital or acquired, caused by the bacterium *Treponema pallidum*. *T. pallidum* is a motile spirochaete that is transmitted either sexually or transplacentally. Acquired syphilis has both early (infectious) and late (non-infectious) stages, each of which has characteristic clinical features. Early syphilis includes the primary, secondary and early latent stages. These typically occur within the two years following acquisition of the infection. Latent syphilis is typically asymptomatic and is diagnosed on the basis of serological testing. Late syphilis occurs years after the primary infection.

    Primary syphilis occurs between 10 and 90 days after exposure to the *T. pallidum*, whereby a painless papule develops at the site of inoculation. This papule soon ulcerates to produce the classic chancre of primary syphilis associated with painless regional lymphadenopathy. The ulcer may be ignored by the patient as it is painless and will usually heal spontaneously within 3–6 weeks or it may go unnoticed if located on the cervix or within the rectum.

    Secondary syphilis occurs weeks to a few months later and causes constitutional symptoms including fever, malaise, lymphadenopathy and arthralgia. The classical rash of secondary syphilis is symmetrical, maculopapular and involves the whole body, including the palms of the hands and soles of the feet. Condylomata lata – large, white, warty lesions – may occur on moist areas, such as the perineum and mouth. 'Snail track ulcers' may be found in the mouth and genitalia.

    Tertiary syphilis is now rare due to effective treatments. Gummas are seen in tertiary syphilis which are granulomas that occur in the skin, mucosa, bones and occasionally viscera. Gummas are sometimes defined as late benign syphilis because of their responsiveness to therapy. Cardiovascular syphilis can cause aortitis, aortic aneurysms and aortic valvulitis leading to aortic regurgitation. Neurosyphilis may cause tabes dorsalis, general paralysis of the insane or meningovascular syphilis. Tabes dorsalis is caused by demyelination in the dorsal roots causing sensory ataxia, lightning pains, Charcot's joints, Argyll–Robertson pupils, extensor plantars and loss of reflexes. General paralysis of the insane causes dementia and psychosis. Meningovascular syphilis causes subacute meningitis associated with cranial nerve palsies and papilloedema.

4. *T. pallidum* cannot be cultured in the laboratory and therefore syphilis is diagnosed either by direct visualization or serological testing. Dark-ground microscopy enables the demonstration of the corkscrew-shaped organism obtained in variable numbers from primary chancres and mucous patches of secondary lesions. Negative dark-ground microscopy does not, however, exclude the diagnosis of syphilis and in clinical practice this test is usually limited to the GUM (genitourinary medicine) clinic.

    The immune response to syphilis involves production of antibodies to a broad range of antigens. These antibodies are both non-specific (e.g. cardiolipin antibodies) and treponemal specific. This immune response forms the basis of the serological tests used to diagnose syphilis. The *T. pallidum* EIA is the screening test of choice and can detect both IgM and IgG antibodies. A positive test is then confirmed with an alternative treponemal specific test, such as the *T. pallidum* haemagglutination assay (TPHA), as well as a treponemal non-specific test such as the rapid plasma reagin (RPR) test. This sequence is recommended due to the potential of false negatives with the non-treponemal tests. The advantage of the non-treponemal tests is that they provide a quantitative result, which is not available with treponemal-specific tests. These quantitative results reflect disease activity and can therefore be used as a guide to treatment response. False positives can occur with endocarditis, autoimmune diseases (especially systemic lupus erythromatosus (SLE)), intravenous drug use and chronic liver disease. The most common cause of a false-negative result occurs with early testing for the infection prior to the development of antibodies.

5. Treatment of syphilis is with penicillin or tetracyclines in those who are penicillin allergic. Early syphilis is usually treated with benzathine penicillin G, 2.4 mU intramuscularly in a single dose (unlicensed in the UK) or doxycycline 100 mg twice a day for 14 days. The antibiotic course should be extended in tertiary syphilis as the treponemes divide more slowly. Measurement of a quantitative non-treponemal-specific test provides evidence of serological response to treatment.

CASE 91: ELDERLY MAN WITH RESPIRATORY DISTRESS

History

You are the surgical F1 called to the ward by the nursing staff. They are concerned about a 75-year-old patient in respiratory distress and have asked you to assess him immediately. He initially presented to hospital 11 days ago with a perforated duodenal ulcer. He was operated on within 24 hours having had an omental patch repair. Postoperatively, he had been progressing well, but recovery had been prolonged due to poorly controlled pain. He has a past medical history of hypertension and chronic kidney disease. The following medications are listed on his drug chart: enoxaparin 40 mg/day, oramorph 10 mg 4 hourly, ramipril 10 mg/day, paracetamol 1 g four times a day, as required oramorph 5 mg up to 2 hourly, intravenous fluids prescribed 8 hourly.

Examination

Examination reveals an elderly man who is drowsy and diaphoretic. Observations show pulse 120 beats per minute regular, blood pressure (BP) 90/60 mmHg, oxygen saturations 86 per cent on air, 95 per cent on 15 litres. Chest examination reveals normal vesicular breath sounds. Auscultation of the heart reveals a sinus tachycardia with a loud pulmonary second sound. Abdominal examination is unremarkable.

Investigations

The previous day's blood results are as follows:

		Reference range
Haemoglobin	10.3 g/dL	13.5–18 g/dL
White cell count	10.3×10^9/L	$4.0–11.0 \times 10^9$/L
Neutrophil count	7.6×10^9/L	$2.0–7.5 \times 10^9$/L
Platelets	323×10^9/L	$150–450 \times 10^9$/L
Sodium	134 mmol/L	135–146 mmol/L
Potassium	3.8 mmol/L	3.2–5.1 mmol/L
Urea	9.5 mmol/L	1.7–8.3 mmol/L
Creatinine	130 mmol/L	62–106 mmol/L
C-reactive protein (CRP)	15 mg/L	<5 mg/L

As you are performing an arterial blood gas, the patient suddenly becomes unresponsive.

QUESTIONS

1. What should you do next?
2. What is your immediate management?
3. Recall the steps involved in in-hospital cardiac-arrest situations.
4. List the potentially reversible causes of cardiac arrest.
5. What are the two most likely explanations for this patient's sudden deterioration?

ANSWERS

1. This patient is clearly extremely unwell and has now become unresponsive. Peri-arrest, your immediate action should be to call for help and assess the patient for signs of life. Many hospitals now have a medical emergency team (MET) that can be summoned to assess and treat patients with sudden physiological deterioration (even in the absence of cardiac arrest). All hospitals share the same emergency phone number '2222' to summon the cardiac arrest team. In the absence of signs of life, cardiopulmonary resuscitation should be commenced.

2. Prior to the arrival of the cardiac arrest team, the patient should be assessed using the ABCDE (airway, breathing, circulation, disability, exposure) approach. Airway management involves head tilt/chin lift and jaw thrust manoeuvres, as well as the use of airway adjuncts, including oropharyngeal or nasopharyngeal airways, bag-valve masks and supplemental oxygen prior to tracheal intubation. Breathing is checked using the look, listen and feel approach for 10 seconds. Circulation is checked simultaneously by palpation of the carotid artery. If there is no pulse or signs of life, then cardiopulmonary resuscitation (CPR) should be commenced immediately. Chest compressions should be given in a ratio of 30 compressions to two ventilations. The depth of compression should be 5–6 cm at a rate of 100–120 per minute. Once intubation has taken place, chest compressions should continue uninterrupted at 100 per minute with ten ventilations per minute.

   During this period of time, monitoring equipment should be attached, including pulse oximetry, blood pressure and electrocardiogram (ECG) monitoring preferably via cardiac defibrillator. Intravenous or intraosseous access should be obtained, as well as sending blood for analysis. Once ECG monitoring is achieved, the cardiac rhythm should be assessed to determine whether a shock should be delivered.

3. In 25 per cent of cases, the first monitored rhythm will be either shockable ventricular fibrillation (VF) or ventricular tachycardia (VT). The remainder will be non-shockable rhythms namely asystole or pulseless electrical activity (PEA). Following a single shock, CPR should immediately be continued for 2 min prior to reassessment of the rhythm. Adrenaline (1 mg) should be given after the third shock in shockable rhythms and as soon as access is obtained in non-shockable rhythms. It is then given every second cycle of CPR, i.e. every 3–5 minutes. Amiodarone 300 mg should also be given after the third shock if the patient is in a shockable rhythm. The patient may switch between both shockable and non-shockable rhythms. The aim is to deliver a shock with minimal disruption to chest compressions.

4. The potentially reversible causes of cardiac arrest can easily be remembered by learning the four 'H's and the four 'T's (see below). Each of the conditions mentioned in the table should be recognized and treated as soon as possible.

Hypoxia	Thromboembolism, cardiac/pulmonary
Hypovolaemia	Tamponade, cardiac
Hypothermia	Toxic/therapeutic disturbances
Hypo-/hyperkalaemia/hypocalcaemia/ metabolic disturbance	Tension pneumothorax

5. There are two likely causes of this patient's cardiac arrest. In the history, it is noted that pain control had been difficult postoperatively and the patient is taking regular doses of opiate analgesia. We are not given information pertaining to the patient's respiratory rate or pupil size in the account of history or examination. The side effects of opiate analgesia are frequently encountered on surgical wards and toxicity is readily treated with intravenous naloxone. If this patient had pinpoint pupils or a low respiratory rate then these would suggest opiate toxicity resulting in respiratory arrest. The other potential cause for deterioration could be massive pulmonary embolism. This was the cause in this case. The patient has developed sudden breathlessness 10 days postoperatively and has recordable hypoxia. In cases of arrest and massive pulmonary embolism, consideration should be made for intravenous thrombolysis (e.g. alteplase). CPR should be continued for up 90 minutes as this is the length of time it may take for thrombolysis to be effective.

CASE 92: YOUNG WOMAN WITH COUGH

History

A 25-year-old woman presents to her GP with a 2-month history of persistent non-productive cough over the summer months. She has had two courses of antibiotics prescribed by the out-of-hours GP with no effect. She finds that the cough is worse in cold weather and with exercise. The cough is particularly troublesome at night.

She has a past history of eczema and hay fever. She is a non-smoker and takes loratidine, as required. She remembers being a 'chesty' child.

Examination

She is comfortable at rest with oxygen saturations of 99 per cent on air. Examination of the chest reveals normal vesicular breath sounds. ENT examination reveals no abnormality.

The GP asks her to record her peak expiratory flow at home for 2 weeks, as well as arranging lung function tests and chest x-ray at the local hospital. She has returned for her results, which are shown in Figures 92.1 and 92.2.

Chest x-ray is reported as normal.

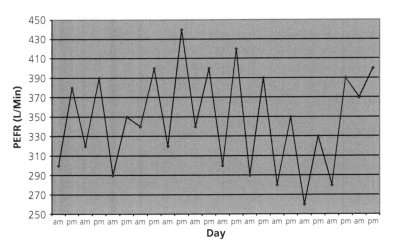

Figure 92.1 Peak expiratory flow rates (L/min).

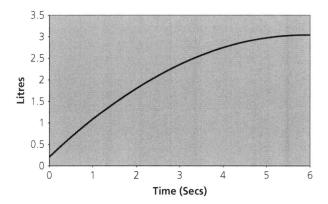

Figure 92.2 Spirometry.

QUESTIONS

1. What is the diagnosis?
2. What is demonstrated in Figure 92.1?
3. What is demonstrated in Figure 92.2?
4. Calculate the FEV_1 (forced expiratory volume in one second), FVC (forced vital capacity) and FEV_1/FVC ratio.
5. Describe the changes in spirometry associated with both an obstructive lung disease and restrictive lung disease.
6. What is meant by the term 'transfer factor'?

ANSWERS

1. The diagnosis here is that of asthma. The history of atopy and nocturnal cough lend weight to the clinical diagnosis. Asthma is characterized by airflow limitation that is usually reversible, airway hyper-responsiveness to a wide range of stimuli – in this case pollen – and inflammation of the bronchi leading to mucus plugging and smooth muscle hypertrophy. Patients with asthma report wheezing attacks and episodes of shortness of breath, often worse at night. Cough can be a predominant feature and therefore asthma is often misdiagnosed as bronchitis.

2. The peak flow pattern in Figure 92.1 shows marked diurnal variation in peak flow. Early morning 'dips' are clearly present. A diurnal variation of greater than 20 per cent on more than 3 days per week for 2 weeks is diagnostic of asthma.

3. (Answers 3, 4 and 5). Spirometry is the most readily available and most useful pulmonary function test. It is cheap, easy to use and carries no risk. Spirometry is the preferred diagnostic investigation in asthma and ideally should be performed when the patient is symptomatic. Spirometers measure the forced expiratory volume in 1 second, as well as the forced vital capacity. The FEV_1 and FVC are related to age, sex and height. The technique involves taking a maximal inspiration followed by a forced expiration for as long as possible.

    FEV_1: the volume of air the patient is able to exhale in the first second of forced expiration.

    FVC: the total volume of air that the patient can forcibly exhale in one breath.

    FEV_1/FVC ratio: the ratio of FEV_1 to FVC expressed as a percentage.

    Figure 92.3 demonstrates the technique used to calculate FEV_1 and FVC. Therefore, in this example:

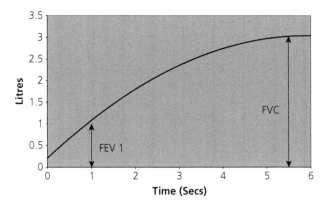

Figure 92.3 Spirometry – calculation of FEV_1 and FVC.

FEV$_1$ = 1.3

FVC = 3.2

FEV$_1$/FVC = 40 per cent

The FEV$_1$/FVC ratio in normal subjects is ~75–80 per cent (Figure 92.4). With airflow limitation, as in chronic obstructive pulmonary disease (COPD) and asthma, the FEV$_1$ falls proportionately more than FVC, therefore the ratio is reduced, i.e. <70. In a patient with airway obstruction, spirometry should be repeated after administration of a bronchodilator to demonstrate airway responsiveness. An increase in FEV$_1$ suggests acute bronchodilator responsiveness and should prompt a therapeutic trial of bronchodilators or steroids. Continued smoking in a patient with COPD will cause an accelerated fall in FEV$_1$ over time. Smoking cessation often results in an increase in FEV$_1$ during the first year followed by a near normal rate of decline of FEV$_1$. The severity of COPD is calculated according to the FEV$_1$ achieved in relation to what is predicted for age, sex and height:

Mild	FEV$_1$ >80 per cent predicted
Moderate	FEV$_1$ 50–79 per cent predicted
Severe	FEV$_1$ 30–49 per cent predicted
Very severe	FEV$_1$ <30 per cent predicted

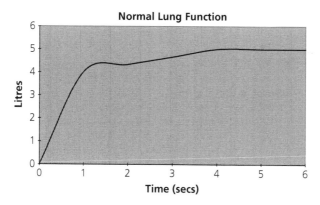

Figure 92.4 Normal spirometry: FEV$_1$, 4; FVC, 5; FEV$_1$/FVC, 80 per cent.

Restrictive lung disease can be divided into three categories: (1) intrinsic lung diseases that cause lung scarring, e.g. interstitial lung disease; (2) extrinsic disorders that affect the chest wall or pleura, e.g. severe kyphosis; or (3) neuromuscular disorders which impair the ability of respiratory muscles to inflate and deflate the lungs, e.g. motor neurone disease (MND). In restrictive lung disease, the FVC is reduced and the FEV$_1$/FVC ratio is normal or raised (see Figure 92.5).

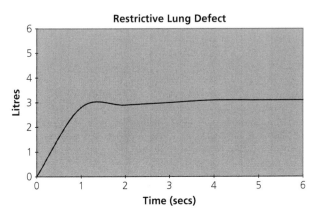

Figure 92.5 Spirometry of a restrictive lung defect: FEV$_1$, 2.8; FVC, 3.1; FEV$_1$/FVC, 90 per cent.

6. The transfer factor is the measurement of the single-breath diffusing capacity of the lung for carbon monoxide (DL$_{CO}$) and acts as a measure of gas exchange. The DL$_{CO}$ is useful in both obstructive and restrictive lung defects. For example, in emphysema the DL$_{CO}$ is reduced and in asthma the DL$_{CO}$ is frequently increased. In restrictive lung disease, the DL$_{CO}$ is generally reduced for intrinsic lung disease, but normal if the cause is due to neuromuscular problems or skeletal deformity.

CASE 93: ELDERLY MAN WITH PROGRESSIVE LEG SWELLING

History

A 66-year-old man presents to his GP complaining of a 3-week history of progressive leg swelling. He has also noticed that his urine has become more frothy. There is no history of shortness of breath or chest pain. He has a past medical history of mild asthma for which he takes a salbutamol inhaler as required. Four weeks ago, he had sustained a back injury for which he had taken over-the-counter ibuprofen for 1 week. He is a non-smoker and drinks 18 units of alcohol per week.

Examination

Examination reveals gross pitting oedema to both legs extending to the mid-thigh. There is also evidence of sacral oedema. He has xanthelasma around both eyelids. His blood pressure is 135/75 mmHg, heart rate 75 beats per minute, oxygen saturations 98 percent on air. He is apyrexial. Cardiovascular examination reveals a normal jugular venous pressure, normal heart sounds and a clear chest. The remainder of his examination is normal.

Investigations

		Reference range
Haemoglobin	14.5 g/dL	13.5–18 g/dL
White cell count	6.6×10^9/L	$4.0–11.0 \times 10^9$/L
Platelets	400×10^9/L	$150–450 \times 10^9$/L
Sodium	137 mmol/L	135–146 mmol/L
Potassium	3.4 mmol/L	3.2–5.1 mmol/L
Urea	5.5 mmol/L	1.7–8.3 mmol/L
Creatinine	80 mmol/L	62–106 mmol/L
Glucose	5.8 mmol/L	3.2–6.0 mmol/L (fasting)
Albumin	18 g/L	34–48 g/L
Bilirubin	15 µmol/L	Up to 21 µmol/L
Alkaline phosphatase (ALP)	80 IU/L	40–129 IU/L
Alanine aminotransferase (ALT)	32 IU/L	Up to 41 IU/L
Cholesterol	9.8 mmol/L	<5 mmol/L

Urinalysis, –; protein, ++++; blood, -ve.
24-hour urinary protein, 8.9 g (0–0.2 g/24 h).

QUESTIONS

1. What do these findings indicate?
2. What is the most likely underlying cause in this case?
3. What further investigations are necessary?
4. What are the management and complications of this condition?

ANSWERS

1. This patient has presented with significant peripheral oedema without evidence
    of cardiac failure. In conjunction with hypoalbuminaemia and heavy proteinuria,
    this is diagnostic of the nephrotic syndrome. Nephrotic syndrome is defined by the
    presence of heavy proteinuria (>3 g/24 h), hypoalbuminaemia (<30 g/L) and periph-
    eral oedema. Severe oedema (anasarca) can also occur due to severe heart failure
    or venous obstruction, or because of hypoalbuminaemia in severe malnutrition or
    chronic liver disease.

    Proteinuria occurs due to an increased leak of protein across the glomerular capil-
    lary membrane and subsequent excretion in the urine. Hence, serum albumin falls
    as a consequence. Peripheral oedema occurs due to a decrease in plasma oncotic
    pressure, as well as increased salt and water retention in the collecting tubules.
    The decreased plasma oncotic pressure is thought to stimulate hepatic lipoprotein
    synthesis (along with albumin synthesis) and thus cause hypercholesterolaemia.

2. In adults, 30 per cent of cases of nephrotic syndrome have an underlying
    pathological cause, such as diabetes mellitus, amyloidosis or systemic lupus
    erythematosus. The remainder of cases are usually due to primary renal disorders,
    such as minimal change disease, membranous nephropathy or focal segmen-
    tal glomerulosclerosis. The history of atopy and the recent use of non-steroidal
    anti-inflammatory drugs (NSAIDs) make minimal change disease the most likely
    underlying cause.

3. Twenty-four-hour urinary protein collection is the reference-standard method to
    measure proteinuria. However, this method is cumbersome and often poorly per-
    formed. An alternative, therefore, is the urine protein–creatinine ratio performed on
    a random urine specimen. This ratio correlates closely with daily protein excretion
    and is a far simpler method of collection. Patients with nephrotic syndrome should
    be referred to a nephrologist for further investigation and management. In adult
    patients, almost all will require a renal biopsy in order to reach a histological diag-
    nosis. This is imperative as treatment of the underlying condition will differ mark-
    edly. The table below summarizes useful blood tests to help establish a diagnosis.

Test	Disease association
Throat swab and ASO (antistreptolysin O) titre	Post-streptococcal glomerulonephritis
Anti-nuclear antibody	Systemic lupus erythematosus
Complement levels	Glomerulonephritis
Anti-neutrophil cytoplasmic antibody (ANCA)	Vasculitis
Anti-glomerular basement membrane (anti-GBM) antibody	Goodpasture's syndrome
Hepatitis B and C serology	Glomerulonephritis

Test	Disease association
Cryoglobulinaemia	Malignant lymphoproliferative disorder
	Hepatitis C
Serum free light chains Immunoglobulins Serum and urine protein electrophoresis	Amyloidosis, myeloma

4. Management of nephrotic syndrome is directed to the underlying aetiology. For example, in minimal change disease, treatment is high-dose immunosupression in comparison to secondary focal segmental glomerulosclerosis in which immunosupression exacerbates the disease.

General measures aim to reduce proteinuria, peripheral oedema and hypercholesterolaemia and avoidance of complications. Proteinuria is treated by lowering intra-glomerular pressure and hence protein excretion. This is best achieved with angiotensin-converting enzyme (ACE) inhibitors or angiotensin receptor blockers (ARBs). Peripheral oedema is treated with dietary sodium restriction and loop diuretics. High doses of diuretic are often required as enteral absorption is often reduced due to gut mucosal oedema, as well as impaired drug delivery to the kidney as a consequence of hypoalbuminaemia. In order to avoid renal impairment associated with these drugs, regular monitoring of kidney function is advocated. The aim should be to achieve 1 kg weight loss per day in order to avoid hypovolaemia/hypotension and subsequent kidney injury, while maintaining adequate diuresis. Hyperlipidaemia is treated in the conventional way with careful dietary modification and the addition of statins or other lipid-lowering drugs.

The nephrotic syndrome is associated with a hypercoagulable state due to loss of fibrinolytic factors in the urine and increased hepatic synthesis of clotting factors. There is subsequently an increased incidence of arterial and venous thrombosis (in particular renal vein and deep vein thrombosis). Patients should therefore receive prophylactic subcutaneous low-molecular-weight heparin. Clinicians should hold a low index of suspicion for the development of any thrombotic condition and early investigation and treatment are imperative.

Patients with nephrotic syndrome are particularly susceptible to infection. This is thought to be due to renal excretion of circulating immunoglobulins. Any infections should be treated promptly with antibiotics. Pneumococcal infection is particularly common, therefore patients should be offered pneumococcal vaccination. Acute kidney injury may occur due to several factors, including overzealous diuresis, hypovolaemia, as well as a complication of the underlying renal disease.

CASE 94: WOMAN SUSPECTED OF ATTEMPTED SUICIDE

History

A 34-year-old woman is brought to A&E by ambulance at 2 a.m. She was found in the bath at home with evidence of cuts to her wrists and with three empty boxes of paracetamol on the floor. On further questioning, she had had an argument with her partner that evening, who found her and called the ambulance. She admitted to taking 36 paracetamol tablets at approximately 8 p.m. She had also been drinking alcohol – approximately half a 1-litre bottle of vodka.

Further details from her partner revealed that she was known to the mental health services with a recent diagnosis of depression. She had recently become unemployed due to mental illness. She lives alone, although her partner stays when he is not away with work. Her medication consists of citalopram 20 mg/day.

Examination

Examination reveals a tearful woman who is difficult to engage and not maintaining eye contact. Pupils are medium-sized, equal and reactive to light. Her wrists reveal superficial cuts with no tendon, nerve or vessel injury. She weighs 60 kg, her observations are within normal limits. Examination reveals mild right upper quadrant pain, but no jaundice, encephalopathy or liver flap.

Investigations

		Reference range
Haemoglobin	13.5 g/dL	13.5–18 g/dL
White cell count	7.5×10^9/L	$4.0–11.0 \times 10^9$/L
Platelets	330×10^9/L	$150–450 \times 10^9$/L
International normalized ratio (INR)	1.1	1.0–1.3
Sodium	140 mmol/L	135–146 mmol/L
Potassium	4.0 mmol/L	3.2–5.1 mmol/L
Urea	3.3 mmol/L	1.7–8.3 mmol/L
Creatinine	44 mmol/L	62–106 mmol/L
Bilirubin	18 µmol/L	<21 µmol/L
Alanine aminotransferase (ALT)	88 IU/L	<31 IU/L
Alkaline phosphatase (ALP)	76 IU/L	35–104 IU/L
Gamma-glutamyl transferase (GGT)	120 IU/L	6–42 IU/L
Paracetamol	160 mg/L	
Salicylate	10 mg/L	

QUESTIONS

1. What is the diagnosis?
2. What is the immediate management?
3. Where can further information be found?
4. What further questions from the history are important to further assess her mental state?

ANSWERS

1. The diagnosis here is an acute paracetamol overdose. Paracetamol overdose is the most common form of poisoning encountered in the UK. Paracetamol is metabolized by the liver and is conjugated with glutathione and subsequently excreted as cysteine and mercapturic conjugates. In overdose, the large amounts of paracetamol exceed the capability of the glutathione conjugation pathway. Paracetamol is then metabolized by oxidation which in the absence of glutathione causes accumulation of the toxic metabolite *N*-acetyl-*p*-benzoquinoneimine (NAPQI) which causes direct hepatotoxicity.

2. (Answers 2 and 3). Immediate management is determined by written guidelines. A 12 g or greater overdose (150 mg/kg) may be fatal if left untreated. Consider activated charcoal if presentation is within 1 hour to bind the paracetamol and hence prevent its absorption by the gastrointestinal tract. Wait until 4 hours from ingestion have elapsed and take blood for urea and electrolytes (U&E), creatinine, liver function tests (LFT), international normalized ratio (INR) and paracetamol level. The risk of severe liver damage is assessed according to the paracetamol concentration/time from ingestion graph (Figure 94.1).

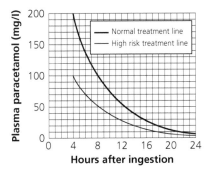

Figure 94.1 Plasma paracetamol concentration/time from ingestion.

The high-risk treatment line should be used if there is history of malnourishment/alcoholism/pre-existing liver disease/chronic debilitating illness (e.g. HIV), as patients are likely to be glutathione deficient. It should also be used if there is a history of concurrent use of liver enzyme-inducing drugs (e.g. carbamezapine, rifampicin, St John's wort).

This patient lies above the treatment line at 6 hours and therefore is at risk of liver toxicity requiring treatment with *N*-acetylcysteine (see table below).

Dose	*N*-acetylcysteine	Volume of 5 per cent dextrose	Duration of infusion
1	150 mg/kg	200 mL	15 min
2	50 mg/kg	500 mL	4 hours
3	100 mg/kg	1 litre	16 hours

Therefore in this case:

Dose 1 = 9 g acetylcysteine in 200 mL of 5 per cent dextrose over 15 min

Dose 2 = 3 g acetylcysteine in 500 mL of 5 per cent dextrose over 4 hours

Dose 3 = 6 g acetylcysteine in 1 litre of 5 per cent dextrose over 16 hours.

If the INR, creatinine, plasma bicarbonate and liver transaminases (should be measured every 12 hours) are in the normal range at the end of the three doses of *N*-acetylcysteine, the patient can be declared medically fit for discharge and no lasting liver damage will be present. If the INR and transaminases remain elevated after this period *N*-acetylcysteine should be continued at dose 3 until improvement in blood results occurs. Discussion with specialist liver teams should be undertaken early, especially if the following are present:

- Encephalopathy, grade III or IV
- INR >2.0 at <48 hours or >3.5 at <72 hours
- Renal impairment
- Blood pH <7.3
- Blood lactate >3.5 mmol/L.

Rash and flushing are common side effects of *N*-acetylcysteine therapy (up to 20 per cent of patients) and can be easily treated with an antihistamine, e.g. chlorpheniramine. An alternative to acetylcysteine is oral methionine, but absorption can be unreliable, particularly if vomiting or there is concurrent use of activated charcoal preparations. The dose of methionine is 2.5 g initially, then 2.5 g 4-hourly for a further three doses. Total methionine dose 10 g over 12 hours. *N*-acetylcysteine may also be given orally. They act by replenishing cellular glutathione stores, *N*-acetylcysteine is also thought to repair oxidation damage caused by NAPQI. If the patient presents greater than 15 hours after ingestion of paracetamol overdose, the efficacy of these treatments is limited.

3. When assessing the patient's suicide intent, the 'SADPERSONS' score can be useful:

S: Male sex
A: Older age (>45 years)
D: Depression
P: Previous attempt
E: Ethanol/substance misuse
R: Rational thinking loss
S: Social supports lacking
O: Organized plan/suicide note

N: No spouse/divorced/widowed

S: Sickness/physical illness

      0–4, Low risk

      5–6, Medium risk

      7–10, High risk.

All patients presenting with attempted suicide should be assessed by the mental health team prior to discharge.

CASE 95: MAN WITH CHEST PAIN AND WEIGHT LOSS

History

A 65-year-old man is referred to the medical assessment unit with a 2-month history of progressive shortness of breath and left-sided chest pain. He has had a chronic cough, but more recently has been coughing up blood-stained sputum. His wife also mentioned that his appetite has diminished and feels he may have lost weight over the preceding months. He has seen the GP previously who started him on an inhaler with little noticeable benefit in symptoms.

His past medical history includes hypertension, gout and recent diagnosis of chronic obstructive pulmonary disease (COPD). Medications include amlodipine 5 mg/day, allopurinol 300 mg/day and 'a purple inhaler'. He recently retired as a taxi driver. He continues to smoke ten cigarettes per day and has a 40 pack-year smoking history. He lives with his wife, they have no pets and, until recently, his exercise tolerance had been miles.

Examination

On general examination, he was thin and gaunt with evidence of clubbing of the finger nails. He was able to complete sentences, but was dyspnoeic on minimal exertion. Observations demonstrated blood pressure (BP) 140/95 mmHg, oxygen saturations 95 per cent on room air, heart rate 80 beats per minute regular, respiratory rate 22 per minute and temperature 36.6°C.

Examination of the respiratory system revealed firm non-tender lymphadenopathy in the cervical chain, decreased expansion on the left with a stony dull percussion note over the left chest and diminished breath sounds.

QUESTIONS

1. What is the diagnosis?
2. What is the next most useful investigation?
3. What is the immediate management?
4. What further tests are necessary?

ANSWERS

1. The clinical diagnosis is that of a left pleural effusion.

2. The next most useful investigation would be a chest x-ray. The PA (posteroanterior) chest x-ray is abnormal in the presence of approximately 200 mL of pleural fluid. The first sign of a pleural effusion may be blunting of the costophrenic angle.

3. (Answers 3 and 4). In this patient, there is no evidence of respiratory compromise, therefore management should be aimed at obtaining a diagnosis. The next most useful step should be to obtain a pleural fluid sample for analysis. Current guidelines are that pleural aspiration should be performed with ultrasound guidance to increase the likelihood of successful pleural fluid aspiration and reduce the risk of organ puncture and iatrogenic pneumothorax. Fluid should be sent for protein, lactate dehydrogenase, Gram stain, cytology and microbiological culture. If there is a diagnostic suspicion of pleural infection, fluid should also be measured for pH. The appearance of the fluid and any odour may assist in the diagnosis, e.g. putrid smell and purulent aspirate is suggestive of empyema.

   The fluid that accumulates may be an exudate or a transudate. Light's criteria should be utilized to distinguish between the two and this requires concurrent measurement of serum lactate dehydrogenase (LDH) and serum protein. (In general terms, a fluid protein >35 g/L is an exudate and <25 g/L is a transudate.)

Light's criteria

Pleural fluid is an exudate if:
- Pleural fluid protein divided by serum protein is >0.5.
- Pleural fluid LDH divided by serum LDH is >0.6.
- Pleural fluid LDH >2/3 the upper limit of laboratory normal serum LDH.

Categorization of pleural fluid into transudates and exudates is an important step in narrowing the differential diagnosis and guiding subsequent investigations. The mnemonic 'PINTS' and 'CHARM' can be a useful aide-memoire for causes of exudates and transudates (see below).

Exudates	Transudates
Pneumonia	Cardiac failure
Infarction (pulmonary embolus)	Hypoalbuminaemia/hypothyroidism
Neoplasia (i.e. malignancy)	Ascites (hepatic hydrothorax)
Tuberculosis	Renal failure (dialysis and nephrotic syndrome)
SLE (systemic lupus erythromatosus)/ other connective tissue disease	Meigs' syndrome (ovarian tumour and right-sided pleural effusion)

Once the cause of the pleural effusion is established, treatment should be directed at the cause. In malignant pleural effusions (the likely cause in this case), pleural fluid cytology is diagnostic in up to 60 per cent of cases. If the pleural fluid pH is <7.2, this suggests on-going pleural infection/empyema and should be treated with chest tube drainage. Pleural fluid amylase can be measured in a suspected case of pleural effusion secondary to oesophageal rupture or pancreatitis. In cases of pleural effusion secondary to rheumatoid arthritis, pleural fluid glucose will be very low (<1.6 mmol/L).

In this case, the most likely cause is a pleural effusion secondary to primary malignant neoplasm. He should be referred urgently to a chest physician for further investigation and management.

CASE 96: YOUNG WOMAN WITH PAIN IN HER LEGS AND BACK

History

A 23-year-old woman is referred to the acute medical unit by her GP. She gives a 5-day history of severe pain in her legs and back. For the last 2–3 days, she has found it increasingly difficult to walk and has noticed paraesthesia in her feet. She is normally fit and well. She had an acute self-limiting, diarrhoeal illness 14 days previously. She takes no regular medication and works as a shop assistant. She does not smoke and drinks 10 units of alcohol per week. There is no history of significant illness in her family.

Examination

On examination, she was apyrexial, blood pressure (BP) 120/75 mmHg, pulse 110 beats per minute sinus rhythm, respiratory rate 23 per minute, oxygen saturations 98 per cent on air. On examination of the chest, breath sounds are equal bilaterally. Neurological examination reveals symmetrical distal weakness of the lower limbs. Upper limb power was normal and no cranial nerve abnormality could be demonstrated. No deep tendon reflexes could be elicited despite reinforcement manoeuvres. Plantar responses were down-going bilaterally. Despite her complaint of paraesthesia in the feet, no objective sensory loss could be demonstrated. The remainder of her cardiovascular and abdominal examination was normal.

QUESTIONS

1. What is the most likely diagnosis?
2. What investigations will confirm the diagnosis? What would you expect to find?
3. What are the treatments for this condition?
4. What is the prognosis?

ANSWERS

1. The most likely diagnosis here is of Guillain–Barré syndrome. Guillain–Barré syndrome typically presents with a progressive, symmetrical ascending muscle weakness with absent or depressed deep tendon reflexes. It is characteristically associated with a preceding respiratory or gastrointestinal infection. The weakness can vary from mild difficulty in walking to severe paralysis of all muscles including facial, respiratory and bulbar muscles. Severe respiratory muscle weakness occurs in 10–30 per cent of patients, often requiring ventilatory support. Sensory symptoms, when reported, are typically not associated with objective sensory signs on examination. Autonomic involvement may lead to cardiac arrhythmias (sinus tachycardia being the most common), urinary retention and disturbance of blood pressure control. The progressive weakness is usually maximal by 1–2 weeks. The Miller–Fischer variant of Guillain–Barré syndrome is associated with opthalmoplegia, ataxia and areflexia.

2. The diagnosis can be confirmed by performing a lumbar puncture. A lumbar puncture will typically reveal an elevated cerebrospinal fluid (CSF) protein with a normal CSF white cell count, normal CSF glucose and a normal CSF opening pressure (see below). Nerve conduction studies and electromyography are also useful to support the clinical diagnosis of Guillain–Barré syndrome and provide information regarding prognosis. Sensory nerve conduction studies typically show slowing of nerve conduction thought to be due to inflammatory demyelination of the nerve. Electromyography will demonstrate denervation. Serial examination over time can assist in determining improvement or deterioration in nerve function.

Cerebrospinal fluid	Guillain–Barré syndrome	Normal
CSF white cell count	<5 cells/mm^3	<5 cells/mm^3
CSF protein	450–2000 mg/L	150–450 mg/L
CSF glucose	2.2–3.9 mmol/L	2.2–3.9 mmol/L
CSF opening pressure	60–150 mm CSF	60–150 mm CSF

3. Treatment can be divided into supportive care and disease-modifying therapies. Most patients can be managed on a general ward, paying close attention to pressure areas, bowel and bladder care, as well as prophylaxis for deep vein thrombosis.

   Since respiratory failure in Guillain–Barré syndrome is common, it is imperative to monitor forced vital capacity (FVC), at least 4 hourly, as a rapid progression of respiratory muscle weakness may require intubation and ventilation. Admission to the intensive therapy unit (ITU) should be considered if: (1) the FVC <1.5 L; (2) arterial blood gases demonstrate hypoxia and hypercapnia; and (3) there is on-going severe muscle weakness. Mechanical ventilatory support, often with tracheostomy, may be required for weeks to months during the recovery phase.

Psychological, physiotherapy and occupational therapy support are an essential component of rehabilitation from Guillain–Barré syndrome, which frequently follows a protracted course. Neuropathic pain is common and may not respond to simple analgesics. In cases of intractable neuropathic pain, gabapentin and carba-mezapine have been shown to be effective.

The disease-modifying therapies for Guillain–Barré syndrome include plasma exchange (plasmapheresis) and intravenous immunoglobulin. The rationale behind both treatments is to alter the immune response that leads to nerve damage. Current evidence suggests that both treatments are equally effective. The choice between plasma exchange and intravenous immunoglobulin depends on local availability, contraindications and preference. There is no evidence that glucocorticoids alter the clinical course of Guillain–Barré syndrome.

4. In general, the prognosis of Guillain–Barré syndrome is good, with 80 per cent of patients making a complete recovery or left with a minor residual deficit. Between 5 and 10 per cent of patients have a prolonged course of illness, often requiring months of ventilator dependence, leading to a delayed and incomplete recovery. Mortality rate from Guillain–Barré syndrome is approximately 5 per cent. Up to 10 per cent of patients may suffer relapse with increased weakness.

Factors suggesting a poor prognosis
• Rapid onset of symptoms
• Older age
• Severe muscle weakness at presentation
• Preceding *Campylobacter jejuni* infection or diarrhoeal illness
• Need for ventilatory support
• Axonal degeneration on nerve conduction studies

CASE 97: MIDDLE-AGED MAN WITH SEVERE HEADACHE

History

A 45-year-old man presents to A&E complaining of a severe headache. The headache started 2 days prior to admission and has rapidly become more unbearable. He describes it as generalized headache associated with nausea and vomiting. He has felt feverish and shivery over the last 24 hours and has preferred to be alone in a dark, quiet room. Over the last week, he had been suffering with earache in his right ear associated with a serous discharge, but had not sought advice from the GP. His past medical history includes recurrent ear infections for which he is being followed up by an ENT surgeon. He takes no regular medication and has no allergies. He lives with his wife and two children all of whom are well. He works as an IT manager, drinks 34 units of alcohol per week and is a lifelong non-smoker.

Examination

On examination, he appears flushed and unwell with no rashes. His temperature is 39.5°C, heart rate 124 beats per minute regular, blood pressure (BP) 110/65 mmHg, oxygen saturations 100 per cent on air. He is in a cubicle with the lights switched off. His neck is stiff and he finds it difficult to move his head. He is drowsy, but rousable, and able to obey commands. There is no focal neurological deficit. Fundoscopy is normal, but he appears a little irritable. Examination of cardiovascular, respiratory and abdominal systems is unremarkable.

Investigations

		Reference range
Haemoglobin	14.5	13.5–18 g/dL
White cell count	18.5×10^9/L	$4.0–11.0 \times 10^9$/L
Neutrophil count	16.4×10^9/L	$2.0–7.5 \times 10^9$/L
Platelets	540×10^9/L	$150–450 \times 10^9$/L
Sodium	128 mmol/L	135–146 mmol/L
Potassium	3.4 mmol/L	3.2–5.1 mmol/L
Urea	12.6 mmol/L	1.7–8.3 mmol/L
Creatinine	99 mmol/L	62–106 mmol/L
Glucose	5.8 mmol/L	3.2–6.0 mmol/L (fasting)
C-reactive protein (CRP)	200 mg/L	<5 mg/L
International normalized ratio (INR)	1.1	1.0–1.3

Lumbar puncture

Cerebrospinal fluid (CSF)		
Appearance	Turbid	Clear and colourless
Opening pressure	22	6–18 cm CSF
White cell count	100 (mainly polymorphs)	<5/mm
Protein	1450	150–450 mg/L
Glucose	1.2	2.2–3.9 mmol/L
Gram stain	Gram-positive cocci	

QUESTIONS

1. What is the diagnosis?
2. What is the differential diagnosis of an acute severe headache?
3. What further examinations would be useful?
4. What is the likely causative organism?
5. What is the management of this patient?

ANSWERS

1. The diagnosis here is of acute bacterial meningitis. He has presented with a sudden-onset headache, photophobia, fever and neck stiffness. The leukocytosis with neutrophilia, tachycardia and raised CRP are more suggestive of bacterial infection than viral meningitis.

2. The differential diagnosis of an acute severe headache includes: meningitis (viral, bacterial, fungal, cryptococcal and tuberculous), subarachnoid haemorrhage, encephalitis, temporal arteritis and acute migraine.

3. Given the history of ear problems, examination of the ears with an otoscope is imperative. Further tests to illicit meningism may also be useful. Kernig's sign is positive if pain and resistance are elicited on passive knee extension with the hips flexed. Brudzinski's sign is positive when hips flex on neck flexion.

    In this case, the history of chronic ear problems suggests direct extension from the ear to the meninges. The most common organisms that cause bacterial meningitis in the UK are *Neisseria meningitis* and *Streptococcus pneumoniae*, accounting for approximately 70 per cent of cases. *Haemophilus influenzae* has virtually been eliminated as a cause of meningitis in the UK due to the childhood immunization programme. The most likely causative organism in this case is *Streptococcus pneumoniae* due to the history of concurrent ear infection and the presence of Gram-positive cocci on Gram stain.

4. (Answers 4 and 5). Bacterial meningitis if left untreated carries a 70–100 per cent mortality rate, therefore, early recognition and rapid treatment is vital. Meningococcal meningitis is suspected clinically by the presence of a characteristic petechial rash, and immediate treatment with antibiotics (prior to lumbar puncture) is imperative. In this case, there is no suggestion of meningococcal infection, localizing neurological signs or papilloedema, therefore lumbar puncture should be performed immediately after CT head scan with contrast has excluded a cerebral abscess. This is important in view of the history of recurrent ear infections. See table below for typical CSF findings in meningitis. Intravenous antibiotics should be administered according to local hospital protocols; usually a third-generation cephalosporin (e.g. ceftriaxone). The subsequent choice and duration of antibiotic therapy should be made in conjunction with a microbiologist. Amoxicillin is often added if the patient is elderly (>55 years old), immunocompromised or alcoholic. In the absence of septic shock, immunocompromise or post-neurosurgical intervention then dexamethasone 10 mg i.v. four times a day should be administered for 4 days. Evidence suggests that steroids reduce the frequency of neurological complications, in particular deafness. This patient should also be referred to the ENT surgeons for review and advice on management of the patient's otitis media. The headache seen in meningitis is often severe requiring adequate analgesia including opiates. This patient has a mild hyponatraemia due to the fever and increased insensible losses, as well as the syndrome of inappropriate ADH (anti-diuretic hormone) secretion and should be treated with intravenous normal saline.

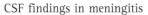

CSF findings in meningitis

	Normal	Pyogenic	Viral	Tuberculous
Appearance	Clear and colourless	Turbid/ purulent	Clear	Turbid/viscous
Cell count	<5 mm^3	>10 mm^3	50–1000	100–300
Predominant cell	Nil	Polymorphs	Mononuclear	Varies
Protein	140–450 mg/L	500–2000 mg/L	400–800 mg/L	500 mg–3 g/L
Glucose	2.2–3.9 mmol/L (>2/3 blood glucose)	<1/2 blood glucose	>1/2 blood glucose	<<1/2 blood glucose

All cases of bacterial meningitis should be reported to the local Health Protection Agency (HPA). The HPA will advise on prophylactic treatment and possible vaccination of contacts with meningococcal disease.

Complications of acute bacterial meningitis and their treatment

- Raised intracranial pressure, treated with steroids and mannitol.
- Hydrocephalus, treated by urgent neurosurgical intervention and interventricular shunting.
- Seizures should be treated in the conventional way.
- Disseminated intravascular coagulation is an ominous sign and suggests overwhelming sepsis. It carries a high mortality rate.

CASE 98: MIDDLE-AGED MAN WITH EPIGASTRIC PAIN

History

A 45-year-old man presented to the acute medical unit with a 48-hour history of grad-ual onset epigastric pain. He described this as 'gnawing' in nature and radiating through to the back. It was associated with vomiting and nausea, while coming and going in waves. The pain was made worse following a meal with partial relief on leaning for-ward. He described the severity as 8 out of 10.

He had recently seen his GP for investigation of high blood sugars. Fifteen years ago, he had a similar problem but had discharged himself from hospital after 3 days. He takes no regular medication and has no allergies. He works as a publican and lives in his pub with his wife. He drinks 40 units of alcohol per week and has recently stopped smoking with a 25 pack-year history. There is no relevant family history.

Examination

On examination, he is overweight and clearly in pain. Observations reveal a low-grade fever of 37.5°C, blood pressure (BP) 135/75 mmHg, pulse 120 per minute regular, res-piratory rate 22 per minute, oxygen saturations 98 per cent on air. Abdominal examina-tion reveals tenderness on palpation of the epigastrium and right hypochondrium with no rebound or guarding. Cardiovascular and respiratory examinations are unremarkable.

Investigations

		Reference range
Haemoglobin	14.5 g/dL	13.5–18 g/dL
White cell count	11.8×10^9/L	$4.0–11.0 \times 10^9$/L
Platelets	476×10^9/L	$150–450 \times 10^9$/L
Sodium	133 mmol/L	135–146 mmol/L
Potassium	3.4 mmol/L	3.2–5.1 mmol/L
Urea	4.5 mmol/L	1.7–8.3 mmol/L
Creatinine	99 mmol/L	62–106 mmol/L
C-reactive protein (CRP)	50 mg/L	<5 mg/L
Amylase	300 IU/L	28–100 IU/L

His abdominal x-ray is shown in Figure 98.1.

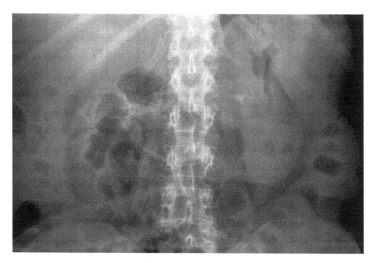

Figure 98.1

QUESTIONS

1. What does the abdominal x-ray show (Figure 98.1)?
2. What is the diagnosis?
3. What are the consequences and complications of this condition?
4. What other investigations may be useful?
5. What is the treatment for this condition?

ANSWERS

1. The abdominal x-ray demonstrates calcification within the pancreatic duct and side branches, this occurs in approximately 30 per cent of cases of chronic pancreatitis. A calcified pancreas is most commonly seen in chronic pancreatitis secondary to alcohol excess. Other causes of a calcific pancreas include pancreatic pseudocyst, hyperparathyroidism, cystic fibrosis and hereditary pancreatitis.

2. Given his occupation and history of excessive alcohol consumption, the most likely diagnosis here is of acute-on-chronic alcoholic pancreatitis. It is likely that the episode of abdominal pain 15 years ago was also related to this. Abdominal pain is usually the dominant feature of chronic pancreatitis and presents in a very similar way to acute pancreatitis as the disease progresses; rather than discrete episodes of pain it tends to become more continuous.

3. The classical triad of pancreatic calcifications, steatorrhoea and diabetes mellitus strongly suggests the diagnosis but are usually only seen with advanced disease. As the disease progresses, pancreatic exocrine deficiency may develop (usually not clinically significant until over 90 per cent of pancreatic function is lost). This leads to fat malabsorption and the passage of steatorrhoea (loose, greasy, foul-smelling stool that is difficult to flush). Diabetes mellitus is usually difficult to treat often requiring insulin therapy.

4. The serum amylase level in this case is only marginally elevated, in comparison to cases of acute pancreatitis where it may reach thousands. This is due to the fact that chronic pancreatitis causes fibrosis of the pancreas resulting in decreased enzyme levels. Pancreatic insufficiency can be assessed by the use of stool tests measuring faecal fat globules and faecal elastase. Further imaging may be useful including ultrasound, computed tomography (CT) and magnetic resonance imaging (MRI) (in particular magnetic resonance cholangiopancreatography (MRCP)) depending on the clinical scenario. CT scanning has the advantage of both ruling out other causes of abdominal pain, such as pancreatic malignancy, as well as assessing for complications of chronic pancreatitis, including pseudocyst formation and splenic vein thrombosis, and is highly sensitive in the detection of pancreatic calcification. Endoscopic retrograde cholangiopancreatography (ERCP) is usually reserved for patients who require therapeutic intervention.

5. The aims of treatment of chronic pancreatitis include adequate pain control, correction of pancreatic insufficiency and management of complications. Abdominal pain can range from mild and occasional postprandial epigastric pain to a severe and debilitating pain with vomiting and weight loss. Where possible, treatment should be aimed at the underlying aetiology of pancreatitis. Alcohol is a frequent precipitant of pain in chronic pancreatitis and therefore abstinence is a key factor in relieving pain. Smoking is recognized to accelerate the natural history of the disease and increase the risk of progression to pancreatic cancer. Smoking cessation should therefore be encouraged.

Excess stimulation of the pancreas should be avoided. Small, low-fat meals may be of benefit with varying degrees of success. Suppression of pancreatic exocrine function by using pancreatic enzyme supplements (e.g. Creon®) may also relieve pain in some patients. Suppression of stomach acid with proton pump inhibitors may also inhibit stimulation of pancreatic secretion.

Pain relief should be administered in a stepwise fashion, starting initially with non-opiate analgesics. Neuropathic pain agents, such as amitriptyline, may be of benefit. However, chronic opioid analgesia is often required in patients with persisting pain. Other methods to treat intractable pain include coeliac plexus blocks (either percutaneous or endoscopic). These methods have varying degrees of success and, due to their potential complications, should be performed by specialists only. Surgery, including pancreatic resection, is seen as a last resort.

Fat malabsorption (steatorrhoea) occurs with severe pancreatic exocrine dysfunction as patients are unable to digest complex foods and fats. The result is the passage of loose, greasy, offensive stools that are difficult to flush. Treatment includes both pancreatic enzyme supplementation and dietary modifications with restriction of fat intake. It may be necessary to supplement fat-soluble vitamins (A, D, E, K). The aim of treatment is to ensure adequate nutrition with control of abdominal symptoms.

Glucose intolerance occurs frequently in chronic pancreatitis, however, overt diabetes mellitus occurs late in the course of the disease. Patients who develop diabetes mellitus usually require insulin therapy and should be managed by specialist diabetologists.

Patients with chronic pancreatitis require long-term follow up as symptoms usually progress with time. There is an increased risk of progression to pancreatic carcinoma, therefore clinicians should be vigilant of this potentially fatal complication.

CASE 99: ELDERLY WOMAN WITH FEVER AND MILD CONFUSION

History

A 70-year-old woman is referred to the acute medical unit with a 3-day history of fever, mild confusion and urinary frequency. Her abbreviated mental test score is 7/10. She is a recently diagnosed type 2 diabetic for which she takes metformin 500 mg three times a day. She has a past medical history of hypertension and hypothyroidism. Her other medication includes lisinopril 5 mg/day and levothyroxine 75 µg/day. She has no allergies. She lives with her husband and is totally independent. She is a non-smoker and drinks 30 units per week.

Examination

On examination, she is pleasantly confused and looks well. Her temperature is 38.2°C, blood pressure (BP) 148/85 mmHg, pulse 77 per minute regular, oxygen saturations 99 per cent on air. Abdominal examination reveals mild suprapubic tenderness with no palpable bladder and no pain on examination of the loins. Chest and cardiovascular examinations are unremarkable.

Investigations

		Reference range
Haemoglobin	13.5 g/dL	13.5–18 g/dL
White cell count	12.0×10^9/L	$4.0–11.0 \times 10^9$/L
Neutrophil count	7.9×10^9/L	$2.0–7.5 \times 10^9$/L
Platelets	400×10^9/L	$150–450 \times 10^9$/L
Sodium	136 mmol/L	135–146 mmol/L
Potassium	4.5 mmol/L	3.2–5.1 mmol/L
Urea	7.0 mmol/L	1.7–8.3 mmol/L
Creatinine	83 mmol/L	62–106 mmol/L
C-reactive protein (CRP)	88 mg/L	<5 mg/L
Glucose	10.1 mmol/L	3.2–6.0 mmol/L (fasting)

Urine dipstick, nitrites positive, leukocytes 2+, blood 1+, glucose 1+.
Urine culture, awaited.

QUESTIONS

1. What is the diagnosis?
2. What is the appropriate management of this case?
3. Describe the steps involved in obtaining a midstream urine.
4. What are the most likely organisms?
5. What is the accuracy of the urine dipstick?
6. What are the causes of a sterile pyuria?

ANSWERS

1. The diagnosis here is of a simple lower urinary tract infection (UTI). Symptoms of lower UTI include urinary frequency, dysuria, urgency, haematuria, strangury (painful, frequent passage of small amounts of urine on straining) and suprapubic tenderness.

2. Prior to commencement of antibiotics, a midstream urine should be obtained and sent to the laboratory for culture. UTIs can be a common cause of acute confusion in the elderly and should be managed as with any other cause of acute delirium. She should be encouraged to drink plenty of fluid (at least 2 litres per day) to help flush bacteria from the urinary tract. Her blood sugars should be tightly controlled. Empirical antibiotic therapy should be given as per local hospital guidelines, based on local sensitivity and resistance patterns. Typical first-line antibiotics are trimethoprim 200 mg twice a day for 3 days or nitrofurantoin 50 mg four times a day for 3 days, remembering men will require a longer 7-day course of antibiotics. Intravenous antibiotics including the use of gentamicin should be considered if there are signs of the systemic inflammatory response syndrome.

3. The reference standard test in diagnosis of UTI is suprapubic aspiration of bladder contents. Clearly, this is impractical and not without risk, and is therefore not routinely used in clinical practice. Urine samples are generally obtained following natural micturition and are therefore subject to artefactual contamination by normal urethral organisms. The likelihood of detecting a UTI by urine culture is highest if the specimen is taken on arising, as the urine is likely to be most concentrated and bacteria in the bladder will have had time to multiply overnight.

Obtaining a midstream urine
• Clean and dry the urethral meatus and adjacent mucosa. • Minimize mucosal contact: spread the labia in females, pull back foreskin in males. • Discard the first voided specimen as it will contain urethral contaminants. • Collect sample of midstream urine in sterile container.

The sample should be sent immediately to the laboratory as the bacteria will continue to proliferate in warm, freshly voided urine leading to increased cell counts.

4. Urinary tract infections are most commonly caused by bacteria from the patient's own bowel flora. These bacteria colonize the periurethral area and are then able to ascend the urethral passage into the bladder. Women are particularly prone as they have a shorter distance between the anus and urethra, as well as a shorter urethra than men. Prostatic fluid also has bactericidal properties that help prevent ascending infection in men. Other risk factors for UTI include use of the diaphragm contraceptive, vaginal atrophy, sexual intercourse, instrumentation of the urinary tract, diabetes mellitus and an anatomically abnormal urinary tract.

> ## The common causative organisms
>
> - *Escherichia coli* (~70 per cent)
> - *Proteus mirabilis* (~11 per cent)
> - *Staphylococcus saprophyticus* or *epidermidis* (~10 per cent)
> - *Enterococcus faecalis* (~7 per cent)
> - *Klebisella aerogenes* (~4 per cent)

5. The diagnosis of UTI is confirmed by laboratory urine culture demonstrating $\geq 10^5$ colony-forming units/mL along with pyuria. Urine dipsticks are a useful screening tool for the diagnosis of UTI prior to obtaining urine culture results. However, they should be used in conjunction with assessment of urinary symptoms. Urine dipsticks are able to detect the presence of leukocyte esterase and nitrites in the urine. Presence of nitrites depends on the conversion of nitrates to nitrites by nitrate-reductase producing bacteria in the bladder. Reasons for a negative nitrite test in the presence of UTI may be due to insufficient bladder incubation time (e.g. <4 hours) to allow conversion of nitrates to nitrites, inability of some organisms to convert nitrates to nitrites and decreased urinary pH (e.g. due to concurrent use of cranberry juice). Leukocyte esterase is produced by neutrophils and corresponds to pyuria most frequently seen in UTI.

   Studies have demonstrated that the presence of nitrites is most predictive of the diagnosis of a UTI, followed by the presence of both leukocytes and blood. A recent study assessed urine dipsticks (nitrites, leukocytes and blood) and clinical criteria (urine cloudiness, dysuria and nocturia) for the diagnosis of UTI in women in the primary care setting (see Little *et al.* 2010). It demonstrated that if all three dipstick results were negative, the negative predictive value of diagnosing a UTI was 76 per cent meaning that 24 per cent of patients who are dipstick-negative will actually have a UTI-based on laboratory culture. If nitrites and either blood or leukocytes were present, this provided a positive predictive value of 92 per cent. Nitrites alone or leukocytes with blood provide a positive predictive value of 81 per cent. These results demonstrate that urine dipsticks are a useful bedside tool to improve immediate diagnostic accuracy in UTI but high false-negative rates need to be considered.

6. The term 'sterile pyuria' refers to the presence of leukocytes in the urine in the absence of bacterial infection. Causes of sterile pyuria are:

   - Concurrent use of antibiotics (often due to self-medication with antibiotics)
   - Sample contamination, e.g. vaginal leukocytes
   - Chronic interstitial nephritis
   - *Chlamydia* infection
   - Nephrolithiasis
   - Uroepithelial tumours
   - Tuberculosis.

CASE 100: ELDERLY WOMAN ADMITTED FOLLOWING A FALL

History

An 85-year-old woman is brought to A&E by ambulance on New Year's bank holiday Monday morning, having been found on the floor by her daughter. She lives alone and had last been seen by her daughter on Friday night. She was found slumped in the lounge by her favourite armchair. She has a past medical history of rheumatoid arthritis, type 2 diabetes, hypothyroidism and hypertension. Her medication includes co-dydramol, gliclazide, levothyroxine and atenolol. She has no allergies. She functions independently at home with the support of her daughter, but has no formal care package. Her mobility is limited to 10 yards due to her arthritis and she walks with the assistance of a stick.

Examination

On examination, she looks frail and has cold peripheries. She is unkempt and covered in urine and faeces. She has mild confusion and her Glasgow Coma Score (GCS) is 13. Examination of the nervous system reveals equal and reactive pupils and no localizing neurological signs. She has globally diminished deep tendon reflexes and keeps trying to undress. Tympanic temperature reading less than 34°C, blood pressure 88/61 mmHg, pulse 64, respiratory rate 13 per minute. Despite best efforts, no reliable saturation trace can be achieved. Chest examination reveals coarse crackles at the right base. Abdominal and cardiovascular examinations are otherwise normal.

Investigations

		Reference range
Haemoglobin	16.5 g/dL	13.5–18 g/dL
White cell count	13.0×10^9/L	$4.0–11.0 \times 10^9$/L
Neutrophil count	11.4×10^9/L	$2.0–7.5 \times 10^9$/L
Platelets	400×10^9/L	$150–450 \times 10^9$/L
Sodium	147 mmol/L	135–146 mmol/L
Potassium	5.0 mmol/L	3.2–5.1 mmol/L
Urea	18.7 mmol/L	1.7–8.3 mmol/L
Creatinine	240 mmol/L	62–106 mmol/L
Glucose	3.6 mmol/L	3.2–6.0 mmol/L (fasting)

Electrocardiogram (ECG) tracing is shown in Figure 100.1.

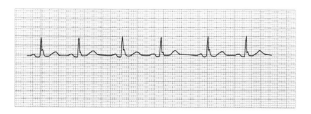

Figure 100.1

QUESTIONS

1. What is the cause of this patient's presentation? What does her ECG rhythm strip show?
2. What further investigations are necessary?
3. What factors in the history are likely to be contributing to the problem?
4. What is the management?

ANSWERS

1. This elderly woman has probably been on the floor for quite some time. There is no clear indication for the cause of her fall. Her ECG clearly demonstrates a J-wave which is characteristic of hypothermia (Figure 100.2, arrows). Hypothermia is defined as a core temperature below 35°C and occurs due to an imbalance between heat production and heat loss as excess heat is lost via evaporation, radiation, conduction and convection. The hypothermic heart is exquisitely sensitive to movement and therefore hypothermic patients should be handled with care. Any rough jostling may result in arrhythmia.

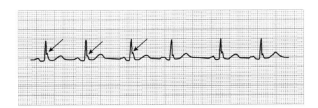

Figure 100.2 Arrows on J wave

2. Tympanic thermometers can be unreliable at measuring temperatures below 34°C, therefore the use of a low-reading thermometer is essential to ensure accurate determination of core body temperature. In practice, a rectal probe thermometer is most often used due to accuracy and ease of use. An oesophageal temperature probe is an alternative, but requires invasive ventilation. Further investigations that are necessary in this case include an arterial blood gas. This will provide an accurate assessment of oxygen levels, as well as acid-base balance. Other essential tests include measurement of serum creatinine kinase, thyroid function tests and a chest x-ray.

Further investigations	Result	Reference range
pH	7.31	7.35–7.45
pO_2	17.2 kPa	11.1–14.4 kPa
pCO_2	3.1 kPa	4.7–6.4 kPa
Lactate	10 mmol/L	0.5–2.2 mmol/L
HCO_3	12 mmol/L	22–29 mmol/L
Creatinine kinase	43 000 IU/L	30–145 IU/L
Thyroid-stimulating hormone (TSH)	3.3 mU/L	0.3–4.2 mU/L
Free thyroxine	16 pmol/L	12–22 pmol/L
Cortisol	380 nmol/L	171–536 nmol/L

Chest x-ray shows consolidation at the right base.

The arterial blood gas reveals a severe metabolic lactic acidosis with partial respiratory compensation. The elevated creatinine kinase is often seen in patients after a long lie and is suggestive of rhabdomyolysis. Normal thyroid function excludes hypothyroidism as a cause of her hypothermia and normal serum cortisol excludes an Addisonian crisis.

3. The elderly are particularly prone to hypothermia as they have a diminished ability to sense the cold and often have loss of insulating fat. Frequently, the elderly suffer from intercurrent illness (in this case, community-acquired pneumonia) which can impair thermoregulatory processes and may cause failure to rewarm. The elderly are also more likely to be socially isolated; in this case, the patient may have been on the floor for anything up to 3 days, thus exacerbating the impact of environmental exposure on temperature control. Drugs can also contribute in the impaired ability to sense cold, as well as inhibiting compensatory mechanisms. This woman's opiate analgesia may be contributory to her decreased level of consciousness, but absence of pinpoint pupils makes opiate toxicity less likely. Beta-blockers cause impaired response to thermoregulatory pathways, thus exacerbating this patient's hypothermia.

This patient's diagnosis is of hypothermia secondary to severe community-acquired pneumonia (CURB score, 4) with acute kidney injury, partially compensated metabolic lactic acidosis and probable rhabdomyolysis.

4. The management of hypothermia in the elderly is with gradual rewarming and careful nursing, given the risk of inducing arrhythmia to the irritable myocardium. The aim should be to increase the core body temperature by 1°C per hour. Rewarming techniques can be divided into passive external rewarming, active external warming and active internal rewarming. Rewarming the trunk should be undertaken prior to the extremities as this will minimize the risk of peripheral arterial vasodilatation and subsequent hypotension, acidaemia and core temperature after-drop. Passive external rewarming involves the use of 'space blankets' to cover and insulate the patient resulting in a reduction in heat loss. In elderly patients, this is often unsuccessful as they lack the normal metabolic and cardiovascular mechanisms to achieve thermoregulation. Therefore, the elderly usually require active rewarming. This is achieved by the use of heated blankets, warm inspired oxygen and warmed intravenous fluids. In severe cases, bladder and peritoneal lavage can be used as well as extracorporeal blood rewarming, e.g. cardiopulmonary bypass.

Alongside rewarming strategies, this patient should be referred to the intensive care physicians (if appropriate) as she will require close monitoring of fluid balance (including catheterization and measurement of hourly urine output) and cardiac rhythm. Broad-spectrum intravenous antibiotics should be used to treat the community-acquired pneumonia in line with local antibiotic policies.

Before discharge, preventing further episodes is essential. Improving home heating and insulation, financial support for heating during the winter months and extra supervision during cold periods are all useful strategies to prevent recurrence. Close liaison with social services and the GP are essential. Any drugs that may predispose to further episodes of hypothermia should be reviewed and stopped if possible. Approximately 30 000 deaths per year in the UK are attributable to hypothermia.

BIBLIOGRAPHY

Akumjee N, Akumjee M. *The Easy Guide to OSCEs for Final Year Medical Students.* Oxford: Radcliffe Publishing, 2007.

Bickle I, Hamilton P, Stockham B. *Data Interpretation for Medical Students,* 2nd edn. Knutsford: Pastest, 2012.

Fuller G. *Neurological Examination Made Easy,* 4th edn. Edinburgh: Churchill Livingstone, 2008.

Ginsberg L. *Lecture Notes: Neurology,* 9th edn. Oxford: Wiley-Blackwell, 2010.

Hampton JR. *The ECG Made Easy,* 7th edn. Edinburgh: Churchill Livingstone, 2008.

Hennessey I, Japp A. *Arterial Blood Gases Made Easy.* Edinburgh: Churchill-Livingstone, 2007.

Herring W. *Learning Radiology: Recognising the Basics,* 2nd edn. Philadelphia, PA: Saunders, 2011.

Hoffbrand V, Moss P. *Essential Haematology,* 6th edn. Oxford: Wiley-Blackwell, 2011.

Howlett D, Ayers B. *The Hands-on Guide to Imaging.* Oxford: Blackwell, 2004.

Kalra P. *Essential Revision Notes in Medicine for Students.* Knutsford: Pastest, 2006.

Koppel C, Naparus A. *Thinking Medicine: Structure your Thoughts for Success in Medical Exams,* 2nd edn. London: Cavaye Publishing, 2011.

Kumar P, Clark M. *Kumar and Clark's Clinical Medicine,* 7th edn. Philadelphia, PA: WB Saunders, 2009.

Lim E, Loke YK, Thompson A (eds). *Medicine and Surgery: An Integrated Textbook,* 1st edn. Edinburgh: Churchill Livingstone, 2007.

Little P, Turner S, Rumsby K *et al. British Journal of General Practice* 2010; 60: 495–500.

Longmore M, Wilkinson I, Davidson E *et al.* (eds). *The Oxford Handbook of Clinical Medicine,* 8th edn. Oxford: Oxford University Press, 2010.

Marshall WJ, Bangert SK. *Clinical Chemistry,* 6th edn. St Louis, MO: Mosby, 2008.

Raby N, Berman L, de Lacey G. *Accident and Emergency Radiology: A Survival Guide,* 2nd edn. Philadelphia, PA: Saunders, 2005.

Ryder B, Mir A, Freeman A. *Medical Short Cases for Medical Students.* Oxford: Wiley-Blackwell, 2000.

Selby C. *Respiratory Medicine: An illustrated Colour Text.* Edinburgh: Churchill Livingstone, 2002.

Sprigings D, Chambers J (eds). *Acute Medicine: A Practical Guide to the Management of Medical Emergencies,* 4th edn. Oxford: Wiley-Blackwell, 2007.

Swanton RH, Banerjee S. *Swanton's Cardiology: A Concise Guide to Clinical Practice,* 6th edn. Oxford: Wiley-Blackwell, 2008.

Thomas J, Monaghan T (eds). *Oxford Handbook of Clinical Examination and Practical Skills.* Oxford: Oxford University Press, 2007.

Travis S, Ahmad T, Collier J, Hillary-Steinhart A. *Gastroenterology (Pocket Consultant),* 3rd edn. Oxford: Wiley-Blackwell, 2005.

West JB. *Respiratory Physiology: The Essentials,* 9th edn. Philadelphia, PA: Lippincott Williams & Wilkins, 2011.

Index

A

Abbreviated Mental Score (AMT), 52
abbreviations, *xiii*
ABCDE approach
  respiratory distress, 412
  shortness of breath, 155
abdominal pain
  chronic diarrhoea, 24–27
  evolving inferior myocardial infarction,
    361–364
  inflammatory bowel disease, 115–121
  toxic colitis, 204–209
abnormal blood test results, 314–317
ACD, *see* Anaemia of chronic
    disease (ACD)
ACE (angiotensin-converting enzyme)
    inhibitors
  aldosterone/PRA, 17
  diabetes, 160
  headache, 90
  kidney disease, 390
  leg swelling, 423
  NT-proBNP levels, 11
  syncope, 360
N-acetylcysteine, 426–427
achalasia of the oesophagus, 127–131
acquired haemolytic anaemia, 256–259
acquired pneumothoraces, 134
ACTH, *see* Adrenocorticotropic
    hormone (ACTH)
activated charcoal, 48
activated partial thromboplastin
    time (APTT)
  bruising, 275
  emergency hip repair, 303
  knees, swollen, 287
  leg pain and swelling, 295
  light-headedness, 248
  panic attacks, 279
  right-sided weakness, 307–309
  swollen knee, 288
  tiredness, 311

acute bacterial meningitis, 436–439
acute cardiac failure, 200–203
acute disseminated encephalomyelitis
    (ADEM), 140
acute inferior myocardial infarction,
    339–340
acute ischaemia, 388–390
acute large bowel obstruction, 229–233
acute leukaemia, 274–277
acute lymphoblastic leukaemia
    (ALL), 276
acute lymphocytic leukaemia (ALL),
    272–273
acute migraine, 438
acute mitral regurgitation, 350
acute myeloid leukaemia (AML)
  bruising, 265–269
  unexplained bruises, 277
acute-on-chronic alcoholic pancreatitis,
    440–443
acute peridarditis, 391–392
acute renal failure
  hyponatraemia, 6
  NT-proBNP levels, 11
acute severe cord compression, 195–199
acute subarachnoid haemorrhage (SAH),
    191–194
acute viral infections
  hip pain, 270–273
  unexplained bruises, 277
Addison's disease
  dysuria, 70–73
  hypercalcaemia, 73
  hyponatraemia, 6
ADEM, *see* Acute disseminated
    encephalomyelitis (ADEM)
adenocarcinomas, 222
ADH, *see* Antidiuretic hormone (ADH)
adjusted calcium, *see also* Calcium
  abdominal pain, 24
  colicky pain, 62
  confusion, 95

cough, 20
depression, 29
dysuria, 70
headache, 13, 90
renal failure, 56
adjusted magnesium
depression, 29
dysuria, 70
headache, 13
adrenal cortex anitbody, 71
adrenal insufficiency, 6
adrenal medullary tissue, 93
adrenocorticotropic hormone (ACTH)
diabetes mellitus, 68
dysuria, 71–72
periods (menstruation), 107
AF, *see* Atrial fibrillation (AF)
age, NT-proBNP levels, 10
AIHA, *see* Autoimmune haemolytic
anaemia (AIHA)
alanine aminotransferase (ALT)
abdominal pain, 204
abnormal blood test results, 314
anaemia, 253, 257
attempted suicide, 424
bloody cough, 161
bruising, 275
cellulitis, 319
chest pain, 242
confusion, 94, 95, 99, 260
constipation, 230
cough, 20
diabetes mellitus, 66
dysuria, 70
emergency hip repair, 303
falls, 82
fatigue, 235
fever and lethargy, 299
hip pain, 271
hypokalaemia, 22
knees, 108, 110, 287
leg swelling, 419
lethargy, 238
light-headedness, 248
nose bleeds, 283
NT-proBNP levels, 10–11
panic attacks, 279
periods (menstruation), 291
right-sided weakness, 307

semi-consciousness, 44
shortness of breath, 8, 78, 80
tiredness, 100, 311
albumin
abdominal pain, 115, 204
abnormal blood test results, 314
anaemia, 253, 257
bloody cough, 161
bruising, 275
cellulitis, 319
chest pain, 242
colicky pain, 62
confusion, 94, 95, 260
constipation, 230
cough, 20, 52, 55
depression, 28
diabetes mellitus, 66
dysuria, 70
emergency hip repair, 303
falls, 82
fatigue, 235
fever and lethargy, 299
headache and vomiting, 34
hips, 271, 303
knees, swollen, 287
leg swelling, 419
lethargy, 238
nose bleeds, 283
panic attacks, 279
periods (menstruation), 291
renal failure, 56
right-sided weakness, 307
semi-consciousness, 44
shortness of breath, 8, 78
tiredness, 100, 311
upper limb weakness, 219
vomiting, 38
alcohol excess
epigastric pain, 442
fatigue, 236
lethargy, 237–240
profound fatigue, 236
alcoholic cirrhosis, 99
alcoholic pancreatitis, acute-on-chronic,
440–443
aldosterone
dysuria, 71–72
headache, 14
hypokalaemia, 16–19

aldosterone/renin ratio, 14
alkaline antiacids, 23
alkaline phosphatase (ALP)
  abdominal pain, 24, 204
  abnormal blood test results, 314
  anaemia, 253, 257
  attempted suicide, 424
  bloody cough, 161
  bruising, 275
  cellulitis, 319
  chest pain, 242
  colicky pain, 62
  confusion, 94, 95, 99, 260
  constipation, 230
  cough, 20
  depression, 29
  diabetes mellitus, 66
  dysuria, 70
  emergency hip repair, 303
  falls, 82
  fatigue, 235
  fever and lethargy, 299
  headache, 90
  headache and vomiting, 34, 37
  hips, 271, 303
  knees, 108, 287
  leg swelling, 419
  lethargy, 237
  light-headedness, 248
  nose bleeds, 283
  panic attacks, 279
  periods (menstruation), 291
  renal failure, 56
  right-sided weakness, 307
  semi-consciousness, 44, 46
  shortness of breath, 8, 78, 80
  tiredness, 100, 311
  upper limb weakness, 219
alkalosis
  abdominal pain, 206
  aspirin overdose, 50
  hypokalaemia, 16, 22
  vomiting, 41
ALL, see Acute lymphoblastic
    leukaemia (ALL); Acute lymphocytic
    leukaemia (ALL)
allopurinal, 301
ALP, see Alkaline phosphatase (ALP)
ALT, see Alanine aminotransferase (ALT)

American trypanosomiasis, 131
amiodarone
  atrial fibrillation, 386
  palpitations, 366
AML, see Acute myeloid leukaemia
    (AML)
ammonium chloride, 65
AMT, see Abbreviated Mental Score
    (AMT)
amylase, 440
ANA, see Anti-nuclear antibody (ANA)
anaemia
  abdominal pain, 206
  autoimmune haemolytic anaemia,
    256–259
  bruising, 268
  causes, 254
  insufficient blood production, 252–255
  renal failure, 56–60
  tiredness, 312
anaemia of chronic disease (ACD),
    254, 255
aneurysms, 194
angiotensin-converting enzyme, see ACE
    inhibitors
angiotensin receptor blockers (ARBs)
  kidney disease, 390
  leg swelling, 423
  NT-proBNP levels, 11
animal thyroxine, 76
anion gap
  aspirin overdose, 50
  colicky pain, 64
  headache and vomiting, 36
  hypokalaemia, 17
antiacids, 23
anticoagulation levels, 282–285
antidiuretic hormone (ADH)
  depression, 32
  headache, 182, 438
anti-gastric parietal antibody, 101
antihistamines, 394
anti-liver/kidney microsomal
    antibody, 101
anti-mitochrondrial antibody, 101
anti-nuclear antibody (ANA), 101
antiphospholipid syndrome, 306–309
antipsychotic drugs, 32
anti-smooth muscle antibody, 101

aortic balloon valvuloplasty, 352
aortic stenosis, severe, 351–352
appendicitis, 118
APTT, *see* Activated partial
   thromboplastin time (APTT)
ARBs, *see* Angiotensin receptor blockers
   (ARBs)
Army medical examination, 376–378
arterial blood gas, *see also* Blood gas
   abdominal pain, 205
   falls, 451
   respiratory distress, 409–413
   shortness of breath, 141, 151–152
asbestos-related chest disease, 122–126
aspartate transaminase (AST)
   abdominal pain, 204
   bloody cough, 161
   confusion, 95
   knees, painful, 108, 110
   NT-proBNP levels, 10
   semi-consciousness, 46
   shortness of breath, 80
   upper limb weakness, 219
aspiration pneumonia, 131
aspirin
   bruising, 268
   salicylate poisoning, 48–51
AST, *see* Aspartate transaminase (AST)
asthma diagnosis, 414–418
asthmatic individuals
   constipation, 232
   cough, 52–55
atherosclerotic disease, 206
atrial fibrillation (AF)
   nose bleeds, 284
   palpitations, 325–330
   treatment options and risks, 384–387
attempted suicide, 424–428
atypical bacterial/fungal infections, 273
autoimmune disorders and malignancies
   cellulitis, 320
   panic attacks, 278–281
autoimmune haemolytic anaemia (AIHA),
   256–259, 256–259
axial FLAIR image, 136

B
back pain, 432–435
bacterial infection, 273

bacterial meningitis, 436–439
barium/contrast studies
   difficulty swallowing, 130
   inflammatory bowel disease, 118
Bartter's syndrome, 18
base excess (BE)
   headache and vomiting, 34
   semi-consciousness, 44
   shortness of breath, 141
BE, *see* Base excess (BE)
Beck's triad, 379–383
bedside spirometry, 141
Behçet's disease, 140
Bence-Jones protein
   confusion, 262
   hypokalaemia, 22
bendrofluazide, 390
beta-blockade, 395
beta-blockers
   aldosterone/PRA, 17
   atrial fibrillation, 386
   depression, 32
   falls, 451
   palpitations, 329, 366
   syncope, 338, 360
BHL, *see* Bilateral hilar
   lymphadenopathy (BHL)
bibliography, 452
bicarbonate
   aspirin overdose, 48
   colicky pain, 62, 64
   diabetes mellitus, 66
   headache, 13
   headache and vomiting, 34
   renal failure, 56, 59
   semi-consciousness, 44
   vomiting, 3, 38
bilateral hilar lymphadenopathy (BHL)
   cough, 176
   panic attacks, 280
bilateral mediastinal adenopathy, 280
biliary cirrhosis, 99
biliary obstruction, 100–103
bilirubin
   abdominal pain, 204
   abnormal blood test results, 314
   anaemia, 253
   attempted suicide, 424
   bloody cough, 161

bruising, 275
cellulitis, 319
chest pain, 242
confusion, 94, 95, 260
constipation, 230
cough, 20
diabetes mellitus, 66
dysuria, 70
emergency hip repair, 303
falls, 82
fatigue, 235
fever and lethargy, 299
hips, 271, 303
knees, 108, 287
lethargy, 237
light-headedness, 248
nose bleeds, 283
panic attacks, 279
periods (menstruation), 291
right-sided weakness, 307
semi-consciousness, 44
shortness of breath, 8, 78, 80
tiredness, 100, 311
upper limb weakness, 219
blood count, full, 219
blood gas, *see also* Arterial blood gas
  aspirin overdose, 50
  cough, 53
  semi-consciousness, 46
blood production, insufficient, 252–255
blood test results, abnormal, 314–317
bone disease, 65
bone marrow
  cellulitis, 320
  confusion, 263
  hypokalaemia, 22
bony metastases, 22
bony sclerotic lesions, 188
Boutonnière's deformity, 212
bowel obstruction, acute large, 229–233
brain lesions, 183–184
brain natriuertic peptide (BNP), *see*
  NT-proBNP
breath, *see* Shortness of breath
breathlessness, 232
British Thoracic Society, 81
broad complex tachycardia, 366
bronchogenic carcinoma, 122–126
bronchoscopy, 67

bronze diabetes, 111
bruising
  acute leukaemia, 274–277
  acute myeloid leukaemia, 265–269
  periods (menstruation), 292
bundle branch block, 328, 366

C
calcium, *see also* Adjusted calcium
  abdominal pain, 115
  abnormal blood test results, 314
  anaemia, 253, 257
  bruising, 275
  chest pain, 242
  chronic diarrhoea, 26
  confusion, 95, 260, 403
  constipation, 230
  cough, 20
  fatigue, 235
  fever and lethargy, 299
  headache, 93, 438
  hip pain, 270
  lethargy, 237
  light-headedness, 248
  nose bleeds, 283
  panic attacks, 279
  periods (menstruation), 291
  right-sided weakness, 307
  tiredness, 310
calcium-channel blockers
  aldosterone/PRA, 17
  atrial fibrillation, 386
calcium gluconate, 390
calcium phosphate stones, 61–65
calprotein, 26
Campylobacter jejuni, 435
Campylobacter sp., 208–209
capacity of lung for carbon dioxide
  (DL_{CO}), 418
Caplan syndrome, 214
carbamezapine, 426
cardiac arrhythmia, 330
cardiac failure, acute, 200–203
cardiac ischaemia, 330
cardiology, *see also* Electrocardiogram
  (ECG)
  abdominal pain, 361–364
  Army medical examination, 376–378
  atrial fibrillation, 384–387

chest pain, 331–335, 339–340,
  348–350, 353–357, 391–392
 fever, 367–371
 kidney disease, 388–390
 light headedness, 341–342
 palpitations, 325–330, 343–347,
  365–366, 393–395
 shortness of breath, 372–375, 379–383
 syncope, 336–338, 351–352, 358–360
 weight loss, 367–371
catecholamine secretion, 93
cavitating lung lesion, 124
cellulitis
 leg pain and swelling, 297
 profound neutropenia, 318–321
central chest pain, 391–392
central nervous system lymphoma, 140
cerebral abscess
 diabetes, 160
 head injury, 216
cerebral aneurysms, 194
cerebral oedema, 184
cerebral tumour, 160
cerebral vasculitis
 diabetes, 160
 vision loss, 140
cerebral venous thrombosis, 160
cerebrospinal fluid (CSF), 436–439
cerebrovascular accident, 216
cerebrovascular disease, 140
CHADS-VASc calculator, 284
Chagas' disease, 131
chest pain
 acute inferior myocardial infarction,
  339–340
 acute peridarditis, 391–392
 community-acquired pneumonia,
  241–246
 inferior STEMI with complete heart
  block, 348–350
 left pleural effusion, 429–431
 left-sided pneumothorax, 132–135
 severe ischaemic heart disease, 331–335
 type A aortic dissection, 353–357
Chlamydia sp., 447
chloride
 aspirin overdose, 48
 colicky pain, 62, 64
 diabetes mellitus, 66

headache, 13
 headache and vomiting, 34
 vomiting, 3, 38
cholestasis, 100–103
cholesterol
 falls, 82
 knees, painful, 108
 leg swelling, 419
 renal failure, 56
 tiredness, 100
cholesterol:HDL ratio, 100, 103
chromogranin A, 90
chronic haemolytic anaemias, 312
chronic hypoxia, 317
chronic kidney disease (CKD), 58–60
chronic lymphocytic leukaemia (CLL),
  272–273
chronic myeloid leukaemia, 313
chronic obstructive pulmonary
  disease (COPD)
 chest pain and weight loss, 429
 cough, 417
 hyperosmolar hyperglycaemic state,
  398–402
 NT-proBNP levels, 10
 shortness of breath, 141–145
cirrhosis
 hyponatraemia, 6
 NT-proBNP levels, 10
CJD, *see* Creutzfeldt-Jakob disease (CJD)
CK, *see* Creatine kinase (CK)
CKD, *see* Chronic kidney disease (CKD)
clinical chemistry
 abdominal pain, 24–27
 aspirin overdose, 48–51
 colicky pain, 61–65
 confusion, 94–99
 cough, 20–23, 52–55
 depression, 28–33
 diabetes mellitus, 66–69
 dysuria, 70–73
 falls, 82–85
 headache, 13–19, 34–37, 90–93
 knees, painful, 108–111
 nocturia, 86–89
 periods, irregular, 104–107
 renal failure, 56–60
 semi-consciousness, 44–47
 shortness of breath, 8–12, 78–81

tiredness, 74–77, 100–103
vomiting, 3–7, 34–37, 38–43
CLL, *see* Chronic lymphocytic leukaemia (CLL)
Clostridrium difficile, 207–209
Clostridrium perfringens, 258
clotting factors, 288
clubbed fingers/fingernails
  bronchogenic carcinoma, 122
  chest pain and weight loss, 429
  fever and weight loss, 146
CMV, *see* Cytomegalovirus (CMV)
coeliac disease, 26, 27
COHb (carboxyhaemoglobin), 44, 47
colicky pain, 61–65
colitis
  abdominal pain, 204–208
  types, 209
colorectal cancer, 171–172
coma, 193
community-acquired pneumonia
  chest pain, 241–246
  falls, 451
computed tomography (CT)
  bloody cough, 170
  chest pain, 356
  constipation, 232
  cough, 176
  diabetes, 158
  dysuria, 70, 71
  epigastric pain, 442
  headache, 179, 182, 183
  head injury, 216–217
  inflammatory bowel disease, 118
  palpitations, 330
  panic attacks, 280
  right-sided weakness, 306
  shortness of breath, 144
computed tomography pulmonary angiography (CTPA), 375
confusion
  acute subarachnoid haemorrhage, 193
  digoxin therapy, 94–99
  head injury, 215–218
  humeral fracture, multiple myeloma, 260–264
  insufficient information, 403–408
  urinary tract infection, 444–447

Conn's syndrome, 16
constipation, 229–233
COPD, *see* Chronic obstructive pulmonary disease (COPD)
corticosteroids, 177–178
cortisol
  cough, 21
  diabetes mellitus, 67
  dysuria, 70
  periods (menstruation), 105
  vomiting, 3, 4
cough
  asthma diagnosis, 414–418
  bronchogenic carcinoma, 122–126
  hypokalaemia, 20–23
  pulmonary metastases, 167–172
  pulmonary tuberculosis, 161–166
  sarcoidosis, 173–178
  sepsis, 52–55
C-reactive protein (CRP)
  abdominal pain, 24, 115, 205
  abnormal blood test results, 314
  anaemia, 253, 257
  bloody cough, 161
  bruising, 275
  cellulitis, 319
  chest pain, 242
  chronic obstructive pulmonary disease, 398
  colicky pain, 61
  confusion, 261, 403
  constipation, 230
  cough, 52
  depression, 29
  diabetes type 2, 156
  emergency hip repair, 303
  epigastric pain, 440
  fatigue, 235
  fever and confusion, 444
  fever and lethargy, 299
  headache, 436
  hips, 271, 303
  knees, 108, 287
  leg pain and swelling, 295
  lethargy, 238
  light-headedness, 248
  nocturia, 86
  nose bleeds, 283

panic attacks, 279
periods (menstruation), 291
renal failure, 56
respiratory distress, 409
right-sided weakness, 307
shortness of breath, 78
swelling, hands and feet, 210
tiredness, 311
upper limb weakness, 220
weight loss, 146
creatine kinase (CK), 82
creatine phosphokinase (CPK), 66
creatinine
  abdominal pain, 24, 115, 204
  abnormal blood test results, 314
  anaemia, 253, 257
  aspirin overdose, 48
  attempted suicide, 424
  bloody cough, 161
  bruising, 275
  cellulitis, 318
  chest pain, 241
  chronic obstructive pulmonary
   disease, 398
  colicky pain, 61
  confusion, 94, 95, 260, 403
  constipation, 229
  cough, 20, 52, 54
  depression, 28
  diabetes, 66, 156
  dysuria, 70
  emergency hip repair, 303
  epigastric pain, 440
  falls, 82, 448
  fatigue, 234
  fever and confusion, 444
  fever and lethargy, 299
  headache, 13, 90, 436
  headache and vomiting, 34
  hips, 270, 303
  knees, swollen, 287
  leg pain and swelling, 295
  leg swelling, 419
  lethargy, 237
  light-headedness, 248
  nocturia, 86
  nose bleeds, 283
  palpitations, 325
  panic attacks, 279

periods (menstruation), 291
renal failure, 56
respiratory distress, 409
right-sided weakness, 307
semi-consciousness, 44
shortness of breath, 8, 9, 78, 151
tiredness, 310
upper limb weakness, 219
vomiting, 3, 38
weight loss, 146
Creutzfeldt-Jakob disease (CJD), 285
Crohn's disease
  chronic diarrhoea, 26
  colitis types, 209
  inflammatory bowel disease,
   118–120
CSF, *see* Cerebrospinal fluid (CSF)
CT, *see* Computed tomography (CT)
CTPA, *see* Computed tomography
   pulmonary angiography (CTPA)
Cushing's type syndrome, 66–69
cytomegalovirus (CMV), 208–209

D
D-dimer, 78, 81, 374
deep ST depression inferiority, 334
deep vein thrombosis (DVT)
  chronic obstructive pulmonary
   disease, 402
  leg pain and swelling, 294–297
defibrillators, 338
depression, 28–33
desmopressin, 289
Devic's disease, 140
DEXA, 103
dexamethasone, 184
dextrocardia, 376–378
DI, *see* Diabetes insipidus (DI)
diabetes (general)
  knees, painful, 108
  NT-proBNP levels, 10
  periods (menstruation), 106
diabetes insipidus (DI), 32
diabetes mellitus
  Cushing's type syndrome, 66–69
  epigastric pain, 442
diabetes type 2
  hypogonadism, 108–111
  intracerebral haematoma, 156–160

diabetic ketoacidosis (DKA)
  chronic obstructive pulmonary
    disease, 401
  headache and vomiting, 36
  semi-consciousness, 44–47
diarrhoea, 24–27
dietary habits
  chronic diarrhoea, 24
  fatigue, 236
difficulty swallowing, 127–131
diffuse bilateral expiratory wheeze, 141
Digibind, 96, 98–99
digoxin
  atrial fibrillation, 386
  confusion, 94–99
  contraindication, 346
  light-headedness, 342
  NT-proBNP levels, 11
  palpitations, 346
DIPJ, *see* Distal interphalangeal
    joint (DIPJ)
direct current cardioconversion
  atrial fibrillation, 386
  chest pain, 334, 340
  palpitations, 366
distal interphalangeal joint (DIPJ), 212
diuretics, 17, *see also* Thiazide diuretics
dizziness, 365
DKA, *see* Diabetic ketoacidosis (DKA)
DL_{CO} (capacity of lung for
    carbon dioxide), 418
DMARDs, 214
dopamine agonists, 7
drug-induced immune thrombocytopenic
    purpura, 305
Duke criteria and classification
  bloody cough, 171–172
  fever and weight loss, 371
DVT, *see* Deep vein thrombosis (DVT)
dysuria, 70–73

E
ear infection, 34–37
ECG, *see* Electrocardiogram (ECG)
ECT, *see* Electroconvulsive therapy (ECT)
effusion, large pleural, 151–155
effusion, left pleural, 429–431

e-GFR (estimated glomerular
    filtration rate)
  confusion, 94, 95
  depression, 28
  nocturia, 86
  NT-proBNP levels, 10
  renal failure, 56, 58
elder abuse, 268
elderly men, *see also* Men;
    Middle-aged men
  atrial fibrillation, 384–387
  blood test results, abnormal, 314–317
  chest pain, 331–335
  confusion, 403–408
  cough, 20–23
  depression, 28–33
  dysuria, 70–73
  headache, 179–184
  hip pain, 185–190, 270–273
  kidney disease, 388–390
  leg swelling, progressive, 419–423
  nocturia, 86–89
  nose bleeds, 282–285
  palpitations, 325–330, 365–366
  respiratory distress, 409–413
  shortness of breath, 8–12, 200–203
  swelling, progressive leg, 419–423
  syncope, 351–352
elderly women, *see also* Middle-aged
    women; Women; Young women
  anaemia, 252–255
  bruising, 265–269
  chest pain, 348–350
  chronic obstructive pulmonary disease,
    398–402
  confusion, 260–264, 444–447
  constipation, 229–233
  diabetes type 2, 156–160
  epigastric pain, 195–199
  falls, 82–85, 448–451
  fever, 298–301, 367–371, 444–447
  lethargy, 298–301
  light-headedness, 247–251
  nasogastric feeding, stroke unit,
    223–225
  shortness of breath, 151–155
  upper limb weakness, 219–222

vomiting, 3–7
weight loss, 146–150, 367–371
electrical cardioconversion, 366
electrical therapy, 329
electrocardiogram (ECG), *see also*
    Cardiology
    chest pain, 132
    confusion, 95, 98, 215
    diabetes mellitus, 67–68
    difficulty swallowing, 127
    falls, 82
    shortness of breath, 141, 151, 200
electroconvulsive therapy (ECT), 28
electrolytes
    abdominal pain, 206, 361
    confusion, 95
    palpitations, 366
    vomiting, 38–43
electrophoresis
    confusion, 263
    hypokalaemia, 22
emergency hip repair, 302–305
encephalitis
    diabetes, 160
    headache, 438
endocarditis, subacute infective, 367–371
endocrine adenomatosis type 1, 68–69
endocrine disturbances, 406
Entamoeba histolytica, 208–209
Enterococcus faecalis, 447
Enterococcus spp., 370
epigastric pain
    acute-on-chronic alcoholic pancreatitis,
        440–443
    acute severe cord compression,
        195–199
epileptic seizure, 159–160
Epstein-Barr virus infection, 270–273
erythema nodosum, 177
erythrocyte sedimentation rate (ESR)
    abdominal pain, 115, 205
    anaemia, 253
    swelling, hands and feet, 210
    upper limb weakness, 220
    weight loss, 146
erythropoisis-stimulating agents
    (ESA), 58

Escherischia coli
    colitis types, 209
    toxic colitis, 208
    urinary tract infection, 447
ESR, *see* Erythrocyte sedimentation
    rate (ESR)
ethanol, 44
euvolaemic status, 6
evolving inferior myocardial infarction,
    361–364
expiratory phase, 141
extradural haematoma, 216
extrahepatic causes, tiredness, 102

F
faecal calprotectin, 24
Fagan's monogram, 27
falls
    diagnosis and therapy, 82–85
    insufficient information, 448–451
    traumatic haemarthrosis, 286–289
familial adenomatous polyposis
    (FAP), 171
FAP, *see* Familial adenomatous polyposis
    (FAP)
fast atrial fibrillation, 325–330
fatigue, profound, 234–236, *see also*
    Tiredness
feeding tubes, *see* Nasogastric feeding
    and tube insertions
feet, swelling, 210–214
Felty syndrome, 214
ferritin
    abdominal pain, 24
    chronic diarrhoea, 26
    cough, 52
    knees, painful, 108
    renal failure, 56
FEV_1
    cough, 416–417
    shortness of breath, 141
fever
    abdominal pain, 206
    haematology, 298–301
    subacute infective endocarditis,
        367–371
    urinary tract infection, 444–447

fingers/fingernails, clubbed
  bronchogenic carcinoma, 122
  chest pain and weight loss, 429
  fever and weight loss, 146
first-degree heart block, 336–338
FLAIR image, 136
flecanide, 386–387
folate
  abdominal pain, 25
  confusion, 403
  fatigue, 236
  lethargy, 240
  renal failure, 57
follicle-stimulating hormone (FSH)
  hyponatraemia, 7
  knees, painful, 109
  periods (menstruation), 104, 107
  tiredness, 74
  vomiting, 4
forced vital capacity, *see* FVC
fraction bicarbonate excretion, 65
free kappa light chain, 21
free lambda light chain, 21
free thyroxine (fT4)
  confusion, 94
  cough, 21, 52, 55
  depression, 28
  falls, 82–85, 83
  fatigue, 235
  periods (menstruation), 104
  tiredness, 74
  vomiting, 4
free tri-iodothyronine (fT3)
  falls, 84
  periods (menstruation), 104
  tiredness, 74
  vomiting, 4
FSH, *see* Follicle-stimulating
    hormone (FSH)
fT3, *see* Free tri-iodothyronine (fT3)
fT4, *see* Free thyroxine (fT4)
full blood count, 219
fundoscopy, 90
fungal infection
  bloody cough, 170
  hip pain, 273
furosemide
  colicky pain, 65
  kidney disease, 390

renal tubular acidosis, 65
FVC (forced vital capacity)
  cough, 416–417
  shortness of breath, 141

G
gall stone obstruction, 99
Gamma-glutamyltransferase
    (GGT; Gamma-GT)
  attempted suicide, 424
  confusion, 95
  cough, 21
  diabetes mellitus, 67
  headache and vomiting, 34, 37
  hypokalaemia, 22
  knees, painful, 108
  semi-consciousness, 44, 46
  tiredness, 100
GCS, *see* Glasgow Coma Score (GCS)
G-CSF, *see* Granulocyte
    colony-stimulating factor (G-CSF)
GGT, 99
Gitelman's syndrome, 18
glandular fever, 278–281, 279
Glasgow Coma Score (GCS)
  confusion, 216
  falls, 448
  semi-consciousness, 44
globulin
  cough, 20, 52
  shortness of breath, 78
glomerular filtration rate, *see* e-GFR
    (glomerular filtration rate)
  NT-proBNP levels, 10
  renal failure, 59
glucocorticoid suppressable
    hyperaldosteronism, 18
glucose
  aspirin overdose, 48
  cellulitis, 319
  chronic obstructive pulmonary
    disease, 398
  confusion, 261
  cough, 52
  diabetes, 66, 156
  falls, 82, 448
  fever and confusion, 444
  headache, 90, 436
  headache and vomiting, 34

knees, painful, 108
leg pain and swelling, 295
leg swelling, 419
periods (menstruation), 104, 106
renal failure, 56
right-sided weakness, 307
glucose tolerance tests, 104–107
gluten-free diet, 24, 27
granulocyte colony-stimulating factor
   (G-CSF), 320
Grave's disease, 76–77
growth hormone, 105, 106
Guillain-Barré syndrome, 432–435

H
haematinic deficiencies, 320
haematocrit (Hct)
   abnormal blood test results, 314
   anaemia, 253, 256
   bruising, 274
   cellulitis, 318
   chest pain, 241
   confusion, 260
   constipation, 229
   emergency hip repair, 302
   falls, 82
   fatigue, 234
   fever and lethargy, 299
   hips, 270, 302
   knees, swollen, 286
   leg pain and swelling, 294
   lethargy, 237
   light-headedness, 247
   nose bleeds, 282
   panic attacks, 279
   periods (menstruation), 290
   right-sided weakness, 306
   shortness of breath, 151
   tiredness, 310
   vomiting, 38
haematological malignancies, 240
haematology
   anaemia, 252–255, 256–259
   blood test results, abnormal, 314–317
   bruising, 265–269, 274–277
   cellulitis, 318–321
   chest pain, 241–246
   confusion, 260–264
   constipation, 229–233

fever, 298–301
hips, 270–273, 302–305
leg pain, 294–297
lethargy, 237–240, 298–301
light-headedness, 247–251
nose bleeds, 282–285
panic attacks, 278–281
periods, heavy, 290–293
profound fatigue, 234–236
right-sided weakness, 306–309
swelling, 286–289, 294–297
tiredness, increasing, 310–313
haematoma, 217
haemochromatosis (HC), 110–111
haemoglobin (Hb)
   abdominal pain, 24, 115, 204
   abnormal blood test results, 314, 317
   anaemia, 252, 256
   attempted suicide, 424
   bloody cough, 161
   bruising, 274
   cellulitis, 318
   chest pain, 241
   chronic obstructive pulmonary
      disease, 398
   confusion, 94, 260, 403
   constipation, 229
   cough, 52
   depression, 28
   diabetes type 2, 156
   emergency hip repair, 302
   epigastric pain, 440
   falls, 82, 448
   fatigue, 234
   fever and confusion, 444
   fever and lethargy, 298
   headache, 436
   hips, 270, 302
   knees, swollen, 286
   leg pain and swelling, 294
   leg swelling, 419
   lethargy, 237
   light-headedness, 247
   nose bleeds, 282
   panic attacks, 278
   periods (menstruation), 290
   renal failure, 56
   respiratory distress, 409
   right-sided weakness, 306

shortness of breath, 8, 78
tiredness, 310
upper limb weakness, 219
weight loss, 146
haemolytic anaemias, 312
haemophilia, 288–289
Haemophilus influenzae, 438
hands, swelling, 210–214
Hartman's fluid replacement, 37
Hashimoto's thyroiditis, 76, 77
hay fever
cough, 414
palpitations, 394
HC, *see* Haemochromatosis (HC)
HCO$_2$, 141
HCO$_3$, 398
Hct, *see* Haematocrit (Hct)
HDL, *see* High-density lipoprotein (HDL)
HDU, *see* High-dependency unit (HDU)
headache
acute bacterial meningitis, 436–439
acute subarachnoid haemorrhage,
191–194
ear infection, 34–37
hypokalaemia, 13–19
multiple intracranial ring enhancing
lesions, 179–184
phaeochromocytoma, 90–93
head injury
confusion, 215–218
headache and vomiting, 37
heart, *see also* Cardiology
dextrocardia, 376–378
first-degree block, 336–338
second-degree block, 341–342
severe ischaemic, disease, 331–335
shortness of breath, 80
heavy periods, 290–293
heparin
bronchogenic carcinoma, 124
palpitations, 329
toxic colitis, 208
heparin-induced thrombocytopenia (HIT),
304–305
hepatitis, 292
hereditary haemochromatosis (HC), 110–111
hereditary non-polyposis colon cancer
(HNPCC), 171
Heyde syndrome, 254

HHS, *see* Hyperosmolar hyperglycaemic
state (HHS)
hidden P-waves, 350
high-density lipoprotein (HDL)
renal failure, 56
tiredness, 100
high-dependency unit (HDU), 207
hips
acute viral infections, 270–273
infection/sepsis, 302–305
sclerotic lesions, 185–190
HIT, *see* Heparin-induced
thrombocytopenia (HIT)
HIV infection, *see also* Sexually
transmitted infections
panic attacks, 280
periods (menstruation), 292
unexplained bruises, 277
HNPCC, *see* Hereditary non-polyposis
colon cancer (HNPCC)
Hodgkin lymphoma
panic attacks, 280–281
unexplained bruises, 277
HONK, *see* Hyperosmolar non-ketotic
coma (HONK)
hormone replacement therapy, 74
humeral fracture, multiple myeloma,
260–264
hydrocortisone, 72–73
hydrogen ion, 38
hydroxyl butyrate, 44
hypercalcaemia
Addison's disease, 73
bronchogenic carcinoma, 122, 124
causes, 33
confusion, 263
depression, 28
hypokalaemia, 22–23
respiratory distress, 413
hyperglycaemia
cough, 54
falls, 82–85
hyperkalaemia
chronic obstructive pulmonary
disease, 401
dysuria, 72
kidney disease, 388–390
NT-proBNP levels, 11–12
respiratory distress, 413

hypernatraemia, 32
hyperosmolar hyperglycaemic state
    (HHS), 398–402
hyperosmolar non-ketotic coma
    (HONK), 401
hyperparathyroidism
    headache, 93
    renal failure, 59
hyperphosphataemia, 59
hypervolaemic status, 6
hypoalbuminaemia, 206
hypocalcaemia
    abdominal pain, 24–27
    chronic diarrhoea, 26
    depression, 33
    renal failure, 60
    respiratory distress, 413
hypoglycaemia, 160
hypogonadism, 108–111
hypokalaemia
    chronic obstructive pulmonary
        disease, 401
    confusion, 98
    cough, 20–23
    diabetes mellitus, 68
    headache, 13–19
    palpitations, 329
    respiratory distress, 413
    vomiting, 41
hypomagnesaemia
    chronic diarrhoea, 26
    confusion, 98
hyponatraemia
    dysuria, 72
    headache, 182
    vomiting, 3–7
hypoperfusion, 206, 361
hypotension
    abdominal pain, 206
    light-headedness, 247–251
hypothermia
    falls, 82–85, 448–451
    respiratory distress, 413
hypothyroidism
    falls, 82–85
    fatigue, 236
    lethargy, 240
    lithium, 32
hypovolaemia, 413

hypovolaemic status, 6
hypoxaemia, 10
hypoxia
    abnormal blood test results, 317
    chest pain, 244
    respiratory distress, 413

I
IgA
    abdominal pain, 24
    cough, 20, 52
    tiredness, 100
IgA endomyseal Ab, 25
IgA TTG, 24
IGF, *see* Insulin-like growth factor (IGF)
IgG
    cough, 20, 52
    hypokalaemia, 22
    tiredness, 100
IgM
    cough, 20, 52
    tiredness, 100
immune thrombocytopenic purpura (ITP)
    emergency hip repair, 305
    heavy periods, 290–293
immunofixation, 21
implantable cardiac defibrillator, 395
infections
    cellulitis, 320
    confusion, 406
    emergency hip repair, 305
    panic attacks, 281
    tiredness, 313
infectious colitis, 209
infective endocarditis, subacute, 367–371
inferior myocardial infarction
    abdominal pain, 361–364
    chest pain, 339–340
inferior STEMI, 348–350, 356
inflammatory bowel disease
    abdominal pain, 115–121, 206
    chronic diarrhoea, 26
inflammatory conditions
    colitis, 209
    tiredness, 313
    upper limb weakness, 220
INR, *see* International normalized
    ratio (INR)
insufficient blood production, 252–255

insufficient information
  confusion, 403–408
  falls, 448–451
insulin, 401–402
insulin-like growth factor (IGF), 104
interferon, 76
international normalized ratio (INR)
  abdominal pain, 204
  anaemia, 257
  attempted suicide, 424
  bloody cough, 161
  bruising, 275
  emergency hip repair, 303
  headache, 436
  hips, 303
  knees, swollen, 287
  leg pain and swelling, 295
  lethargy, 238
  light-headedness, 248
  nose bleeds, 284
  panic attacks, 279
  right-sided weakness, 307
  tiredness, 100, 311
intra-abdominal infection, 118
intracerebral haematoma, 156–160
intracerebral hemorrhage, 193
intracranial disturbances, 406
intracranial ring enhancing lesions,
  179–184
intrahepatic causes, 102
intravascular localized
  thrombolysis, 296
iron
  abdominal pain, 25
  bronze diabetes, 111
  cough, 52
  knees, painful, 108
  renal failure, 56
ischaemic colitis, 209
ischaemic heart disease
  chest pain, 331–335
  falls, 84
  light-headedness, 342
ischaemic stroke, 308
ischaemic ventricular septal defect, 350
isotonic fluid loss, 40–43
ITP, *see* Immune thrombocytopenic
  purpura (ITP)

J
JAK2 V617F mutation, 312
Janus kinase 2 (JAK2)
  abnormal blood test results, 316
  diagnosis, 316
  tiredness, 312
jaundice, 100
joints, 210–214
jugular venous pressure (JVP)
  abdominal pain, 361
  atrial fibrillation, 384
  central chest pain, 391
  chest pain, 348
  confusion, 94
  diabetes mellitus, 66
  palpitations, 365, 393
  shortness of breath, 78, 141, 379, 382
JVP, *see* Jugular venous pressure (JVP)
J-wave, 450

K
kappa:lambda ratio, 21
Ketostix, 46
kidney disease
  acute ischaemia, 388–390
  hyperkalaemia, 388–390
  normal variant, 388–390
Klebsiella sp.
  bronchogenic carcinoma, 124
  urinary tract infection, 447
knees, painful, 108–111
Kussmaul's sign, 382

L
lactate
  aspirin overdose, 48
  cough, 55
  falls, 82
  semi-consciousness, 44
lactate dehydrogenase (LDH)
  anaemia, 253, 257
  bruising, 275
  causes of raised, 281
  chest pain, 242
  lethargy, 238
  panic attacks, 279
  shortness of breath, 80
  tiredness, 311

lactic acidosis, 47
large bowel obstruction, acute, 229–233
large pleural effusion, 151–155
LBBB, *see* Left bundle branch block (LBBB)
LDH, *see* Lactate dehydrogenase (LDH)
LDL, *see* Low-density lipoprotein (LDL)
left axis deviation, 325–330
left bundle branch block (LBBB), 328
left pleural effusion, 429–431
left-sided pneumothorax, 132–135
left ventricular function, 350
left ventricular hypertropy, 10
leg pain
   deep vein thrombosis, 294–297
   Guillain-Barré syndrome, 432–435
leg swelling
   deep vein thrombosis, 294–297
   nephrotic syndrome, 419–423
lethargy, *see also* Fatigue; Tiredness
   macrocytic anaemia, 237–240
   neutropenic sepsis, 298–301
leukaemia, 274–277, *see also* Acute myeloid leukaemia (AML)
leukocytosis, 312
LH, *see* Luteinizing hormone (LH)
light-headedness
   second-degree heart block, 341–342
   shock, hypotension and tachycardia, 247–251
Light's criteria, 430
limb weakness, upper, 219–222
lipid abnormalities, 103
lithium
   depression, 28, 33
   hypothyroidism, 32
liver, kidney microsomal (LKM) antibodies, 103
liver disease, 236
liver function
   abdominal pain, 361
   knees, painful, 108
   semi-consciousness, 46
   upper limb weakness, 219
liver toxicity, 426–427
LMWH, *see* Low-molecular-weight heparin (LMWH)
long QT syndrome, 393–395
Lo-Salt, 8, 11

low-density lipoprotein (LDL)
   renal failure, 57
   tiredness, 100
low-molecular-weight heparin (LMWH)
   bronchogenic carcinoma, 124
   palpitations, 329
lumbar puncture
   acute subarachnoid haemorrhage, 193
   headache, 437
   leg and back pain, 434
lung cancer
   cough and weight loss, 122–126
   lesions in brain, 184
luteinizing hormone (LH)
   hyponatraemia, 7
   knees, painful, 109
   periods (menstruation), 104
   tiredness, 74
   vomiting, 4
Lyme disease, 342
lymphocytes
   abnormal blood test results, 314
   anaemia, 252, 256
   bruising, 274
   cellulitis, 318
   chest pain, 241
   constipation, 229
   emergency hip repair, 302
   fatigue, 234
   fever and lethargy, 298
   hips, 270, 302
   knees, swollen, 286
   leg pain and swelling, 294
   lethargy, 237
   light-headedness, 247
   nose bleeds, 282
   panic attacks, 278
   periods (menstruation), 290
   right-sided weakness, 306
   tiredness, 310
lymphoma
   panic attacks, 280
   vision loss, 140
lytic bone lesions, 189

M
macrocytic anaemia
   alcohol excess, 240
   lethargy, 237–240

macrolytic anaemia, 234–236
magnesium, *see* Adjusted calcium
magnetic resonance imaging (MRI)
  diabetes, 67, 158–159
  dysuria, 71
  epigastric pain, 199, 442
  head injury, 217
  inflammatory bowel disease, 118
  knees, painful, 108
  periods (menstruation), 105
  right-sided weakness, 308
  upper limb weakness, 222
  urgency, 199
  vision loss, 136, 138
malignant neoplasm, 431
Marcus-Gunn pupil, 138
Marfanoid characteristics, 93
MCH, *see* Mean corpuscular
  haemoglobin (MCH)
MCHC, *see* Mean corpuscular hemoglobin
  concentration (MCHC)
MCV, *see* Mean cell volume (MCV); Mean
  corpuscular value (MCV); Mean
  corpuscular volume (MCV)
mean cell volume (MCV)
  abdominal pain, 115, 204
  diabetes type 2, 156
  shortness of breath, 151
mean corpuscular haemoglobin
  concentration (MCHC)
  abdominal pain, 24
  renal failure, 56
mean corpuscular haemoglobin (MCH)
  abdominal pain, 24
  anaemia, 252
  constipation, 229
mean corpuscular value (MCV), 24
mean corpuscular volume (MCV)
  abnormal blood test results, 314
  anaemia, 252, 256
  bloody cough, 161
  bruising, 274
  cellulitis, 318
  chest pain, 241
  confusion, 260
  constipation, 229
  emergency hip repair, 302
  fatigue, 234
  fever and lethargy, 299

hips, 270, 302
knees, swollen, 286
leg pain and swelling, 294
lethargy, 237
light-headedness, 247
nose bleeds, 282
panic attacks, 279
periods (menstruation), 290
renal failure, 56
right-sided weakness, 306
tiredness, 310
upper limb weakness, 219
weight loss, 146
medial longitudinal fasciculus (MLF), 140
medication
  erratic use, 85
  fatigue, 236
MEN, *see* Multiple endocrine neoplasia
  (MEN)
men, *see also* Elderly men;
    Middle-aged men
  chest pain, 429–431
  cough, 52–55, 167–172
  diabetes mellitus, 66–69
  headache, 90–93
  knees, painful, 108–111
  renal failure, 56–60
  semi-consciousness, 44–47
  vomiting, 38–43
  weight loss, 429–431
meningitis, acute bacterial, 436–439
menopause, 74, 76, *see also* Periods
  (menstruation)
mesothelioma, 122–126
metabolic alkalosis
  abdominal pain, 206
  hypokalaemia, 16, 22
  vomiting, 41
metabolic bone disease, 65
metabolic causes, head injury, 216
metabolic disturbances
  confusion, 406
  respiratory distress, 413
metabolic syndrome, 111
metanephrine, 92
metastatic malignancies, 313
metastatic prostatic carcinoma, 189
methoxytyramine, 92
MIBI, 29, 33

microcytic anaemia, 232–233
microcytic hypochromic anaemia, 58
middle-aged men, *see also*
    Elderly men; Men
  abdominal pain, 361–364
  confusion, 215–218
  cough, 173–178
  epigastric pain, 440–443
  headache, 436–439
  lethargy, 237–240
  light headedness, 341–342
  shortness of breath, 78–81, 141–145
  syncope, 336–338
  tiredness, increasing, 310–313
middle-aged women, *see also* Elderly
    women; Women; Young women
  anaemia, 256–259
  chest pain, 339–340, 353–357
  cough, 161–166
  right-sided weakness, 306–309
  swallowing difficulty, 127–131
  swelling, hands and feet, 210–214
  tiredness, 74–77
middled-aged men, 318–321
midstream specimen of urine (MSU)
  nocturia, 86
  obtaining, 446
migraine, 438
milk, 23
mitral regurgitation, acute, 350
MLF, *see* Medial longitudinal fasciculus
    (MLF)
monoclonal bands, 22
M-protein, 263
MRI, *see* Magnetic resonance imaging (MRI)
MS, *see* Multiple sclerosis (MS)
MSU, *see* Midstream specimen of urine
    (MSU)
M2-type mitrochondial antibody, 101
multiple endocrine adenomatosis type
    1, 68–69
multiple endocrine neoplasia (MEN)
  diabetes mellitus, 69
  headache, 93
multiple intracranial ring enhancing
    lesions, 179–184
multiple myeloma, humeral fracture
    secondary to, 260–264
multiple sclerosis (MS), 138–140

muscular tear/strain, 297
Mycobacterium tuberculosis, 165
Mycoplasma pneumoniae, 258
myelodysplastic syndrome, 236
myelofibrosis, 310–313
myeloid leukaemia, *see* Acute myeloid
    leukaemia (AML)
myeloma
  confusion, 262–264
  hypokalaemia, 22
myeloma, humeral fracture secondary to
    multiple, 260–264
myocardial infarction, *see also* STEMI
    (ST evaluation myocardial infarction)
  acute inferior, 339–340
  central chest pain, 392
  evolving inferior, 361–364
  shortness of breath, 80
myocardial ischemia, 10

N
N-acetylcysteine, 426–427
NAFLD, *see* Non-alcoholic fatty liver
    disease (NAFLD)
naloxone, 413
narrow complex tachycardia, 346
nasogastric feeding and tube insertions,
    223–225
neck fracture, 304
neck stiffness
  acute subarachnoid haemorrhage, 193
  headache and vomiting, 37
Neisseria meningitis, 438
nephrolithiasis, 65
nephrotic syndrome, 419–423
neutropenia, profound, 318–321
neutropenic sepsis, 298–301
neutrophils
  abdominal pain, 115
  abnormal blood test results, 314
  anaemia, 252, 256
  bruising, 274
  cellulitis, 318
  chest pain, 241
  chronic diarrhoea, 26
  chronic obstructive pulmonary
    disease, 398
  confusion, 94, 260, 403
  constipation, 229

diabetes type 2, 156
emergency hip repair, 302
falls, 448
fatigue, 234
fever and confusion, 444
fever and lethargy, 298
headache, 436
hips, 270, 302
knees, swollen, 286
leg pain and swelling, 294
lethargy, 237
light-headedness, 247
nose bleeds, 282
panic attacks, 278
periods (menstruation), 290
respiratory distress, 409
right-sided weakness, 306
shortness of breath, 78, 151
tiredness, 310
upper limb weakness, 219
weight loss, 146
nocturia, 86–89
non-alcoholic fatty liver disease
    (NAFLD), 10
non-dihydropyridine calcium-channel
    antagonists, 338
non-Hodgkin lymphoma
  fever and lethargy, 298
  unexplained bruises, 277
non-steroidal anti-inflammatory
    medication, *see* NSAID
normcytic anaemia, 254, 255
nose bleeds, 282–285
NSAID (non-steroidal anti-inflammatory
    medication), 214, 422
NT-proBNP, 8–12, 78

O
obesity, 10
oedema, 78
oesophagus, achalasia of, 127–131
oestradiol, 104
oestrogens, 17
OGTT, *see* Oral glucose tolerance test
    (OGTT)
oligoclonal bands, 140
opiate-induced respiratory depression, 47
opiates, 360

opiate screen, 45
oral corticosteroids, 177–178
oral glucose tolerance test (OGTT), 104
osmolality
  headache and vomiting, 34
  vomiting, 3
osteoporosis, 103
osteroarthritis, 213–214
ovarian pathology, 118
Oxford Community Stroke Project
    classification, 159
oxygen saturation
  headache and vomiting, 34
  semi-consciousness, 44

P
pack-years (smoking), 330
$PaCO_2$
  aspirin overdose, 48
  diabetes mellitus, 66, 68
  headache and vomiting, 34
  semi-consciousness, 44, 46
  shortness of breath, 141, 152
  vomiting, 38
Paget's disease
  confusion, 99
  hip pain, 188–189
palpitations
  atrial fibrillation, 325–330
  long QT syndrome, 393–395
  ventricular tachycardia, 365–366
  Wolff-Parkinson-White syndrome,
    343–347
Pancoast tumors, 219–222
pancreatic calcifications, 442
pancreatitis, acute-on-chronic alcoholic,
    440–443
pancytopenia, 268–269
panic attacks, 278–281
PaO_2
  aspirin overdose, 48
  diabetes mellitus, 66
  headache and vomiting, 34
  semi-consciousness, 44
  shortness of breath, 141, 152
  vomiting, 38
papillary muscle rupture, 350
paracetamol

aspirin overdose, 48, 51
attempted suicide, 424–428
semi-consciousness, 45
paraneoplastic disorders
bronchogenic carcinoma, 124
diabetes mellitus, 68
parasympathetic response, 342
parathyroid hormone (PTH)
abdominal pain, 25
bronchogenic carcinoma, 122
cough, 21
depression, 28–29
renal failure, 56
PBC, see Primary biliary cirrhosis (PBC)
pCO$_2$, 398
PCOS, see Polycystic ovary syndrome
(PCOS)
PE, see Pulmonary embolism (PE);
Pulmonary embolus (PE)
penicillin allergy
lethargy, 237
nose bleeds, 284
pericardial effusion, 379–383
pericarditis, acute, 391–392
peridarditis, 391–392
periods (menstruation), see also
Menopause
glucose tolerance tests, 104–107
immune thrombocytopenic purpura,
290–293
pernicious anaemia, 236
phaeochromocytoma
headache, 90–93
pH levels
aspirin overdose, 48
chronic obstructive pulmonary
disease, 398
colicky pain, 65
diabetes mellitus, 66
headache and vomiting, 34
renal tubular acidosis, 65
semi-consciousness, 44, 46
shortness of breath, 141, 152
phosphate
abdominal pain, 24
abnormal blood test results, 314
anaemia, 253, 257
bruising, 275
chest pain, 242

colicky pain, 62
confusion, 95, 260
constipation, 230
depression, 29
fatigue, 235
fever and lethargy, 299
headache, 90
hip pain, 271
lethargy, 237
light-headedness, 248
nose bleeds, 283
panic attacks, 279
periods (menstruation), 291
renal failure, 56
right-sided weakness, 307
tiredness, 310
pigmentation, 72
pitting ankle oedema, 78
placental alkaline phosphatase, 61
plasma potassium, 65
plasma renin activity (PRA)
headache, 14
hypokalaemia, 17–18
platelets
abdominal pain, 115, 204
abnormal blood test results, 314
anaemia, 253, 256
attempted suicide, 424
bloody cough, 161
bruising, 274
cellulitis, 318
chest pain, 241
chronic obstructive pulmonary
disease, 398
confusion, 94, 260, 403
constipation, 229
diabetes type 2, 156
emergency hip repair, 303
epigastric pain, 440
falls, 448
fatigue, 234
fever and confusion, 444
fever and lethargy, 299
headache, 436
hips, 270, 303
knees, swollen, 286
leg pain and swelling, 294
leg swelling, 419
lethargy, 237

light-headedness, 247
nose bleeds, 282
panic attacks, 279
periods (menstruation), 290
respiratory distress, 409
right-sided weakness, 306
shortness of breath, 78, 151
tiredness, 310
upper limb weakness, 219
platelet transfusion, 292
pleural effusion, large, 151–155
pleural effusion, left, 429–431
pleuritic chest pain, 246
pleurodesis, 150
pneumonia
   community-acquired, 241–246
   falls, 451
   palpitations, 330
pneumothoraces, 134–135
pneumothorax, 144
pneumothorax, left-sided, 132–135
pO_2, 398
polycystic ovary syndrome (PCOS),
   104, 106
polycythaemia, 314–317
Portacath, 286, 288
potassium
   abdominal pain, 24, 115, 204
   abnormal blood test results, 314
   anaemia, 253, 257
   aspirin overdose, 48
   attempted suicide, 424
   bloody cough, 161
   bruising, 274
   cellulitis, 318
   chest pain, 241
   chronic obstructive pulmonary
      disease, 398
   colicky pain, 61
   confusion, 94, 95, 260, 403
   constipation, 229
   cough, 20, 52
   depression, 28
   diabetes mellitus, 66
   dysuria, 70
   emergency hip repair, 303
   epigastric pain, 440
   falls, 82, 448
   fatigue, 234

fever and confusion, 444
fever and lethargy, 299
headache, 13, 90, 436
headache and vomiting, 34
hips, 270, 303
hypokalaemia, 16–19
kidney disease, 390
knees, swollen, 287
leg pain and swelling, 295
leg swelling, 419
lethargy, 237
light-headedness, 248
nocturia, 86
nose bleeds, 283
palpitations, 325
panic attacks, 279
periods (menstruation), 290
renal failure, 56
renal tubular acidosis, 65
respiratory distress, 409
right-sided weakness, 307
semi-consciousness, 44
shortness of breath, 8, 9, 78, 151
tiredness, 310
upper limb weakness, 219
vomiting, 3, 38
weight loss, 146
PRA, *see* Plasma renin activity (PRA)
prescription medications, 236
primary biliary cirrhosis (PBC), 102–103
primary malignant neoplasm, 431
profound fatigue, 236, *see also* Tiredness
profound neutropenia, 318–321
progressive leg swelling, 419–423
prolactin
   depression, 28
   hyponatraemia, 7
   periods (menstruation), 104, 105
   vomiting, 4
prostate-specific antigen (PSA)
   cough, 21
   dysuria, 70
   hip pain, 189
   nocturia, 86–89
prostatic carcinoma, 189
proteinuria, 422
Proteus mirabilis, 447
proton pump inhibitors, 93
PSA, *see* Prostate-specific antigen (PSA)

pseudohyperkalaemia, 316
Pseudomembranous colitis, 209
PTH, *see* Parathyroid hormone (PTH)
PTH-related peptide (PTHrP)
  cough, 21
  hypokalaemia, 23
pulmonary embolism (PE)
  chronic obstructive pulmonary
    disease, 402
  NT-proBNP levels, 10
  palpitations, 330
  shortness of breath, 372–375
pulmonary embolus (PE), 294–297
pulmonary metastases, 167–172
pulmonary oedema, 200–203
pulmonary tuberculosis (TB),
  161–166
"purple inhaler," 429
P-waves
  chest pain, 350
  palpitations, 366

Q
QT syndrome, 393–395

R
radiofrequency ablation, 386
radiology
  abdominal pain, 115–121, 204–209
  chest pain, 132–135
  confusion, 215–218
  cough, 161–166, 167–172, 173–178
  diabetes type 2, 156–160
  epigastric pain, 195–199
  headache, 179–184, 191–194
  hip pain, 185–190
  nasogastric feeding, stroke unit,
    223–225
  shortness of breath, 141–145, 151–155,
    200–203
  swallowing difficulty, 127–131
  swelling, hands and feet, 210–214
  upper limb weakness, 219–222
  vision loss, 136–140
  vomiting, 191–194
  weight loss, 122–126, 146–150
radiotherapy
  mesothelioma, 150
  periods (menstruation), 107

RAPD, *see* Relative afferent pupillary
  defect (RAPD)
RAS, *see* Renal artery stenosis (RAS)
RBBB, *see* Right bundle branch block
  (RBBB)
relative afferent pupillary defect (RAPD),
  136–140
renal artery stenosis (RAS), 18
renal dysfunction
  abnormal blood test results, 317
  dysuria, 72
  hypokalaemia, 16–17
  NT-proBNP levels, 10
renal failure
  anaemia, 56–60
  hyponatraemia, 6
  NT-proBNP levels, 11
renal function, 219
renal stones, 61–65
renal tubular acidosis (RTA), 64–65
renin secreting tumour, 18
respiratory alkalosis, 50
respiratory distress, 409–413
reversed tick phenomenon, 98
rheumatoid arthritis (RhA)
  cellulitis, 318
  periods (menstruation), 292
  swelling, 210–214
rheumatoid nodules, 170
rifampicin, 426
right bundle branch block, 325–330
right coronary artery occlusion, 350
right-sided weakness, 306–309
right ventricular overload, 10
R on T phenomenon, 340
RTA, *see* Renal tubular acidosis (RTA)
R-waves
  dextrocardia, 378
  palpitations, 366

S
salbutamol nebulizers
  kidney disease, 390
  leg swelling, 419
salicylate
  aspirin overdose, 48–51
  attempted suicide, 424
  semi-consciousness, 45
Salmonella sp., 208–209

sarcoidosis
  cough, 173–178
  light-headedness, 342
  vision loss, 140
SCC, *see* Squamous cell carcinoma (SCC)
Schwachman-Diamond syndrome, 320
sclerotic lesions, 185–190
second-degree heart block, 341–342
seizures, 193
semi-consciousness, 44–47
sepsis
  clinical indicators, 54
  cough, 54
  emergency hip repair, 305
  laboratory indicators, 54
  NT-proBNP levels, 10
serum osmolality
  depression, 29
  vomiting, 38
serum potassium levels, 390
serum protein electrophoresis, 21
severe aortic stenosis, 351–352
severe cord compression, acute, 195–199
severe ischaemic heart disease, 331–335
sex hormone binding globulin
    (SHBG), 104
sexually transmitted infections, 278–281,
    see also HIV infection
SHBG, *see* Sex hormone binding
    globulin (SHBG)
Shigella sp., 208–209
shock, hypotension and tachycardia,
    247–251
shortness of breath
  acute cardiac failure and pulmonary
    oedema, 200–203
  Beck's triad, 379–383
  chronic obstructive pulmonary disease,
    141–145
  large pleural effusion, 151–155
  NT-proBNP levels, 8–12
  pericardial effusion, 379–383
  pulmonary embolism, 372–375
  troponin T concentrations, 78–81
SIADH, *see* Syndrome of inappropriate
    antidiuretic hormone (SIADH)
    secretion
sickle cell disease, 244–246

sinus tachycardia, 346
Sipple's syndrome, 93
SLE, *see* Systemic lupus erythromatosus
    (SLE)
sodium
  abdominal pain, 24, 115, 204
  abnormal blood test results, 314
  anaemia, 253, 257
  aspirin overdose, 48
  attempted suicide, 424
  bloody cough, 161
  bruising, 274
  cellulitis, 318
  chest pain, 241
  chronic obstructive pulmonary
    disease, 398
  colicky pain, 61
  confusion, 94, 95, 260, 403
  constipation, 229
  cough, 20, 52
  depression, 28
  diabetes mellitus, 66
  dysuria, 70
  emergency hip repair, 303
  epigastric pain, 440
  falls, 82, 448
  fatigue, 234
  fever and confusion, 444
  fever and lethargy, 299
  headache, 13, 90, 436
  headache and vomiting, 34
  hips, 270, 303
  knees, swollen, 287
  leg pain and swelling, 295
  leg swelling, 419
  lethargy, 237
  light-headedness, 247
  nocturia, 86
  nose bleeds, 283
  palpitations, 325
  panic attacks, 279
  periods (menstruation), 290
  renal failure, 56
  respiratory distress, 409
  right-sided weakness, 306
  semi-consciousness, 44
  shortness of breath, 8, 9, 78, 151
  tiredness, 310

upper limb weakness, 219
vomiting, 3, 38
weight loss, 146
sotalol, 386
spironolactone
    aldosterone/PRA, 17
    kidney disease, 390
spontaneous pneumothoraces, 134–135
squamous cell carcinoma (SCC)
    bronchogenic carcinoma, 124–125
    upper limb weakness, 222
St. John's wort, 426
Staphylococcus aureus
    bronchogenic carcinoma, 124
    fever and weight loss, 370
Staphylococcus epidermidis, 447
Staphylococcus saprophyticus, 447
steatorrhoea, 442
STEMI (ST elevation myocardial
    infarction), 348–350, 356, *see also*
    Myocardial infarction
sterile pyuria, 447
steroid treatments, 177–178
Streptococcus pneumoniae, 438
Streptococcus viridans, 370
stress, 92
stroke
    diabetes, 159–160
    right-sided weakness, 308
subacute infective endocarditis,
    367–371
subarachnoid haemorrhage (SAH)
    headache, 438
    vomiting, 191–194
subdural haematoma
    diabetes, 160
    head injury, 216
suicide, attempted, 424–428
superior sulcus lung carcinoma, 219–222
supraventricular tachycardia, 366
swallowing difficulty, 127–131
swan neck deformity, 212
swelling
    falls, traumatic haemarthrosis, 286–289
    haematology, 294–297
    nephrotic syndrome, 419–423
    rheumatoid arthritis, 210–214
synacthen, 70, 72

syncope
    first-degree heart block, 336–338
    severe aortic stenosis, 351–352
    vasovagal response, 358–360
syndrome of inappropriate antidiuretic
    hormone (SIADH) secretion
    headache, 182
    hyponatraemia, 6
syphilis, 407–408
systemic anticoagulation, 296
systemic lupus erythromatosus (SLE)
    periods (menstruation), 292
    right-sided weakness, 306

T
tachycardia
    abdominal pain, 206
    light-headedness, 247–251
    NT-proBNP levels, 10
    palpitations, 346, 365–366
tamponade
    central chest pain, 392
    shortness of breath, 382
TAVI, *see* Transcatheter valve implant
    (TAVI)
TB, *see* Pulmonary tuberculosis (TB)
TCER, *see* Transcapillary escape rate (TCER)
teenagers
    bruising, 274–277
    chest pain, 241–246
    colicky pain, 61–65
    headache, 34–37
    panic attacks, 278–281
    swelling, 286–289
    vomiting, 34–37
temporal arteritis, 438
testosterone
    knees, painful, 109, 111
    periods (menstruation), 104
thiazide diuretics, *see also* Diuretics
    confusion, 94
    diabetes, 160
    hypokalaemia, 22
    hyponatraemia, 6
third-degree heart block, 338
thrombocytopenia
    bruising, 268
    emergency hip repair, 302–305

thrombocytosis
  abdominal pain, 206
  causes, 251
thyroid disease, 342
thyroid function, 32
thyroiditis, 76
thyroid peroxidase (TPO) antibody
  falls, 82–85
  tiredness, 74
thyroid-simulating hormone (TSH)
  confusion, 94, 403
  cough, 21, 52
  depression, 28
  falls, 82, 83
  fatigue, 235
  hyponatraemia, 7
  periods (menstruation), 104, 107
  tiredness, 74
  vomiting, 4
thyrotoxicosis, 76
thyroxine replacement therapy, 74
tilt table testing, 358, 360
tiredness, see also Fatigue; Lethargy
  bruising, 268
  cholestasis, 100–103
  diagnosis, 74–77
  myelofibrosis, 310–313
TNM classification, 172
Todd's paresis, 159–160
total protein
  abdominal pain, 204
  abnormal blood test results, 314
  anaemia, 253, 257
  bloody cough, 161
  bruising, 275
  cellulitis, 319
  chest pain, 242
  confusion, 94, 95, 260
  constipation, 230
  cough, 20, 52
  depression, 28
  diabetes mellitus, 66
  dysuria, 70
  emergency hip repair, 303
  falls, 82
  fatigue, 235
  fever and lethargy, 299
  headache and vomiting, 34
  hips, 271, 303

  knees, swollen, 287
  lethargy, 238
  nose bleeds, 283
  panic attacks, 279
  periods (menstruation), 291
  right-sided weakness, 307
  semi-consciousness, 44
  shortness of breath, 8, 78
  tiredness, 100, 311
  upper limb weakness, 219
  vomiting, 38
toxic colitis, 204–209
TPO, see Thyroid peroxidase (TPO)
    antibody
transcapillary escape rate (TCER), 55
transcatheter valve implant
    (TAVI), 352
transcutaneous pacing, 338
transferrin
  abdominal pain, 25
  cough, 52, 54
  knees, painful, 108
  renal failure, 56
transferrin saturation
  abdominal pain, 25
  cough, 52
  knees, painful, 108
  renal failure, 56
transoesophageal echocardiogram, 370
Treponema pallidum, 407–408
triglycerides
  falls, 82
  knees, painful, 108
  renal failure, 57, 60
  tiredness, 100
troponin T
  diabetes mellitus, 66
  palpitations, 325, 330
  shortness of breath, 78–81
Truelove and Witt's Classification of
    Acute Colitis, 207–208
TSH, see Thyroid-simulating hormone
    (TSH)
tube insertions, see Nasogastric feeding
    and tube insertions
tuberculosis
  bronchogenic carcinoma, 124
  cough, 161–166
  shortness of breath, 382

T-waves, 390
tympanic temperature, 448, 450

U
ulcerative colitis
  chronic diarrhoea, 26
  colitis types, 209
  inflammatory bowel disease, 118, 120
ultrasound
  epigastric pain, 442
  inflammatory bowel disease, 118, 120
unconjugated hyperbilirubinaemia, 80
upper gastrointestinal bleeding, 251
upper gastrointestinal fluid loss, 40
upper limb weakness, 219–222
urate, 299
urea
  abdominal pain, 24, 115, 204, 361
  abnormal blood test results, 314
  anaemia, 253, 257
  aspirin overdose, 48
  attempted suicide, 424
  bloody cough, 161
  bruising, 275
  cellulitis, 318
  chest pain, 241
  chronic obstructive pulmonary
    disease, 398
  colicky pain, 61
  confusion, 94, 95, 260, 403
  constipation, 229
  cough, 20, 52
  depression, 28
  diabetes, 66, 156
  dysuria, 70
  epigastric pain, 440
  falls, 82, 448
  fatigue, 234
  fever and confusion, 444
  fever and lethargy, 299
  headache, 13, 90, 436
  headache and vomiting, 34
  hip pain, 270
  hips, 303
  knees, swollen, 287
  leg pain and swelling, 295
  leg swelling, 419
  lethargy, 237

  light-headedness, 248
  nocturia, 86
  nose bleeds, 283
  palpitations, 325
  panic attacks, 279
  periods (menstruation), 290
  renal failure, 56
  respiratory distress, 409
  right-sided weakness, 307
  semi-consciousness, 44
  shortness of breath, 8, 9, 78, 151
  tiredness, 310
  vomiting, 3, 38
  weight loss, 146
urinalysis, 406
urinary tract infection (UTI), 444–447
urine, 41
urine albumin:creatinine ratio, 57
urine anion gap, 65
urine calcium, 65
urine citrate, 65
urine metanephrine, 90
urine methoxytyramine, 90
urine normetanephrine, 90
urine osmolality
  depression, 29
  vomiting, 38
urine pH, 65
urine potassium, 13
urine sodium
  depression, 29
  vomiting, 38
UTI, see Urinary tract infection (UTI)

V
vascular colitis, 209
vasculitits, 206
vasovagal response, 358–360
vasovagal syncope, 360
vegan diets, 236
venous thromboembolism (VTE)
  chronic obstructive pulmonary
    disease, 402
  leg pain, 294–297
ventricular arrhythmia, 350
ventricular fibrillation (VF)
  chest pain, 334, 340
  respiratory distress, 412

ventricular septal defect (VSD), 361
ventricular tachycardia
  palpitations, 365–366
  respiratory distress, 412
verapamil
  light-headedness, 342
  syncope, 338
very-low-density lipoprotein (VLDL), 60
VF, *see* Ventricular fibrillation (VF)
viedo-assisted thoracoscopic (VATS)
  decortication, 150
viral colitis, 209
viral infections, 320
viral infections, acute, 270–273
vision loss, 136–140
visual field testing, 3, 6
vitamin B12
  abdominal pain, 25
  confusion, 403
  fatigue, 236
  lethargy, 240
  renal failure, 57
vitamin D
  abdominal pain, 25
  cough, 21
  depression, 29
  tiredness, 100
vitamin deficiencies
  confusion, 406
  profound fatigue, 236
VLDL, *see* Very-low-density lipoprotein
  (VLDL)
volume depletion, 84
vomiting
  acute subarachnoid haemorrhage,
    191–194
  ear infection, 34–37
  electrolytes, 38–43
  hyponatraemia, 3–7
von Willebrand factor (VWF), 289
VSD, *see* Ventricular septal defect (VSD)
VTE, *see* Venous thromboembolism (VTE)

W
warfarin
  atrial fibrillation, 384, 386
  bronchogenic carcinoma, 124
  emergency hip repair, 302

nose bleeds, 284–285
right-sided weakness, 308–309
WBC, *see* White blood cells (WBC); White
  blood count (WBC)
WCC, *see* White cell count (WCC)
Wegener's granulomatosis, 170
weight loss
  bronchogenic carcinoma, 122–126
  left pleural effusion, 429–431
  lung cancer, 122–126
  mesothelioma, 146–150
  subacute infective endocarditis, 367–371
Well's score
  leg pain and swelling, 297
  shortness of breath, 375
wheezing
  chronic obstructive pulmonary
    disease, 398
  shortness of breath, 141
white blood cells (WBC)
  bloody cough, 161
  depression, 29
  diabetes type 2, 156
  falls, 82
  renal failure, 56
  weight loss, 146
white cell count (WCC)
  abdominal pain, 115, 204, 206
  abnormal blood test results, 314
  anaemia, 252, 256
  attempted suicide, 424
  bruising, 274
  cellulitis, 318
  chest pain, 241
  chronic obstructive pulmonary
    disease, 398
  confusion, 94, 260, 403
  constipation, 229
  cough, 52
  emergency hip repair, 302
  epigastric pain, 440
  falls, 448
  fatigue, 234
  fever and confusion, 444
  fever and lethargy, 298
  headache, 436
  hips, 270, 302
  knees, swollen, 286

leg pain and swelling, 294
leg swelling, 419
lethargy, 237
light-headedness, 247
nose bleeds, 282
panic attacks, 278
periods (menstruation), 290
respiratory distress, 409
right-sided weakness, 306
shortness of breath, 78
tiredness, 310
upper limb weakness, 219
Wolff-Parkinson-White (WPW)
    syndrome, 343–347
women, *see also* Elderly women;
    Middle-aged women; Young women
abdominal pain, 24–27, 115–121,
    204–209
confusion, 94–99
cough, 122–126
headache, 13–19, 191–194
hip repair, emergency, 302–305
periods, 104–107, 290–293

shortness of breath, 379–383
suicide, attempted, 424–428
weight loss, 122–126
WPW, *see* Wolff-Parkinson-White
    (WPW) syndrome

Y
young men
Army medical examination, 376–378
chest pain, 132–135, 391–392
palpitations, 393–395
shortness of breath, 372–375
young women, *see also* Elderly women;
    Middle-aged women; Women
aspirin overdose, 48–51
back pain, 432–435
cough, 414–418
leg pain, 294–297, 432–435
palpitations, 343–347
profound fatigue, 234–236
swelling, 294–297
syncope, 358–360
vision loss, 136–140

Printed and bound by CPI Group (UK) Ltd, Croydon, CR0 4YY

23/10/2024

01777672-0019